FIFTH ED

Echocardiographer's
POCKET REFERENCE

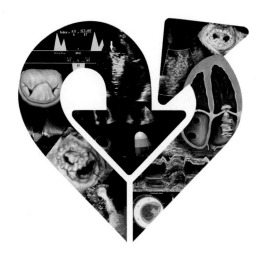

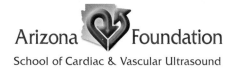

Arizona Foundation

School of Cardiac & Vascular Ultrasound

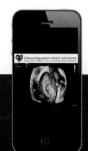

For updates or corrections to this edition,
use the the QR code below.

 QR codes can be found throughout this book, which will allow you to view video clips of various pathology or duplex findings using your smartphone or tablet. To access these files, use the camera on your device and a QR code reader. Your device must have internet to use this feature. There are many free QR code readers available for download, please check your app store for more information.

DEDICATED TO

Edward B. Diethrich, M.D.

Echocardiographer's Pocket Reference Fifth Edition

Fifth Printing 08/2022

Arizona Heart Foundation
Phoenix, Arizona
602-200-0437

ISBN 978-0-578-68717-9

Printed in the United States of America

Table of Contents

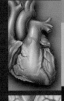

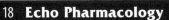

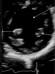

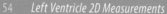

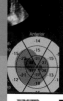

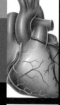

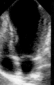

9

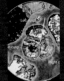

10

11

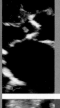
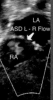

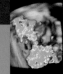

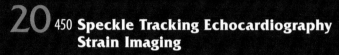
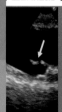

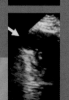

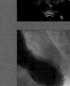

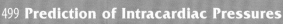

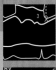

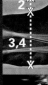

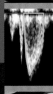

Acknowledgements

This book is dedicated to my wife Terri, and 3 children, Chloe, Lucas, and Sydney. Without their love and support I would not have been able to accomplish everything I wanted to in my career. This edition was an inspiration from all my past and future students. I have been blessed to have so many outstanding mentors and colleagues throughout my career. Thank you, Marilyn Riley RDCS, FASE and Lisa Carl BA, RDCS, the first cardiac sonographers who introduced me to the field of cardiac ultrasound at Beth Israel Hospital in Boston, MA. To Joan Gardiner RN for having so much patience with me, as she taught me all my hands-on skills at Bristol Hospital, in Bristol CT. To the all the physicians that were my mentors, teaching me so many aspects of echocardiography, specifically Bernard Clark III MD and especially Anita Kelsey MD for her friendship and guidance which has been instrumental throughout my career.

To the many talented and brilliant sonographers that have contributed to this edition, it would not have been possible without their expertise. To the amazing editing team Steven Walling, Jason Kendrick, Joy Guthrie and Christie Jordan, your patience, expertise, and skills are the best!

I would like to give a special thanks to Gail Size who was the project manager and Chellie Buzzeo who put all her magic into creating this Edition. And Finally, a big thank you to Paula Banahan, President of the Arizona Heart Foundation – School of Cardiac and Vascular Ultrasound for giving me this opportunity to create this 5th edition.

~ Richard Palma

I would like to acknowledge Pamela Kidd (RDCS), for her original outline and concept for this book, and recognition of Terry Reynolds' (BS, RDCS) efforts to design and update the first four editions. Their efforts led to this significant upgrade to the pocket reference which is still considered the "Gold Standard" around the world. We have taken their idea and matured it into what you are holding today. Enjoy!

~ Paula Banahan, RN CVNS
President, CEO
Arizona Heart Foundation, Inc.

Author and Contributors

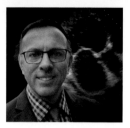

Richard Palma BS, ACS, RCS, RDCS, FACVP, FSDMS, FASE

Richie has worked in the profession since 1990. An Advanced Cardiac Sonographer who currently is the Program Director and Clinical Coordinator of the Duke School of Medicine Cardiac Sonography Certificate Program. He is the only sonographer to receive Fellowship from the American Society of Echocardiography, Society of Diagnostic Medical Sonography and Alliance of Cardiovascular Professionals. A dedicated Educator for over 20 years and recipient of the Distinguished Educator award from the SDMS. Richie is married with 3 children and resides in the city of Durham, NC.

Steven Walling BS, RCS, RDCS, FASE
Co-editor

David Adams
ACS, RCS, RDCS, FASE
Sonographer Emeritus
Duke University Health System
Durham, NC

Dennis Atherton
RDCS, FASE
Technical Director of Cardiac Imaging and Diagnosis
Maine Medical
Portland, ME

Alicia Armour
MA, BS, ACS, RDCS, FASE
Duke Private Diagnostic Clinic-Triangle
Heart Associates
Duke University Health System
Durham, NC

J. Todd Belcik
BS, ACS, RDCS (AE) (PE), FASE
Sr. Research Associate/Research Sonographer
Oregon Health & Science University
Portland, OR

S. Michelle Bierig
PhD, ACS, RCS RDCS, RDMS, CPHQ, FSDMS, FASE
Director, Cardiovascular Services
Hillcrest South
Tulsa, OK

Daniel P. Bourque
MS. RCS, FASE
Orlando Regional Medical Center
Orlando, FL

Merri L. Bremer
Ed.D., RN, ACS, RDCS, FASE
Quality Improvement and Education Coordinator/ACS
Program Director
Mayo Clinic Division of Cardiovascular Ultrasound
Assistant Professor, Mayo Clinic College of Medicine and Science
Rochester, MN

Brigid Culey
BS, RDCS, FASE
Cardiac Sonographer
Meritas Health Cardiology
North Kansas City, MO

Ashlee Davis
BSMI, ACS, RDCS, FASE
Duke University Health System
Durham, North Carolina

Joy Guthrie
PhD., ACS, RDMS, RDCS, RVT, FSDMS, FASE
Community Regional Medical Center
Fresno, CA

Jeffrey C. Hill
BS, ACS, FASE
Department Chair, Assistant Professor, Diagnostic Medical Sonography
School of Medical Imaging and Therapeutics
Boston, MA

Kenneth Horton
ACS, RCS, FASE
Echo Research Coordinator
Intermountain Heart Institute
Intermountain Medical Center
Salt Lake, UT

Christie H. Jordan
BS, RCS, RDCS, RCIS, FASE
Program Director, Cardiovascular Technology
Program Director
Florida State College at Jacksonville
Jacksonville, FL

Eric Kallstrom
MBA, ACS, RDCS, FACVP, FASE
Baylor Scott & White Health
Dallas, TX

Christopher J. Kramer
BA, ACS, RDCS, FASE
Advocate Aurora Health
Milwaukee, Wisconsin

Jason Kendrick
RDCS (AE), RVT
Director of Education
Program Director, Cardiac Ultrasound Program
Arizona Heart Foundation
Phoenix, AZ

Jon Owensby
ACS, RDCS, RRT
Duke University Health System
Durham, North Carolina

Robert W. McDonald
RCS, RDCS, RCCS, ACS, FASE
Doernbecher Children's Hospital
Oregon Health and Sciences University
Portland, OR

Rick Meece
ACS, RDCS, RCS, RCIS, FASE
Advanced Cardiac Imaging Specialist
Perioperative and Structural Heart
Hilton Head Island, SC

Sally J. Miller
BS, RDCS, RT(R), FASE
Program Director, Echocardiography,
Mayo Clinic School of Health Sciences
Assistant Professor of Medicine,
Mayo Clinic College of Medicine and Science
Mayo Clinic
Rochester, MN

Carissa Marsiglio
BS, RDCS
Duke University Health System
Durham, NC

Carol Mitchell
PhD, ACS, RDMS, RDCS, RVT, RT(R), FASE, FSDMS
Associate professorUniversity of Wisconsin-Madison
Madison, WI

Margaret M. Park
BS, ACS, RDCS, RVT, FSDMS, FASE
Lead Imaging Specialist
Heart, Vascular and Thoracic Institute
C5 Imaging Research, Imaging Core
Cleveland Clinic
Cleveland, OH

Sue Phillip
RCS, FASE
Johns Hopkins University, School of Medicine
Baltimore, MD

Laura J Phillips
BS, RDCS, RVT
Lawrence & Memorial Hospital at Yale New
Haven Health
Program Director, School of Vascular Sonography
Hoffman Heart and Vascular Institute School of
Cardiovascular Technology
Saint Francis Hospital and Medical Center
Hartford, CT

Michael Rampoldi
ACS, RDCS, RVT, FASE
The Baylor Scott and White Heart and Vascular Hospital
Dallas and Ft. Worth, TX

Brad J. Roberts
BS, ACS, RCS, FASE
Baylor Scott & White
Program Director, Cardiovascular Institute
The Heart Hospitals
Cardiovascular Institute
Plano, TX

Marsha L. Roberts
BS, ACS, RCS, RDCS (AE/PE), FASE
President, Inside Echo LLC
Mansfield, TX

Danny Rivera
RCS, ACS
Duke University Health System
Durham, NC

Steven Walling
BS, RCS, RDCS, FASE
Program Director and Clinical Coordinator
Hoffman Heart and Vascular Institute School of
Cardiovascular Technology
Saint Francis Hospital and Medical Center
Hartford, CT

Foreword

Since 1993, The Echocardiographer's Pocket Reference has been the primary reference for sonographers and all students of Echocardiography. Now in a 5th edition, this textbook has been completely redesigned to allow for integrated learning. Entirely written by sonographers, 24 chapters of Echocardiographic pearls are available at your fingertips. This edition has added four additional chapters, including anatomy and physiology in cardiac development, cardiac medications, instrumentation, and the comprehensive echo exam.

Designed as a reference text with the user in mind, educational content has been optimized with videos and color images that cover a broad spectrum of complex cardiac disease states. The author, Richard Palma (Richie), has done an excellent job providing all the basic concepts of echocardiographic evaluation of the heart in a format that is comprehensive and easy to access. Any student of Echocardiography can use this text as an educational tool and a primary reference text.

I have had the pleasure of working with Richie for 16 years as Medical Director of the School for Cardiac Ultrasound at the Hoffman Heart and Vascular Institute. He has a passion for teaching and a love of echo that is second to none. Richie works to distill complicated concepts for his students, launching them on successful careers in Echocardiography. As a Physician Echocardiographer myself, I appreciate the skill required to perform and interpret an echocardiogram. All students of Echocardiography using this book can benefit from Richie's years of expertise and skillful content delivery. I know you will find this reference textbook an invaluable resource. I am pleased to say that Richie has joined me now at Duke where we will share in the education of many new sonographers at the Duke Cardiac Ultrasound Certificate Program.

~ **Anita M. Kelsey, MD, MBA**
Vice Chief, Non-Invasive Cardiac Imaging
Division of Cardiology
Duke University Health System

Cardiac Anatomy and Physiology
Joy Guthrie, PhD., ACS, RDMS, RDCS, RVT, FSDMS, FASE

Embryology

Formation of the Heart and Blood Vessels

The cardiovascular system is the first major system to develop and function in the embryo. The first structure is the early embryonic pole with a cardiogenic primordium at the superior pole along with primitive blood vessels at approximately 18 days. The next structure to develop within the cardiovascular system are two paired angioblastic cords. These cords are composed of an endoderm, mesoderm, and ectoderm. The two cords fuse to form a single heart tube by the end of the 3rd week. The heart starts to beat on day 23 of gestation. The heart is completely formed by the 8th week of gestation.

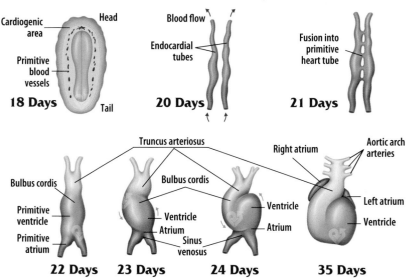

Figure 1.1: The timing of events in the formation of the heart

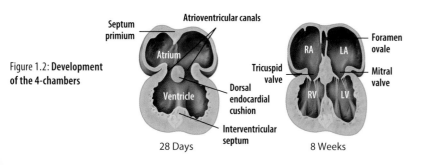

Figure 1.2: Development of the 4-chambers

The development of the embryonic heart includes the following:

- Vitelline veins
- Umbilical veins
- Sinus Venosus
- Cardinal Veins
- Primitive atria
- Atrioventricular (AV) canal
- Primitive ventricle
- Bulbus cordis
- Truncus arteriosus
- Aortic sac and arches

Vitelline Veins

The vitelline veins become the definitive hepatic and portal veins. They return poorly oxygenated blood from the umbilical vesicle (yolk sac). The vitelline veins enter the sinus venosus.

Umbilical Veins

The right and left umbilical veins carry highly oxygenated blood from the chorionic sac (will become the placenta) through the umbilical cord to the fetus. Only the left umbilical vein persists.

Sinus Venosus

The sinus venosus consists of both a right and left horn. The sinus venosus will eventually form the inferior and superior vena cava, the coronary sinus, and the posterior wall of the atria. The distal end of the left horn usually regresses, however, if it does not there will be a persistent left superior vena cava to the coronary sinus.

Cardinal Veins

The cardinal veins provide the main venous drainage of the embryo. The anterior cardinal veins drain the cranial portion of the embryo and the posterior cardinal veins drain the caudal portion. The cardinal veins become the innominate (also known as the brachiocephalic) and superior vena cava (SVC). The subcardinal veins form the suprarenal and renal veins as well as the gonadal veins and a portion of the inferior vena cava (IVC). The supracardinal veins form the azygous and hemiazygous veins above the level of the kidneys. Below the renal level the left supracardinal vein regresses allowing the inferior IVC to form.

Primitive or Primordial Atrium

The primordial atrium is divided into the right and left atria. The atrium starts as a single atrium and then is divided into two atria by the formation of the atrial septum. Towards the end of the 4th week of development the septum primum grows toward the fusing endocardial cushions from the superior aspect of the atrium partially dividing into right and left halves. As the septum primum develops a large opening the ostium primum forms between the endocardial cushion and the free edge of the septum primum. The ostium primum disappears as it fuses with the endocardial cushion to become the AV septum. Before the ostium primum disappears (5th week) perforations appear in the central portion of the septum primum. The perforations coalesce to form the ostium secundum. The opening in the septum secundum is called the foramen ovale. The remaining portion of the septum primum attached to the endocardial cushion forms the valve of the foramen ovale (foraminal flap).

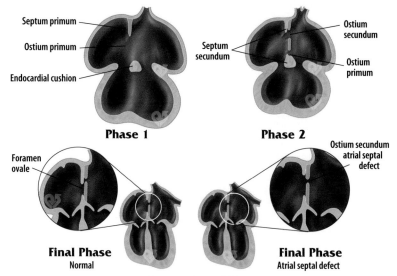

Figure 1.3: **Primordial Atrium**

Atrioventricular (AV) Canal

The atrioventricular canal is a large communication between the primitive atria and primitive ventricle. The endocardial cushions will divide the AV canal into two separate mitral and tricuspid annuli. This will also contribute to the closure of the ostium primum (inferior) portion of the atrial septum as well as the membranous portion of the interventricular septum. Complete absence of the endocardial cushions will result in a complete atrioventricular septal defect. This is the most common intracardiac defect associated with Trisomy 21 (Down's Syndrome).

Bulbus Cordis

During the fifth week of development mesenchymal cells proliferate and form bulbar ridges at the same time truncal ridges are formed. The bulbus cordus is divided into three sections: primitive right ventricle, ventricular outflow tracts (conus cordus) and the trunctus arteriosus. The Bulbus cordus connects the great vessels to the ventricles. Conotruncal abnormalities such as Tetralogy of Fallot, truncus arteriosus and double outlet right ventricle result from disruption of formation or migration of cells in this region.

Truncus Arteriosus

The truncal ridges and bulbar ridges are derived from neural crest cells. The aortopulmonary trunk starts as a single vessel. Within the truncus arteriosus the bulbar and truncal ridges undergo a 180 degree spiraling resulting in the aortopulmonary septum. The septum divides the bulbus cordus and truncus arteriosus into the definitive aorta and pulmonary trunk. Failure of the aortopulmonary septum to form will result in persistent truncus arteriosus.

Aortic Sac and Arches

The aortic arches arise from the aortic sac. Embryologically, the aortic arches start as six pairs although they are not all present at the same time. By the time the sixth pair have formed the first two have nearly regressed with very few arterial tributaries. The final aortic arterial arrangement is completed by the eighth week. Aortic arch derivatives include the following:

- 1st pair- maxillary arteries and external carotid arteries
- 2nd pair- stapedial arteries
- 3rd pair- common carotid and internal carotid arteries
- 4th pair- left forms the transverse aortic arch, right forms the proximal part of the right subclavian artery
- 5th pair- rudimentary vessels that will regress
- 6th pair- left forms the left pulmonary artery and ductus arteriosus, right forms the right pulmonary artery

Segmental Notation of Cardiac Position

Van Praagh's segmental notation has long been accepted as the appropriate method for determining cardiac segmentation and position. This notation is divided into three segments including atria, ventricles, and great artery orientation. The groups are separated by commas and confined by brackets to determine the set. This nomenclature will be seen in all congenital echocardiographic reports with symbols such as (S, D, S). The most efficient way to learn this notation is to take each segment at a time.

Visceroatrial Designation

This is the first symbol in the set.

Visceralatrial situs
- "S" solitus: Largest lobe of liver is on the right and stomach and spleen are on the left
- "I" inversus: Largest lobe of the liver in the left and stomach and spleen are on the right.
- "A" ambiguous: Visceral organs do not fit into either of the other categories

Thoracoabdominal situs
- "S" solitus: Right lung and largest lobe of the liver are on the right side
- "I" inversus: Right lung and largest lobe of liver are on the left side
- "A" ambiguous: Duplicated sidedness or does not meet the other categories

Atrial situs
- "S" solitus: Morphologic right atrium is on the patient's right side
- "I" inversus: Morphologic right atrium is o the patient's left side
- "A" ambiguous: Sidedness of the atrium cannot be determined.

If any of the letters are recorded as **A** then the visceralatrial arrangement is denoted ambiguous. If all are recorded as **S** then it is situs solitus or normal orientation. If all are recorded as **I** the visceralatrial arrangement is denoted as situs inversus.

Ventricular Loop Designation

Ventricular loop designation defines which side of the body the morphologic right or left ventricle are placed.

This is the second symbol in the set.

- "D" Dextroloop: The morphologic right ventricle is to the right of the left ventricle.
- "L" Levoloop: The morphologic right ventricle is to the left of the left ventricle.
- "X" Neither: The ventricle location does not meet either classification

Great Vessel Orientation and Relationship

This designation defines the orientation and relationship of the great arteries at the level of the aortic and pulmonary valves.

This is the third symbol in the set.

- "S" The aorta is posterior and to the right of the pulmonary artery
- "I" The aorta is posterior and to the left of the pulmonary artery
- "D-TGA" The aorta is anterior and right of the pulmonary artery
- "L-TGA" The aorta is anterior and to the left of the pulmonary artery
- "D-MGA" The great vessels are juxtaposed next to each other but the aorta is to the right
- "L-MGA" The great vessels are juxtaposed next to each other but the aorta is to the left

The normal orientation in a patient with normal anatomy is {S, D, S}. This classification defines a stepwise approach to determining the exact orientation of the heart and great vessels.

Comparison of Fetal and Postnatal Circulation

The understanding of uteroplacental flow helps to define the expected location and type of flow from placenta to fetus. Fetal circulation depends on placental oxygenation of fetal blood, three intrafetal shunts, and the fetal heart to provide blood pressure.

In the normal pregnancy the blood supply to the uterus increases significantly from 50ml/min to approximately 500ml/min at term. This transformation occurs between 18-20 weeks when there is a trophoblastic invasion of the myometrium. The trophoblastic cells invade the placental bed destroying the elastic lamina of the spiral arteries and replaces them with smooth muscles cells. This transformation increases the radius of the spiral arteries allowing for a larger volume and lower resistance system. If there is an interruption or retardation of this process a high resistance system can continue to exist. This can lead to intrauterine growth restriction and/or maternal hypertension.

Placenta Oxygenation

The fetal lungs are collapsed and only 20% of the blood flows into the fetal lung parenchyma. This flow is primarily used to perfuse the fetal lungs as tissue not as a functioning organ. The placenta acts as the fetal lungs. Placental oxygen transfer is approximately 8 mL O_2/minute/kg of fetal weight. This is sufficient oxygenation of the fetus as long at the flow is continuous.

Intrafetal Circulatory Shunts

The flow from mother to fetus is continuous and is a closed system. Oxygenated blood flow enters the fetus through the **umbilical vein**. This contains the highly oxygenated blood directly from the placenta. About 50% of from the umbilical vein flows into the portohepatic system and the other 50% flows into the first fetal shunt, the **ductus venosus.** The radius of the ductus venosus is smaller than the umbilical vein, allowing the velocity and pressure to increase. The ductus venosus is met with the IVC and enters the right atrium. At the junction of the right atrium there is a valve (Eustachian valve) that diverts the highly oxygenated placenta flow across the **foramen ovale** (second fetal shunt). This allows the highly oxygenated blood to enter the left atrium and provide flow to the fetal systemic circulation. The flow in the right atrium passes through the tricuspid valve and out through the pulmonary artery to the lungs. The fetal lungs provide high vascular resistance (we cannot breathe under water) so only 20% of blood flows to the fetal lungs.

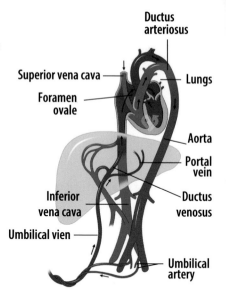

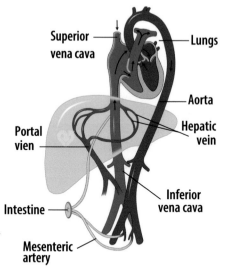

The rest of the right ventricular outflow goes through the **ductus arteriosus** (Third fetal shunt). The ductus arteriosus joins the descending aorta providing blood to the abdominal organs and the returns to the placenta through the paired umbilical arteries.

Postnatal Circulation

The ductus venosus, foramen ovale, and ductus arteriosus usually close shortly after birth. In premature infants, the ductus arteriosus and foramen ovale may not spontaneously close. This is called a patent foramen ovale and patent ductus arteriosus. In term infants the ductus arteriosus usually closes within 48 to 72 hours. Upon closure the ductus arteriosus becomes the ligamentum arteriosum, and the ductus venosus becomes the ligamentum venosum between the caudate lobe and left lobe of the liver. After delivery when the pulmonary vascular resistance decreases and left sided pressures increase, the foramen ovale typically closes and becomes the fossa ovalis in the adult.

Cardiac Anatomy

The heart is composed to two receiving chambers (atria) and two pumping chambers (ventricles). The right and left atria are separated by the interatrial and interventriculuar septum, respectively. In order to fully understand each chamber morphologically, each will be discussed separately.

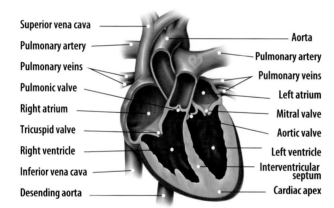

Right Atrium (RA)

The right atrium receives deoxygenated blood from the superior and inferior vena cava and the coronary sinus. This process occurs during ventricular systole. The blood entering the right ventricle flows through the tricuspid valve into the right ventricle in diastole. The right atrial appendage differs from the left atrial appendage as it has a broader base and is triangular shaped. The left atrial appendage has been described as a "dog ear" appearance.

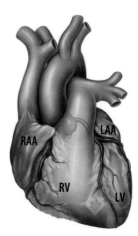

The right atrium has two components including the posterior smooth walled portion which is formed from the embryologic sinus venosus and the right atrial appendage. Along the RA free wall are a number of pectinate muscles that extend into the right atrial appendage. The right atrium has a thin muscular wall that is very compliant. This allows for a very low right atrial pressure (usually between 0-4mmHg).

The interior ridge of the SVC-right atrial junction is called the crista terminalis. This can be prominent and mimic an intraatrial thrombus. The crista terminalis is the internal component of the external ridge between the SVC and IVC called the sulcus terminalis.

At the IVC-right atrial junction there is a vestigial valve called the **eustachian valve**. The role of the eustachian valve is limited to prenatal blood flow where it serves to divert the highly oxygenated flow from the ductus venosus and IVC across the foramen ovale. Beyond fetal life, it has no function but still exists at the right atrial -IVC junction. The fenestrated portion of the eustachian valve that extends from the SVC to IVC is referred to as the Chiari network. The vestigial valve that guards the incoming flow from the coronary sinus to the right atrium is called the **thebesian valve.**

Left Atrium (LA)

The left atrium receives highly oxygenated blood via the four pulmonary veins from the lungs during ventricular systole. The pulmonary veins enter the posterior aspect of the left atrium. The left atrium is separated from the right atrium medially by the interatrial septum. The left atrium consists of the main chamber and the left atrial appendage. The left atrial appendage and left atrial free wall contain pectinate muscle. The left atrial appendage has been described as a "dog ear" appearance.

The left atrium is the most posterior cardiac chamber and is immediately anterior to the descending aorta and the esophagus. The walls of the left atrium and slightly thicker than the right atrial walls. The normal left atrial pressure is approximately 5mmHg. During ventricular diastole the oxygenated blood flows into the left ventricle through the mitral valve. Two thirds of the blood flows during early diastole and the last third flows into the left ventricle during atrial contraction in late diastole.

Interatrial Septum (IAS)

The interatrial septum divides the common atrium into equal halves. There are three distinct portions of the interatrial septum. The central portion is thin and fibrous and was the site of the foramen ovale during fetal life. This becomes the fossa ovalis after birth. The primitive septum primum and the limbus fossa ovalis form the fossa ovalis borders. The central region of the atrial septum is called the ostium secundum. This is the most common site of an atrial septal defect. A patent foramen ovale occurs in approximately 25% of the adult population and can be detected by echocardiography or with a bubble study, or with agitated saline. A patent foramen ovale may be a relative benign finding or may contribute to neurological deficit secondary to the potential for a right to left shunt across the defect.

The superior portion of the interatrial septum is referred to as the sinus venosus. Atrial defects in this region may allow flow from the right upper pulmonary vein to flow anomalously into the right atrium instead of the left atrium. This is termed partial anomalous pulmonary venous return (PAPVR). The inferior ridge of the atrial septum is the ostium primum. This portion of the atrial septum is in direct contact with the cardiac crux at the level of the atrioventricular valves. Defects in this region are common in the setting of atrioventricular septal defects (AVSD). These type of atrial defects are common in individuals with Trisomy 21 (Downs Syndrome). Any significant defect in the atrial septum will result in a right ventricular volume overload (RVVO). Qp/Qs calculation will assist in grading the severity of the intracardiac shunt.

Right Ventricle (RV)

The right ventricle is the most anterior chamber of the heart. It is triangular in shape. The right ventricle receives deoxygenated blood from the inferior and superior vena cava and pumps blood out through the pulmonary artery to the lungs for oxygenation. The right ventricular pressure is lower than the left ventricle (approximately 25mmHg). The right ventricle is divided into three segments: RV inflow tract, apex, and outflow tract.

The RV inflow tract includes the atrioventricular valve referred to as the tricuspid valve that allows blood to flow between the right atrium and the right ventricle. The tricuspid leaflets include the septal, anterior, and posterior leaflets. The RV inflow tract also includes the chordae tendinae, and three papillary muscles including the anterior, posterior, and medial (conal).

The RV apex differs from the LV in that it is heavily trabeculated. There is a distinct muscular band, the moderator band, that spans across the lower 1/3 of the right ventricular walls. The right ventricle has trabeculated walls in comparison with the left ventricular smooth walls. The right ventricular outflow tract extends superiorly toward the pulmonic valve and main pulmonary artery. The atrioventricular valve follows the ventricle. The atrioventricular valve aligned with the right ventricle is the tricuspid valve. A distinguishing feature of the right ventricle is the septal leaflet of the tricuspid valve inserts more apically into the interventricular septum compared to the mitral valve.

The right ventricular outflow tract is smooth walled and extends from the right ventricle toward the pulmonic valve. This region is called the infundibulum. The anterior muscle bundle, crista supraventricularis, divides the RV inflow from the RV outflow tract. Externally, the conus arteriosus is a ridge that divides the right ventricular outflow tract from the main pulmonary artery.

Left Ventricle (LV)

The left ventricle is the systemic pump of the heart. The left ventricle is three times thicker than the right ventricle and occupies approximately 75% of the hearts total mass. The thicker ventricular wall allows the blood to flow at systemic pressure. The normal LV pressure is approximately 120mmHg at rest. The endocardial border of the left ventricle is smooth and the chamber is bullet shaped. The left ventricle forms the cardiac apex. The left ventricle pumps oxygenated blood to the body in ventricular systole. The left ventricle is divided into an inflow tract, apex, and left ventricular outflow tract.

The atrioventricular valve aligned with the left ventricle is the mitral valve. There are two mitral valve leaflets, anterior and posterior. The left ventricular inflow tract includes the mitral valve annulus, mitral valve leaflets, chordae tendinae, anterolateral and posteromedial papillary muscles.

There is fibrous communication of the posterior aortic root and the anterior mitral leaflet. Any disruption in this fibroannular connection will cause the cardiac axis to be deviated leftward. The left ventricular outflow tract extends from the mitral valve annulus to the aortic valve annulus.

Interventricular Septum (IVS)

The interventricular septum is the dividing wall between the left and right ventricle. Due to higher left sided pressures the septum typically bows towards the right ventricle. The left ventricle should define the shape of the septum. The majority of the ventricular septum is thick and muscular with the exception of the thin membranous septum that lies beneath the aortic valve. The muscular portion of the septum is divided into three distinct regions:

Inlet

The inlet region of the interventricular septum is located between the atrioventricular (MV and TV) valves and inferior to the membranous septum. This comprises the posterior and superior one-third of the ventricular septum. Defects in this region are associated with atrioventricular septal defects previously referred to as endocardial cushion defects.

Trabecular or Muscular

The trabecular or muscular region of the interventricular septum is the largest portion and extends inferiorly from the membranous septum to ventricular apex. Defects in this region of the septum have an increased opportunity of spontaneous closure due to muscular growth aiding closure. Thickening of the septum occurs with systemic hypertension, hypertrophic cardiomyopathy, diabetic cardiomyopathy, and any condition with increased afterload including aortic stenosis.

Infundibular or Outlet

The infundibular or outlet septum lies anterior-superior to the trabecular septum and inferior to the aortic and pulmonary valves. This is the muscular division between the subaortic and subpulmonic region. Conotruncal abnormalities such as Tetralogy of Fallot, Double Outlet Right Ventricle, and Truncus Arteriosus have defects in this region.

Intracardiac Valves

There are four intracardiac valves. The two atrioventricular (AV) valves are the tricuspid valve and the mitral valve and two semilunar valves, the aortic and pulmonary.

Atrioventricular Valves

The two atrioventricular valves allow inflow from the atria to the ventricles in ventricular diastole.

Tricuspid Valve

The tricuspid valve is the inlet valve between the right atrium and right ventricle. As the name implies, there are three leaflets of the tricuspid valve including the anterior (largest), septal, and posterior. The tricuspid valve inserts slightly more apically into the interventricular septum compared to the mitral valve.

The components of the tricuspid valve apparatus include the TV annulus, three leaflets, chordae tendinae, and three papillary muscles.

Mitral Valve

The mitral valve is the inlet valve between the left atrium and left ventricle. The mitral valve leaflets include both the anterior and posterior leaflets and medial and lateral commissures.

The components of the mitral valve apparatus include the mitral valve annulus, two leaflets , chordae tendinae, and two papillary muscles. The anterior and posterior leaflets each have these scallops

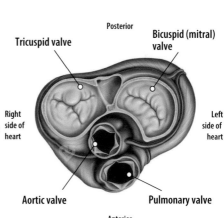

Semilunar Valves

The aortic and pulmonary valves are two semilunar valves located at the base of the aortic and pulmonary artery respectively. The semilunar shape of these valves prevent backflow of blood into the ventricles.

Aortic Valve

The aortic valve is located at the base of the aorta and is the outflow valve of the left ventricle. During ventricular systole the left ventricle pressure exceeds the aortic pressure and the aortic valve opens. During ventricular diastole the aortic valve is closed.

There are three cusps of the aortic valve including the right coronary, left coronary and noncoronary cusps.

The components of the aortic valve apparatus include the cusps, nodule of Arantius, sinus of Valsalva, and the lunula. The nodules of Arantius are thickening of the intima media on the ventricular surface of the aortic valve cusps. The aortic valve is in fibrous continuity with the anterior mitral valve leaflet.

Pulmonary Valve

The pulmonary valve is located anteriorly and is the outflow valve of the right ventricle. During ventricular systole the right ventricular pressure exceeds the pulmonary artery pressure and the pulmonary valve opens. During ventricular diastole the pulmonary valve is closed.

There are three cusps of the pulmonary valve including the right, left (posterior) and anterior.

The components of the pulmonary valve structure include the cusps, nodule of Arantius, lunula, and pulmonary sinus. The commissure is the region of the cusps that come together with the adjacent cusp.

Systemic and Pulmonary Veins

Systemic Veins

The systemic veins return deoxygenated blood from the body and return to the right atrium. Both the arteries and veins have the same three layers; intima (inner layer), media (middle layer), and adventitia (outer layer). The walls of the veins are thinner than arterial walls. There are three major and one minor systemic venous veins including the superior and inferior vena cava, coronary sinus, and azygous veins.

Superior Vena Cava (SVC)

The superior vena cava drains blood from the head and arms to the right atrium.

Inferior Vena Cava (IVC)

The inferior vena cava drains blood from the trunk and legs below the diaphragm to the right atrium. The valve at the junction of the right atrium and the IVC is the eustachian valve and has a netlike fenestrated portion termed the Chiari network.

Coronary Sinus

The coronary sinus drains deoxygenated blood from the coronary arteries and returns to the right atrium. The thebesian valve guards the entrance of the coronary sinus to the right atrium.

Azygous Vein

The azygous vein is a vein beginning in the abdomen as a continuation of the ascending lumbar vein. The azygous vein and it's tributaries serve as a connecting link to return blood to the superior vena cava and becomes an important conduit in the setting of obstruction of the IVC or SVC.

Pulmonary Veins

The pulmonary veins deliver highly oxygenated blood from the lungs to the left atrium. There are four pulmonary veins: right upper, right lower, left upper, and left lower. Because embryologically the pulmonary veins do not arise from the left atrium, there is a potential for them to drain anomalously into the right atrium.

Arteries

The arterial network delivers oxygenated blood from the heart to the vital organs and extremities. The largest conduit in the arterial system is the aorta. The aorta is divided into the following sections:

- Aortic annulus
- Aortic root
- Sinotubular junction
- Ascending aorta
- Aortic arch (transverse arch)
- Aortic isthmus
- Descending aorta
- Thoracic aorta
- Abdominal aorta

Right common carotid artery · Left common carotid artery · Right subclavian artery · Left subclavian artery · Innominate artery · Aortic arch · Ascending aorta · Descending aorta · Left main coronary artery · Right coronary artery · Thoracic aorta

There are three branches of the aortic arch: innominate artery (also referred to as brachiocephalic) which gives rise to the right subclavian and right common carotid artery, the left common carotid artery, and the left subclavian artery. The abdominal aortic branches to supply the vital organs in the abdominal and pelvic cavity and then bifurcates into the common iliac arteries leading towards the legs.

Coronary Arteries

The coronary arteries perfuse the ventricular myocardium. They provide oxygenated blood to other structures of the heart such as the atria and SA, AV nodes.

Left Coronary Artery

The left coronary artery arises from the aortic root and gives rise to the left anterior descending artery and the left circumflex artery. The left anterior descending and circumflex arteries provide oxygenated blood to the anterior, anteroseptal, anterolateral, and inferolateral aspect of the heart, respectively.

Right Coronary Artery

The right coronary artery arises from the aortic root and provides oxygenated blood flow to the right atrium, sinoatrial and atrioventricular nodes, and the right ventricle. The posterior descending artery is a branch of the right coronary artery and provides blood flow to the inferior surface of the heart.

Pulmonary Artery

The pulmonary artery arises from the right ventricle and branches into the right and left pulmonary artery branches. The pulmonary artery takes deoxygenated blood to the lungs for oxygenation.

Cardiovascular Physiology

Systemic and Pulmonary Circulation

The circulatory system is made up of both the systemic and pulmonary circulation. The pulmonary circulation takes blood from the heart to the lungs and back to the heart. The systemic circulation takes blood from the heart to the arteries, arterioles, capillaries, venules, veins, and back to the heart.

Pulmonary circulation
- Right ventricle
- Main and branch pulmonary arteries
- Pulmonary capillaries
- Pulmonary veins

Systemic circulation
- Left ventricle
- Aorta
- Systemic capillaries
- Systemic venules and veins
- Superior and Inferior vena cava

Cardiac Hemodynamics

Several factors contribute to the filling and contraction of the heart. The following terms define these factors:

Stroke Volume (SV)

Stroke volume is the amount of blood ejected out of the heart per beat. Normal values are between 70cc-100cc. The Doppler formula for measuring the stroke volume is Cross Sectional area x Velocity Time Integral (CSA x VTI).

The stroke volume can be measured on both the right and left side.

Right stroke volume = RVOT CSA x RVOT VTI

Left stroke volume = LVOT CSA x LVOT VTI

Heart Rate (HR)

The normal heart rate in adults is between 60-100 beats per minute. The heart rate contributes to the overall cardiac output.

Cardiac Output (CO)

Cardiac output is the amount of blood ejected by the heart per minute. The normal range is between 4-8 L/min. The formula for calculating the cardiac output is Stroke volume x heart rate.

Cardiac Index (CI)

Cardiac index is the cardiac output adjusted by body surface area. Normal values range between 2.4 lpm/m² to 4.2 lpm/m². The formula for calculating cardiac index is: Cardiac output/ body surface area.

Frank Starlings Law

Frank Starlings Law states that the greater the stretch of the myocardial fibers (preload) the stronger the contraction. This is true up to a point. With excessive myocardial fiber stretching ventricular contraction can decrease leading to ventricular failure.

Preload

Preload is the volume in the ventricles at end diastole. Some factors affecting preload include the following:

- Aortic or pulmonary valve insufficiency
- Mitral or tricuspid valve regurgitation
- Ventricular septal defects
- Fluid overload
- Dilated cardiomyopathy

Afterload

Afterload is the resistance the ventricle faces upon ejection. Interventricular pressure and the resulting tension the myocardium must generate to overcome the resistance or pressure within the ventricle. Some factors affecting afterload include the following:

- Aortic or pulmonary valve stenosis
- Coarctation of the aorta
- Renal arterial stenosis
- Systemic hypertension

Increased afterload can cause ventricular hypertrophy. Prolonged and sustained increased afterload will result in ventricular failure.

Electrophysiology

The cardiac cells are unique. They have potential for spontaneous electrical depolarization. Terms associated with the heart include the following:

- **Automaticity:** The heart can beat and maintain rhythm without the assistance of the nervous system.

- **Excitability:** The cardiac muscle spontaneously accepts and responds to electrical impulses.

- **Conductivity:** The cardiac cells have the ability to transfer an electrical impulse to the next cardiac cell.

- **Contractility:** The heart contracts as a response to an electrical impulse.

- The cardiac conduction system is composed of the following components:

- **Sinoatrial (SA) node:** The SA node is located in the upper right atrial chamber near the entrance of the SVC. It has the highest degree of automaticity and is considered the pacemaker of the heart. The SA node fires electrical impulses at a rate of 60-100 beats per minute. This rate of firing is the rate of depolarization.

- **Internodal tracts:** From the SA node the cardiac impulse is carried to both atria via the internodal pathways or tracks. This causes the atria to depolarize and then contract.

- **Atrioventricular (AV) node:** The AV node receives the cardiac impulse from the internodal tracks and provides a slight 0.10 second delay before sending the impulse to the Bundle of His.

- **Bundle of His:** The Bundle of His is a thin bundle connecting the AV node with the bundle branches. The Bundle of His can also provide an intrinsic beat; however, the rate is much slower than the SA node. The Bundle of His fires at a rate between 40-60 beats per minute.

- **Left and Right Bundle branches:** The right and left bundle branches course along the right and left side of the interventricular septum and deliver the cardiac impulse to the right and left ventricle.

- **Perkinje Fibers:** The perkinje fibers are the terminal end of the bundle branches and deliver the cardiac impulse to the right and left ventricles causing ventricular depolarization. The left ventricle depolarization occurs slightly before the right ventricle. Biventricular contraction occurs after depolarization.

Phases of the Cardiac Cycle

Wigger's Diagram

- **Phase 1:** AV valves open; semilunar valves close – atrial systole. Denoted as P wave on ECG. S4 heart sound. Atrial contraction accounts for the remaining 30% of ventricular filling and is also known as the atrial "kick".

- **Phase 2: Isovolumic contraction** – time between the AV valve closure and semilunar valve opening. All valves are closed in this phase. Denoted by QRS complex on the ECG. S1 heart sound. Rapid increase in interventricular pressure.

- **Phase 3: Rapid ejection** – aortic and pulmonary valves are open; AV valves closed. The interventricular pressure exceeds the pressure in the aorta and pulmonary artery causing the semilunar valves to open. The ventricles eject blood into the great arteries. In normal valves there is usually no heart sound associated with ventricular ejection. Systolic mumurs are heard with valvular disease or intracardiac shunts.

- **Phase 4: Reduced ejection** – ventricular repolarization occurs and is denoted by the T wave on ECG. The rate of ventricular emptying falls.

- **Phase 5: Isovolumic relaxation** – time period between semilunar valve closure and AV valve opening. This represents early ventricular relaxation as ventricular pressures drop with no change in ventricular volume.

- **Phase 6: Rapid filling** – The atrioventricular valves open. The ventricular pressure falls below the atrial pressure. When this occurs rapid early filling occurs. There is usually no heart sound with ventricular filling. When a third sound (S3) is heard it may be related to ventricular dilatation.

- **Phase 7: Reduced filling** – The atrioventricular valves remain open. The rate of filling falls during this stage. Approximately 90% of atrial filling occurs before atrial contraction and is still considered passive filling.

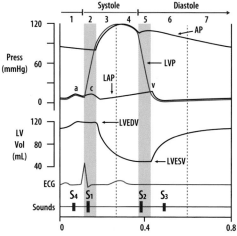

References

1. Reynolds, T. (1997). *Cardiovascular Principles. A Registry exam preparation guide.* Arizona Heart Foundation.

2. Otto, C. (2018). *Textbook of Clinical Echocardiography,* 6th edition. Elsevier.

3. Klein, A., Asher, C. (2017). *Clinical Echocardiography Review, A Self-Assessment Tool.* Wolters Kluwer

4. Guthrie, J. (2010). *Fetal Cardiac Sonography, National Certification Educational Review (NCER),* Society of Diagnostic Medical Sonography.

5. Klabunde, R. Cardiovascular Physiology Concepts. Downloaded on 01/03/2020 at https://www.cvphysiology.com

6. Schallert, E., Danton, G., Kardon, R., & Young, D. Describing Congenital Heart Disease by Using Three-Part Segmental Notation, RadioGraphics, March-April 2013.

7. Moore, K., Persaud, T.V.N., Torchia, M. (2013). Before we are Born. Essentials of Embryology and Birth Defects, 8th edition. Elsevier Saunders.

8. Bulwer, B. (2015). Transthoracic Echocardiography. Foundations of image Acquisition and Interpretation, Echo Stethoscope.

Echo Pharmacology
Christie H. Jordan, BS, RCS, RDCS, RCIS, FASE

A cardiac sonographer is not licensed to administer any type of drug. The information contained in this chapter pertains to helpful information about common cardiac medications that may be administered to cardiovascular patients or during a diagnostic or interventional cardiac examination.

Generic vs. Trade (Brand) Names

In pharmacology, all drugs have two names, a trade name and a generic name. For example, the generic name of Acetaminophen has a trade name of Tylenol, Acetaminophen (Tylenol). Naproxen is the generic name for Aleve, Naproxen (Aleve). For the purpose of this chapter, drugs will be listed as: Naproxen (Aleve) with the trade name in parenthesis.

Generic drugs are copies of brand-name drugs that have the exact dosage, intended use, effects, side effects, route of administration, risks, safety, and strength as the original drug. The pharmacological effects of the generic drug are the same as those of their brand-name counterparts.

Agonist vs. Antagonist

Most drugs work by binding to the target receptor site. They can either block the physiological function of the protein or mimic its effect. If a drug causes the protein receptor to respond in the same way as the naturally occurring substance, then the drug is referred to as an agonist. Antagonists are drugs that interact selectively with receptors but do not lead to an observed effect. Instead they reduce the action of an agonist at the receptor site involved.

Cardiovascular Medications / Agents

Beta Blocking Agents

Common Medications

- Propranolol (Inderal)
- Metoprolol (Toprol, Lopressor)
- Atenolol (Tenormin)

Mechanism of Action

Blocks beta adrenergic receptor sites causing a decrease in heart rate, afterload and contractility

Indications

- Angina Pectoris
- Acute coronary syndrome
- Hypertension
- Arrhythmias
- Heart Failure
- Other cardiac disease states (HOCM, MS, MVP, Aortic dissections)

Side Effects

- Bronchospasm and cold extremities
- Exaggeration of bradycardia
- Heart block

Contraindications

- Severe bradycardia
- High grade AV block
- Sick sinus syndrome

Calcium Channel Blockers

Common Medications

- Verapamil (Calan)
- Diltiazem (Cardizem)
- Nifedipine (Procardia)
- Amlodipine (Norvasc)

Mechanism of Action

Inhibits the flow of calcium into channels causing a decrease in heart rate, contractility and reduction of myocardial demand

Indications

- Stable and unstable angina
- Coronary spasm
- Hypertension
- Supraventricular tachycardia
- Post myocardial infarction protection

Side Effects

- Headaches
- Facial flushing
- Dizziness

Contraindications

- Sick sinus syndrome
- Preexisting AV block

ACE Inhibitors (angiotensin-converting enzyme)

Common Medications

- Captopril (Capoten)
- Enalapril (Vasotec)
- Lisinopril (Zestril, Prinivil)

Mechanism of Action

- Reduction of the effects of angiotensin

Indications

- Heart failure
- Hypertension
- Post myocardial infarction protection

Side Effects

- Cough
- Angioedema
- Transient renal failure

Contraindications

- Renal artery stenosis
- Systemic hypotension
- Pregnancy

ARBs (Angiotensin II Receptor Blockers)

Common Medications

- Losartan (Cozaar)
- Irbesartan (Avapro)
- Telmisartan (Micardis)

Mechanism of Action

- Inhibiting the formation of angiotensin II

Indications

- Heart Failure
- Hypertension

Side Effects

- Dizziness
- Hyperkalemia
- Angioedema

Contraindications

- Pregnancy

Antiarrhythmics

Common Medications

- Quinidine (Quinidex)
- Lidocaine (Xylocaine)
- Adenosine (Adenocard)
- Verapamil (Calan)
- Amiodarone (Cordarone)
- Sotalol (Betapace)

Mechanism of Action

- Used to alleviate life threatening or symptomatic arrhythmias

Indications

- **Supraventricular arrhythmias**
    - Adenosine (Adenocard)
    - Verapamil (Calan)
    - Diltiazem (Cardizem)
- **Atrial arrhythmias**
    - Rapid ventricular rate control with Beta blocker
    - Amiodarone for conversion of fibrillation
    - Ibutilide for conversion of flutter
- **Ventricular arrhythmias**
    - Amiodarone
    - Beta blocker
    - Verapamil (Calan)

Table 2.1: Classifications for Antiarrhythmics		
	Mechanism of Action	**Common Medications**
1A	Prolongs repolarization	Quinidine, Procainamide
1B	Shortens repolarization	Lidocaine, Mexiletine
1C	Positive sodium channel inhibitors	Flecainide
II	Blocks beta receptor and inhibition of current I_f	IV Beta blocking agents such as Propranolol, Sotalol, Acebutolol, Esmolol
III	Blocks sodium, calcium and repolarizing potassium channel	Amiodarone, Sotalol, Ibutilide
IV & IV	Slows conduction through the AV node	Calcium channel blockers such as Verapamil and Diltiazem and Class V Adenosine

Anticholinergic Agent

Common Medication

- Atropine (Atropine)

Mechanism of Action

- Inhibits muscarinic acetylcholine receptor sites producing an anticholinergic effect

Indications

- Bradycardia

Side Effects

- Blurred vision
- Tremors

Contraindications

- Pregnancy

Nitrates and Antianginal

Common Medications

- Nitroglycerin (Nitro-dur, Nitrostat)
- Isosorbide dinitrate (Isordil)
- Amyl nitrite (Amyl nitrite)

Mechanism of Action

- Coronary and peripheral vasodilation, reduction of oxygen demand

Indications

- Angina

Side Effects

- Hypotension
- Headaches
- Syncope

Contraindications

- Systolic BP of >90mmHg
- HOCM
- Patients taking sildenafil (viagra) sildenafil (Cailis)
- Acute Inferior MI
- Cor pulmonale

Diuretics

Common Medications

- Loop diuretics include Furosemide (Lasix)
- Thiazide diuretics include Hydrochlorothiazide, also known as HCTZ (HydroDiuril)
- Thiazide-like diuretics Chlorthalidone (Thalitone)

Mechanism of Action

- Alters physiologic renal mechanism to increase the flow of urine with great excretion of sodium

Indications

- Treatment of symptomatic heart failure with fluid retention, used as first line of therapy for hypertension with some vasodilation effects

Side Effects

- Hypokalemia
- Ventricular arrhythmia
- Hypovolemia

Contraindications

- Heart failure without fluid retention
- Dehydration

Acute or Chronic Heart Failure

Common Medications

- Dobutamine Hydrochloride (Dobutamine)
- Dopamine Hydrochloride (Dopamine)
- Epinephrine (Adrenaline)
- Norepinephrine (Noradrenaline)
- Isoproterenol (Isoprenaline)
- Nitroprusside (Nitropress)
- Vasopressin (Pitressin)

Mechanism of Action

- **Dobutamine:** β adrenergic stimulating agent, major characteristic is positive inotropic effect
- **Dopamine:** Catecholamine like agent, at higher doses causes a significant vasoconstriction effect
- **Epinephrine (Adrenaline):** mixed $\beta_1\beta_2$ stimulation with some added α mediated effects at high doses
- **Norepinephrine:** prominent β_1 and α-effects with less β_2
- **Isoproterenol:** Pure B stimulant (B1 >B2)
- **Vasopressin:** Antidiuretic hormone synthesized in the hypothalamus
- **Nitroprusside:** Strong vasodilator

Indications

- **Dobutamine:** Heart failure, Severe Acute MI, Cardiogenic Shock
  - Also given to mimic exercise in pharmacologic stress testing
- **Dopamine:** Severe Heart Failure, Cardiogenic shock
- **Epinephrine:** Cardiac arrest
- **Norepinephrine:** Cardiogenic shock
- **Isoproterenol:** Cardiogenic shock
- **Vasopressin:** Septic shock, intraoperative hypotension
- **Nitroprusside:** Hypertensive Crisis, Dissecting Aortic Aneurysm

Lipid Modifying (Statins)

Common Medication

- Atorvastatin (Lipitor)
- Pravastatin (Pravachol)
- Simvastatin (Zocor)

Mechanism of Action

- Slow the progression of coronary atherosclerosis, reduces total cholesterol, LDL and triglycerides

Indications

- Reduction of LDL levels in patients at risk for cardiovascular heart disease

Contraindications

- Advanced liver disease
- Pregnancy

Antithrombotic Agents

Platelet Inhibitors
- Acts as an arterial thrombogenesis/antithrombotic effect

Common Medication
- Aspirin (Bayer)
- Abciximab (ReoPro)

Mechanism of Action
- Blocks aggregation of thrombin

Indications
- Reduction of embolic events with patients with history of CV events
- Reduces mortality after CABG
- Prevention of stroke in atrial fibrillation
- Decreases thrombosis in patients with AV shunts

Side Effects
- Bleeding
- Gastric irritation
- GI Issues

Contraindications
- Aspirin intolerance
- History of GI bleed

Anticoagulants
- Limit further formation of thrombus, when given chronically helps prevent thromboembolism

Common Medication
- Heparin (Heparin (IV)
- PO medications:
    - Warfarin (Coumadin)
    - Dabigatran etexilate (Pradaxa)
    - Rivaroxaban (Xarelto)

Mechanism of Action
- Interaction with antithrombin and thrombin to prevent thrombin induced platelet aggregation, interferes with the formation of Vitamin K

Indications
- AMI
- Atrial fibrillation
- Protective agent for PCI

Side Effects
- Bleeding

Contraindications
- Recent Stroke
- History of GI bleed
- Uncontrolled Hypertension
- First trimester pregnancy

Fibrinolytic agents

Common Medication

- Alteplase (tPA, Tissue Plasminogen Activator)
- Tenecteplase (Tnkase)
- Reteplase (Retavase)
- Streptokinase (Streptase)

Mechanism of Action

- Rapidly dissolve thrombus by binding to fibrin

Indications

- STEMI
- Acute ischemic stroke

Side Effects

- Relate chiefly to hemorrhage

Contraindications

- Risk of hemorrhage or hemorrhagic stroke

References

1. Opie L, Gersh B: *Drugs for the Heart.* Philadelphia, Elsevier Saunders, 2013.

2. Otto, C. *Textbook of Clinical Echocardiography.* Philadelphia, Elsevier, 2018.

Cardiac Sonography Instrumentation
Jon Owensby, ACS, RDCS, RRT

Basic Echo Physics

An Ultrasound imaging system uses electrical current to vibrate piezoelectric crystals within the transducer causing them to emit ultrasound waves into the body. The crystals also receive some of the sound waves emitted as reflections or "echoes" which are sent to scan converters within the system converting the returning sound waves into a visual display for diagnostic purposes.

Diagnostic Ultrasound normally uses a frequency range of 2-15 Megahertz (MHz).

Wavelength

Table 3.1: Frequency Comparisons	
Low frequency	High frequency
Longer wavelength	Shorter wavelength
Inferior resolution	Superior resolution
Less attenuation	More attenuation
Better penetration	Worse penetration

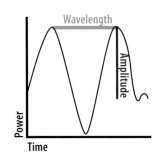

Amplitude

Ultrasound pulses are rapidly submitted into the body tissue for imaging with only a fraction of the pulses returning for display.

- Attenuation (heat distribution) is the most common loss of sound transmitted

- Scatter (Non-specular) occurs when imaging a structure with different tissue properties changing the impedance and minimal reflection returns to the probe

- Refraction is when imaging a structure at a non-perpendicular angle and the beam reflects back at a non-specular angle to the probe diluting the sample

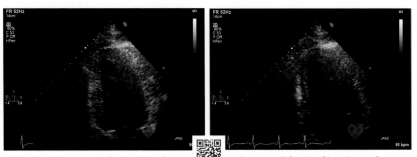

Figure 3.1: **Optimal imaging angle**   Figure 3.2: **Suboptimal imaging angle**

Two-Dimensional Echo (2D)

- Most commonly used modality

- Limited by body habitus

- Temporal resolution and frame rate are most affected by imaging depth, and air lung interference sector width, and number of focal zones

- Operator dependent

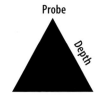

Figure 3.3: **2D echo image of the PLAX**

Optimizing Image

- Because depth is one of the most important factors in frame rate, it is recommended to image as shallow as possible.

- When receiver gain is increased it will amplify weak signals and decrease image resolution.

- Frequency and penetration are inversely related.

Table 3.2: Gain Comparison	
Overall Gain	**Time gain control (TGC)**
Adjust entire depth	Customize where needed
Post processing adjustable	Supplement weak reflectors in far field

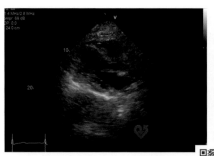

Figure 3.4: **Optimal TGC settings**

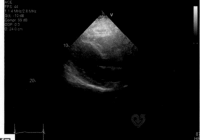

Figure 3.5: **Suboptimal TGC settings**

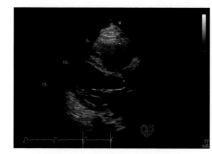

Figure 3.6: **Optimal overall gain**

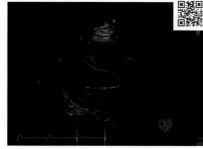

Figure 3.7: **Low overall gain**

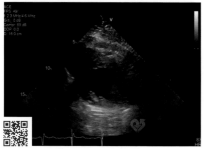

Figure 3.8: **Highest frequency**

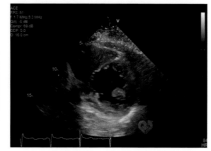

Figure 3.9: **Lowest frequency**

There is a trade off between resolution and depth of penetration when adjusting transmit frequency *(Table 3.1)*. It is recommended to use the highest frequency available in order to obtain the best resolution. Lower, high frequency has greater attenuation which leads to less penetration

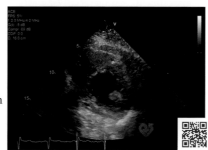

Figure 3.10: **Optimal frequency**

M-mode

- Highest temporal resolution
- Single scan line
- Excellent for timing of events. Best if you are perpendicular to the structure.

Since the machine is continuously refreshing a single scan line and not writing the whole sector the temporal resolution is excellent; the pitfall is the angle of incidence to the structure of interest.

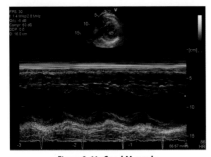 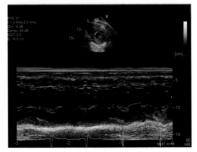

Figure 3.11: **Good M-mode**   Figure 3.12: **Poor M-mode**

Spectral Doppler

Pulse Wave (PW) Doppler

- Capability to sample at an exact location (range resolution)
- Limited velocity capability (aliasing)
- Adjustable sample size (millimeters)
- Pulse wave Doppler has the capability of pinpointing a velocity at an exact location. Normal pulse wave Doppler envelope has a very specific appearance called a modal frequency with a clean "window" beneath the modal frequency

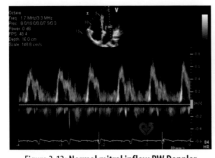 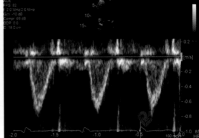

Figure 3.13: **Normal mitral inflow PW Doppler**   Figure 3.14: **Normal LVOT PW Doppler**

- As the flow within the sample starts to get turbulent the clean "window" of the pulsed Doppler starts to fill in giving it the look of continuous wave Doppler

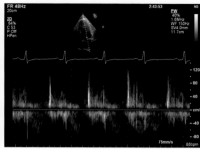

Figure 3.15: **Turbulent mitral inflow**

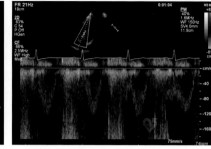

Figure 3.16: **Turbulent LVOT PW Doppler**

- Once the measured velocity exceeds what pulsed wave is capable of processing the velocity will alias or "wrap around" the baseline undermining the accuracy of the sample

- Another valuable feature of pulsed Doppler is the capability of adjusting the size of the sample gate to acquire more flow. Most machines have a adjustable range of 1-10 millimeters.

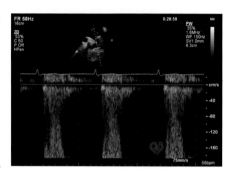

Figure 3.17: **Aliased PW Doppler**

Continuous Wave (CW) Doppler

- Displays all velocities along a scan line
- Will not alias
- CW has range ambiguity
- May pickup proximal flow interference from nearby flow
- Continuous wave Doppler is constantly sending and receiving pulses all along the dedicated scan line so the display is a representation of the entire scan line

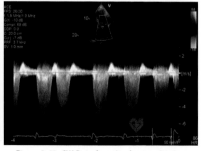

Figure 3.18: **CW Doppler mitral regurgitation**

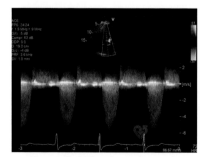

Figure 3.19: **CW Doppler aortic stenosis**

- As the heart contracts and the patient breathes it is easy to pick up multiple flows along the same sample line

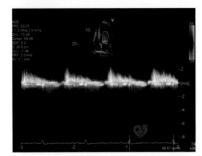

Figure 3.20: **Mitral inflow with aortic regurgitation**   Figure 3.21: **Dynamic LV gradient with MR**

• These are examples of picking up multiple significant flows along the scan line. The peak velocity is always displayable but quantifying the point of origin is the pitfall of Continuous Wave Doppler

Color Doppler

• Superimposed on 2D image

• Aliases at the Nyquist limit

• Added demand on processor decreases refresh "frame" rate

• Commonly used modality to evaluate appropriate blood flow. Used to verify the competency of the valves and interatrial/interventricular shunts. Operator can easily miss underlying pathology with too low of frame rate. Color Doppler display is dependent on the red blood cells flowing parallel to the transducer to fill the display; if no blood flow was moving then there would be nothing to display.

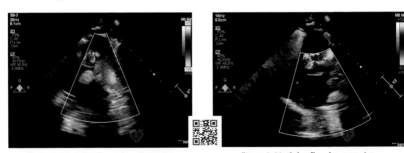

Figure 3.22: **Color flow normal nyquist**   Figure 3.23: **Color flow low nyquist**

With the size of the color box roughly the same size. The image on the right is at a deeper depth which slows the frame rate. The frame rate is displayed in the upper left hand corner of the image (Frames Per Second). Also notice that the color scale bar graph (right) shows darker colors towards the middle of the bar and lighter colors towards the edges of the bar graph indicating that the higher velocity flows are displayed as a lighter, brighter color. When the velocity of the color flow exceeds the number at the ends of the bar scale then the color wraps around the scale with flow coming towards the transducer turning red to blue and flow traveling away from the transducer turning from blue to red (color aliasing).

Echo Views / Comprehensive Echo Exam
Carol Mitchell, PhD, ACS, RDMS, RDCS, RVT, RT(R), FASE, FSDMS

This chapter will discuss the echocardiography views and images to be acquired when performing the comprehensive transthoracic echocardiogram (TTE).[1]

Definition of Protocol

Formal method for obtaining standard views when performing a comprehensive transthoracic echocardiogram (TTE).

The comprehensive adult TTE typically begins with imaging in the parasternal window in the long axis plane with the patient positioned in the left lateral decubitus position.[1] Usually this is a parasternal left window as in most patients the cardiac apex is directed towards the left side of the body (levocardia) with normal situs (situs solitus). After images are acquired from the parasternal long axis views, parasternal short axis views are acquired followed by apical, subcostal and suprasternal notch views.[1-6] The apical window is located on the left side of the body aligned to the midaxillary line and the transducer is placed over the area with maximum apical impulse (usually the fourth or fifth intercostal space).[1] The orientation index marker is positioned to the left side of the patient and the beginning view will demonstrate the apical 4-chamber view.[1] For the subcostal and suprasternal notch image acquisition, the patient is positioned in the supine position.[1-6] For subcostal imaging it may help to have the patient bend their knees to relax the stomach muscles. For subcostal imaging the transducer orientation index marker is positioned to the left side of the body (3 o'clock position) and tilted superior to demonstrated the subcostal 4-chamber view.[1] After imaging the subcostal 4-chamber view, the orientation index marker is rotated to the 12 o'clock position to image the inferior vena cava in a longitudinal plane. When acquiring suprasternal notch images, the patient is positioned in the supine position with a pillow behind the shoulders allowing for extension of the head and neck. The head is turned slightly to the left and the transducer is placed just above the manubrium with the orientation index marker positioned at the 1 o'clock position to demonstrate the ascending aorta, aortic arch and descending aorta.[1] For each imaging window, there are a series of recommended views and measurements to be acquired to follow the American Society of Echocardiography comprehensive TTE protocol.[1] This chapter will outline the image acquisition windows, cardiac imaging axis planes, 2D and color Doppler views to be acquired, 2D measurements, M-mode images to acquire and Doppler measurements.[1]

The term "window" refers to the anatomic position where the transducer is placed. There are four imaging windows used for acquiring TTE images. [1, 7]

• Parasternal (right and left)
• Apical
• Subcostal
• Suprasternal Notch

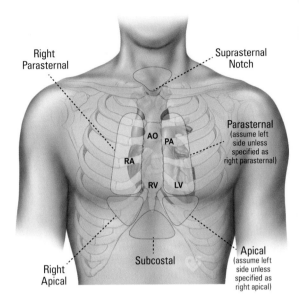

Echocardiography windows

Cardiac Imaging Planes

The term "plane" refers to the orientation of the image. There are three planes used to describe TTE images. [1, 3, 5]

• Long axis
• Short axis
• Apical

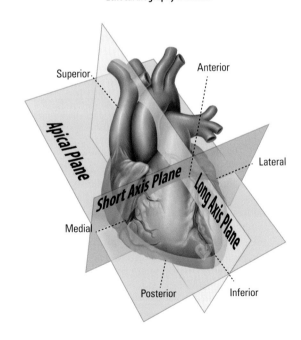

Cardiac axis planes. Yellow (long axis), blue (apical plane), pink (short axis plane)

Maneuvers listed below are described in detail in the *Guidelines for Performing a Comprehensive Transthoracic Echocardiographic Examination in Adults: Recommendations from the American Society of Echocardiography. J Am Soc Echocardiogr. 2019;32:1-64.* [1]

Tilt movement

- Transducer stays in the same imaging axis
- Face of the transducer is manipulated to demonstrate different imaging planes [1,8]
- Clinical example: tilting the transducer posterior to demonstrate the coronary sinus and anterior to image the great vessels [1]

Rotate movement

- Transducer stays in the same position
- Orientation index marker is rotated to a different position [1,8]
- Clinical example: rotating index orientation marker from a parasternal long axis to a parasternal short axis view [1]

Slide movement

- Physically changing the location of the transducer [1,8]
- Clinical example: sliding the transducer from one rib space to another rib space [1]

Rock (small) movement

- Transducer stays in the same imaging plane
- Moved towards or away from the orientation marker [1]
- Clinical example: rocking to center a structure [1,8]

Angle (small) movement

- Transducer stays in same location
- Sound beam directed towards a specific structure
- Clinical example: angling from the focused tricuspid valve to the focused pulmonic valve view in the short axis plane at the level of the aortic valve [1]

Transthoracic Echocardiography
2D and Color Doppler Imaging Views

The term "views" for this chapter, refer to a name for standard images that should be acquired as part of the comprehensive TTE examination. [1] There are a series of views acquired from each image acquisition window. [1,7] Views are described and labeled based on the image acquisition window, axis plane and anatomy demonstrated. [1] The windows and axis planes from which they are acquired are listed below. A corresponding color Doppler image clip should be taken after each grayscale image clip.

- Parasternal long axis (PLAX)
- Parasternal short axis (PSAX)
- Apical (A)
- Subcostal (SC)
- Suprasternal notch (SSN)

Parasternal Window

Long Axis Plane (PLAX) Views

4

Echo Views / Comprehensive Echo Exam / Transthoracic Echocardiography 2D and Color Doppler Imaging Views / Parasternal Window

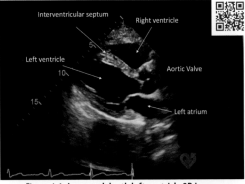

Figure 4.1: **Increased depth left ventricle 2D image**

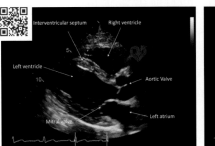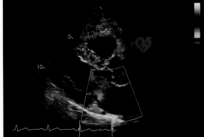

Figure 4.2: **Left ventricle 2D and color Doppler**

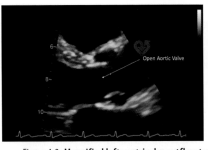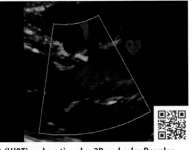

Figure 4.3: **Magnified left ventricular outflow tract (LVOT) and aortic valve 2D and color Doppler**

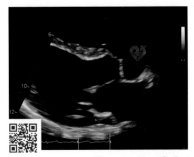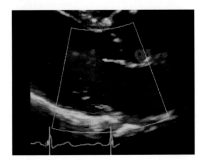

Figure 4.4: **Magnified mitral valve 2D and color Doppler**

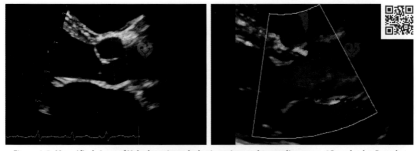

Figure 4.5: **Magnified sinus of Valsalva, sinotubular junction and ascending aorta 2D and color Doppler**

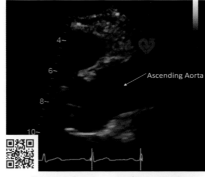

Figure 4.6: **Focus on ascending aorta 2D**

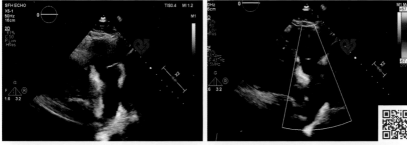

Figure 4.7: **Right ventricular outflow tract (RVOT), pulmonic valve, pulmonary artery 2D and color Doppler**

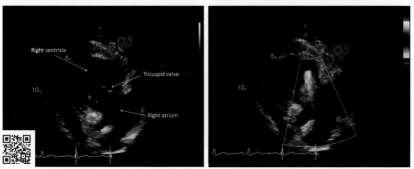

Figure 4.8: **Right ventricular inflow tract (tricuspid valve) 2D and color Doppler**

4

Echo Views / Comprehensive Echo Exam / Transthoracic Echocardiography 2D and Color Doppler Imaging Views / Parasternal Window

Short Axis Plane (PSAX) Views

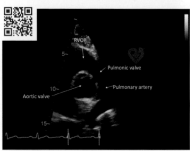
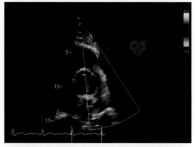

Figure 4.9: **Level of great vessels (aortic valve and pulmonic valve) 2D and color Doppler**

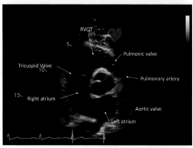
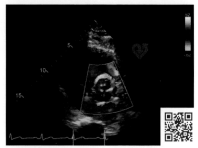

Figure 4.10: **Level of aortic valve 2D and color Doppler**

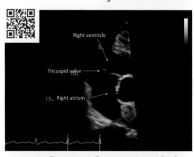
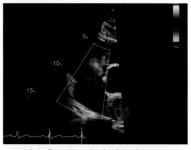

Figure 4.11: **Focus on tricuspid valve, right ventricle inflow 2D and color Doppler**

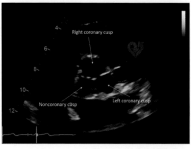
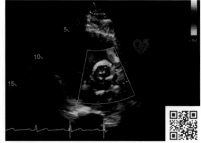

Figure 4.12: **Magnified aortic valve 2D and color Doppler**

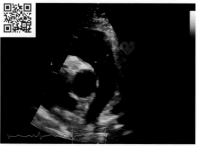
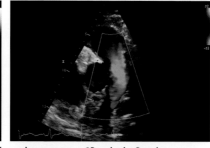

Figure 4.13: **Focus on RVOT, pulmonic valve, pulmonary artery 2D and color Doppler**

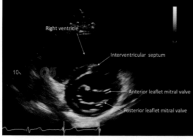
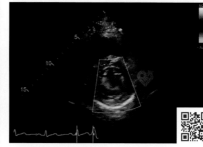

Figure 4.14: **Level of mitral valve (anterior leaflet mitral valve and posterior leaflet mitral valve) 2D and color Doppler**

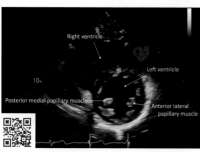
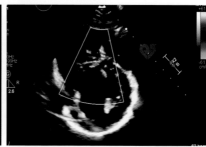

Figure 4.15: **Level of papillary muscles (posterior medial papillary muscle and anterior lateral papillary muscle) 2D and color Doppler**

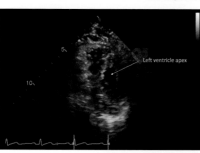
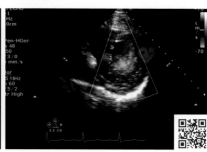

Figure 4.16: **Level of left ventricle apex 2D and color Doppler**

4

Echo Views / Comprehensive Echo Exam / Transthoracic Echocardiography 2D and Color Doppler Imaging Views / Parasternal Window

Apical Window

Apical Views

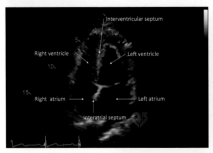
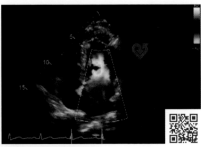

Figure 4.17: **4-chamber 2D and color Doppler**

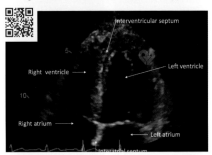

Figure 4.18: **4-chamber focus on left ventricle 2D**

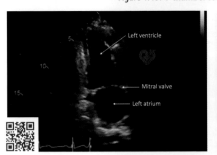
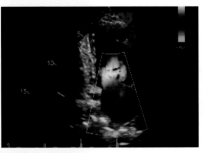

Figure 4.19: **2-chamber 2D and color Doppler**

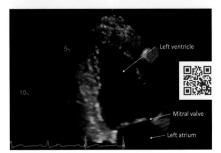

Figure 4.20: **2-chamber focus on left ventricle 2D**

4

Echo Views / **Comprehensive Echo Exam** / Transthoracic Echocardiography 2D and Color Doppler Imaging Views / Apical Window

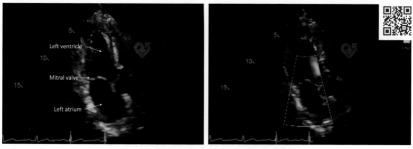

Figure 4.21: **3-chamber 2D and color Doppler**

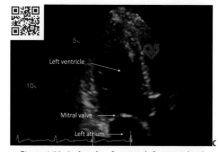

Figure 4.22: **3-chamber focus on left ventricle 2D**

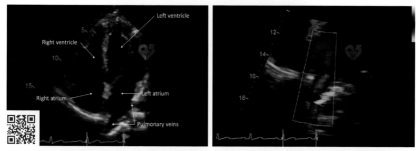

Figure 4.23: **Pulmonary veins 2D and magnified view of pulmonary veins with color Doppler**

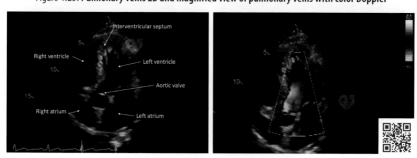

Figure 4.24: **5-chamber 2D and color Doppler**

4

Echo Views / Comprehensive Echo Exam / Transthoracic Echocardiography 2D and Color Doppler Imaging Views / Apical Window

4

Echo Views / Comprehensive Echo Exam / Transthoracic Echocardiography 2D and Color Doppler Imaging Views / Subcostal Window

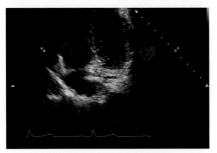

Figure 4.25: **Coronary sinus 2D**

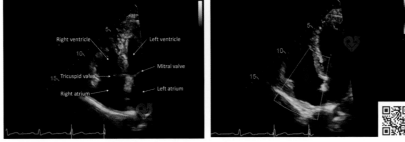

Figure 4.26: **Focus right ventricle 2D and color Doppler**

Subcostal Window

Subcostal Views

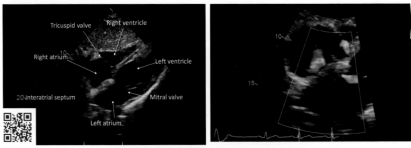

Figure 4.27: **4-chamber (Right: Magnified view of interatrial septum with color Doppler image – an alternative view) 2D and color Doppler**

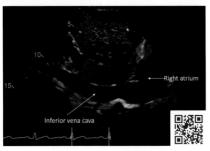

Figure 4.28: **Inferior vena cava 2D**

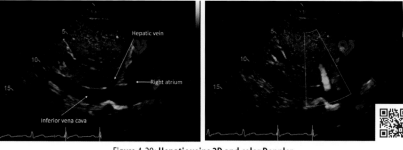

Figure 4.29: **Hepatic veins 2D and color Doppler**

Suprasternal Notch Window

Suprasternal Views

Aortic Arch

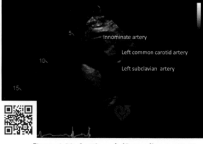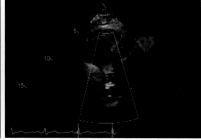

Figure 4.30: **Aortic arch (Ascending aorta, transverse arch, descending aorta) and branches (Innominate artery, left common carotid artery, left subclavian artery) 2D and color Doppler**

4

Echo Views / Comprehensive Echo Exam / Transthoracic Echocardiography 2D and Color Doppler Imaging Views / Suprasternal Notch Window

2D Transthoracic Echocardiography Measurements

2D measurements described below are from the *Guidelines for Performing a Comprehensive Transthoracic Echocardiographic Examination in Adults: Recommendations from the American Society of Echocardiography.* [1]

Parasternal Window

Long Axis Plane (PLAX) Measurements

Left Ventricle View

End-Diastole Measurements

- Right ventricle
- Interventricular septum
- Left ventricle
- Left ventricle posterior wall
- RVOT proximal portion

Technique

- Structures are measured at end-diastole
- Right ventricle – measure from the interface of the compacted myocardium to the leading edge of the interventricular septum [1, 9]
- Interventricular septum measure from the blood septal tissue interface of the right ventricle cavity to the blood tissue interface of the left ventricle cavity Include only compacted tissue [1, 9]
- Left ventricle measure from the blood compact myocardium interface to the leading edge of the posterior wall. The measurement is made at the level of the tips of the mitral valve leaflets. [1, 9]
- Left ventricle posterior wall measure from the blood compacted myocardium interface to the interface of the posterior wall and pericardium [1, 9]
- RVOT proximal portion measure from the compacted myocardium of the right ventricle anterior wall to the aortic septal junction [1, 9, 10]

End-Systole Diameters

- Left ventricle end-systole
- Left atrium end-systole

Technique

- Measure just inferior to the mitral valve leaflet tips from the blood compacted myocardium interface to the leading edge of the interventricular septum [1, 9]
- Measure the left atrium leading edge to leading edge from the level of the aortic sinuses to the leading edge of the posterior left atrial wall. The measurement should be made perpendicular to the long axis of the left atrium. [1, 9]

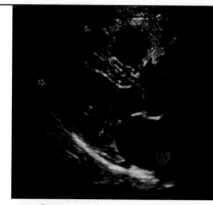

Figure 4.31: **Left ventricle end systole**

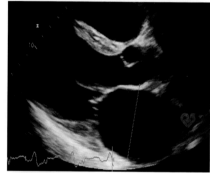

Figure 4.32: **Left atrium end-systole**

LVOT Diameter

Technique

Inner edge to inner edge at mid-systole [1, 9]

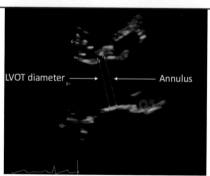

Figure 4.33: **LVOT diameter 2D**

Sinus of Valsalva

Technique

Leading-edge to leading-edge end diastole [1, 9]

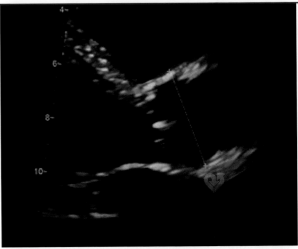

Figure 4.34: **Sinus of Valsalva 2D**

Ascending Aorta

Technique

Leading-edge to leading-edge end diastole [1, 9]

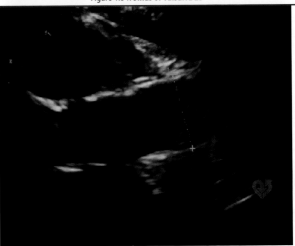

Figure 4.35: **Ascending aorta 2D**

Parasternal Window
Short Axis Plane Views

RVOT Proximal,
RVOT Distal,
Pulmonary Artery Diameters

Technique

- RVOT proximal and distal measured at end-diastole
- Pulmonary artery measured midway between the pulmonary valve and the bifurcation into the right and left pulmonary arteries at end-diastole (inner edge to inner edge) [1, 9, 10]

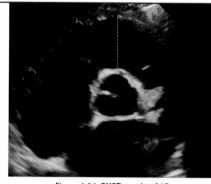

Figure 4.36: **RVOT proximal 2D**

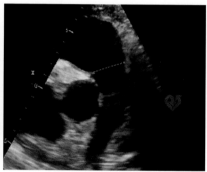

Figure 4.37: **RVOT distal 2D**

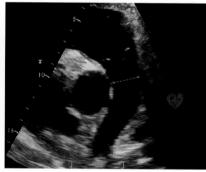

Figure 4.38: **Pulmonary artery 2D**

Apical Window

Apical Views

Left Atrium Volume

Measured at end systole in the apical 4-chamber and apical 2-chamber

Technique

• Measure maximum volume at end-systole

• Trace the left atrium borders along the endocardial borders

• Do not include the atrial appendage or pulmonary veins

• Complete the tracing by drawing a line across the annulus [1, 9]

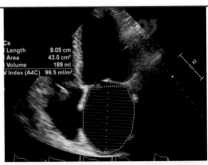

Figure 4.39: **End systole in the apical 4-chamber**

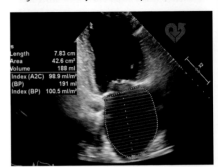

Figure 4.40: **End systole in the apical 2-chamber**

Right Atrium Volume

Technique

• Measure maximum volume at end-systole

• Trace the right atrium borders along the endocardial borders

• Do not include the atrial appendage, inferior vena cava or superior vena cava

• Complete the tracing by drawing a line across the annulus [1, 9]

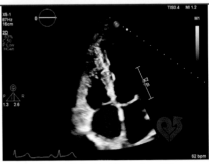

Figure 4.41: **Right atrium volume 2D**

Left Ventricle Volume 2D

Technique

- Measure the left ventricle volumes at end-diastole an end-systole in the apical 4-chamber and apical 2-chamber views

- Trace the left ventricle along the border of the compacted and noncompacted myocardium [1, 9]

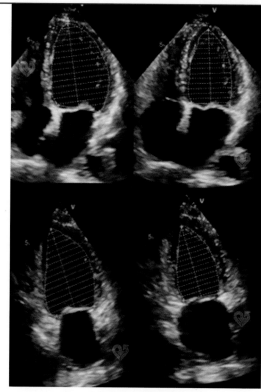

Figure 4.42: **Left ventricle volume 2D**

Left Ventricle Volume 3D

Technique

If 3D imaging is available, volumes and function should be measured and assessed using 3D algorithms [1, 9, 11]

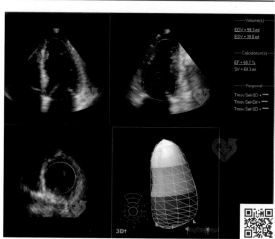

Figure 4.43: **Left ventricle volume 3D**

4

Right Ventricle Diameters (Basal and Mid-Cavity) and Length

Technique
Measurements are made at end-diastole [1, 9]

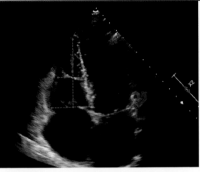

Figure 4.44: **Right ventricle diameters (basal and mid-cavity) and length 2D**

Right Ventricle Area

Technique
- Measurements are made by tracing the compacted myocardium border in end diastole and end systole to calculate the fractional area change
- Trabeculae and papillary muscles are considered part of the right ventricle cavity [1, 9, 10, 12]

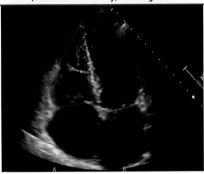

Figure 4.45: **Right ventricle area 2D**

Subcostal Window
Subcostal Views

Inferior Vena Cava

Technique
Measure diameter in longitudinal plane of inferior vena cava [1, 9, 10]

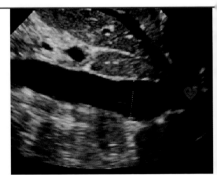

Figure 4.46: **Inferior vena cava**

Transthoracic Echocardiography
M-mode Views and Measurements

M-mode views and measurements described below are from the *Guidelines for Performing a Comprehensive Transthoracic Echocardiographic Examination in Adults: Recommendations from the American Society of Echocardiography. J Am Soc Echocardiogr. 2019;32:1-64.* [1]

Parasternal Window
Long Axis Plane Left Ventricle View

Structure
- Aortic valve M-mode

Technique
- Recommended sweep speed is 100mm/second [1]

Evaluate
- Motion of the aortic root and aortic leaflets

Structure
- Left atrium M-mode

Technique
- Recommended sweep speed is 100mm/second [1]
- Measurement of the left atrium anterior to posterior diameter can be made with M-mode (2D is preferred)
- Diameter measured from sinuses of Valsalva to the left atrium posterior wall
- Measurement is made using the leading edge to leading edge technique

Evaluate
- Left atrium size

Structure
- Mitral valve M-mode

Technique
- Recommended sweep speed is 100mm/second [1]

Evaluate
- Motion mitral valve leaflets, E point septal separation distance

Structure
- Left ventricle M-mode

Technique
- Recommended sweep speed is 100mm/second [1]

Evaluate
- Motion of right ventricle anterior wall, interventricular septum, left ventricle posterior wall

4

Echo Views / Comprehensive Echo Exam / Transthoracic Echocardiography M-mode Views and Measurements / Parasternal Window

Apical Window
Apical Plane 4-chamber Views

Structure
• Tricuspid annular plane systolic excursion (TAPSE) M-mode

Technique
• Recommended sweep speed is 100mm/second [1]
• Measurement is the distance from the trough to the peak and represents the distance traveled by the tricuspid annulus from end-diastole to end-systole [1]

Evaluate
• TAPSE distance measurement

Subcostal Window
Subcostal Inferior Vena Cava Long Axis View

Structure
• Inferior vena cava M-mode

Technique
• Recommended sweep speed is 100mm/second [1]

Evaluate
• Diameter changes with respiration

Important to Note

M-mode is useful to see the timing of structure movement. M-mode is not recommended for routine linear measurements of structure and chamber size. [1] M-mode is recommended for TAPSE, maybe helpful for IVC diameter changes with respiration and for evaluation of AV leaflet motion in individuals with left ventricle assist devices.[1]

Transthoracic Echocardiography
Doppler Views and Measurements

Doppler measurements described below are from the Guidelines for Performing a Comprehensive Transthoracic Echocardiographic Examination in Adults: Recommendations from the American Society of Echocardiography. J Am Soc Echocardiogr. 2019;32:1-64. [1]

Parasternal Window
Long Axis Plane Views

Right ventricle inflow -Tricuspid valve
- Continuous wave Doppler of tricuspid valve regurgitation if present [1]
- Measure peak velocity [1, 13]

Short Axis Plane Views

RVOT

- Pulsed wave Doppler RVOT peak velocity [1]
- Pulsed wave Doppler RVOT velocity time integral [1]

RVOT, Pulmonary Valve

- Continuous wave Doppler pulmonary valve peak velocity [1]
- Continuous wave Doppler pulmonary valve velocity time integral [1]
- Continuous wave Doppler of pulmonary valve regurgitation if present; measure end-diastolic pulmonary regurgitation velocity [1]

Apical Window

Apical Views

Apical 4-Chamber

- Pulsed wave Doppler mitral valve inflow
- Measure peak E-wave velocity, deceleration slope, deceleration time and peak A-wave velocity [1]
- Patient Valsalva maneuver and evaluate mitral valve inflow pulsed wave Doppler pattern [1]
- If tachycardia is present the mitral valve deceleration time may be interrupted and fusion of the E and A wave may be present. If fusion of the E and A wave (A wave starts on the E deceleration slope line at an E velocity >20cm/sec), deceleration time should not be measured. [1, 14, 15]
- Continuous wave Doppler of mitral valve inflow should be performed if stenosis, other pathology or prosthetic valves are present. [1]
    - Continuous wave Doppler of mitral valve inflow to measure mean gradient, pressure half-time, velocity time integral and peak velocity [1]
- Continuous wave Doppler of mitral valve regurgitation if present. Measure peak regurgitant velocity and velocity time integral. [1]
- **Focused pulmonary veins:** Doppler flow in pulmonary vein. Evaluate S-wave, D-wave and A-wave [1]
- **Doppler tissue imaging:** Perform Doppler tissue imaging of the tricuspid lateral annulus and mitral valve lateral and medial annulus and measure s', e' and a' velocities at each location [1, 14]

Apical 5-Chamber

LVOT: Pulsed wave Doppler LVOT and measure LVOT peak velocity and velocity time integral [1, 16, 17]

Aortic valve:

- Continuous wave Doppler through aortic valve. Measure aortic valve peak velocity and velocity time integral [1, 16, 17]
- Continuous wave Doppler aortic valve regurgitation if present. Measure peak velocity (used to calculate proximal isovelocity surface area) and measure aortic regurgitation slope (used to calculate pressure half-time) [13]

Subcostal Window
Subcostal Views

Hepatic Vein View
• Pulsed wave Doppler hepatic vein. Evaluate S, D, and A waves. [1, 15]

Suprasternal Notch Window
Suprasternal Notch Views

Aortic Arch
- Pulsed wave Doppler of the ascending aorta, measure the peak velocity [1]
- Pulsed wave Doppler of the descending aorta, measure the peak velocity [1]
- Pulsed wave Doppler of the descending aorta if aortic regurgitation is present. Measure the velocity time integral of the aortic regurgitant flow. [1]

Important to Note

Full Imaging Protocol can be referenced to the *Guidelines for Performing a Comprehensive Transthoracic Echocardiographic Examination in Adults: Recommendations from the American Society of Echocardiography.* [1]

References

1. Mitchell C, Rahko PS, Blauwet LA, Canaday B, Finstuen JA, Foster MC, Horton K, Ogunyankin KO, Palma RA and Velazquez EJ. Guidelines for Performing a Comprehensive Transthoracic Echocardiographic Examination in Adults: Recommendations from the American Society of Echocardiography. *J Am Soc Echocardiogr.* 2019;32:1-64.

2. Otto CM. Principles of echocardiographic image acquisition and Doppler analysis. In: Otto CM, editor. Textbook of clinical echocardiography. 5th Ed. Philadelphia: Elsevier Saunders; 2013. pp. 1-30.

3. Otto CM. Normal anatomy and flow patterns on transthoracic echocardiography. In: Otto CM, editor. Textbook of clinical echocardiography. 5th Ed. Philadelphia: Elsevier Saunders; 2013. pp. 31-64.

4. Otto CM. The echo exam: quick reference guide basic principles. In: C.M. Otto, editor. Textbook of clinical echocardiography. 5th Ed. Philadelphia: Elsevier Saunders; 2013. pp. 500-503.

5. Anderson B. The two-dimensional echocardiographic examination. In: B. Anderson, ed. *Echocardiography the normal examination and echocardiographic measurements.* 3rd Edition. Australia: Echotext Pty Ltd; 2017. pp. 33-70.

6. Anderson B. The spectral Doppler examination *Echocardiography The normal examination and echocardiographic measurements.* 3rd edition. Australia: Echotext Pty Ltd; 2017. pp. 105-128.

7. Henry WL, DeMaria A, Gramiak R, King DL, Kisslo JA, Popp RL, Sahn DJ, Schiller NB, Tajik A, Teichholz LE and Weyman AE. Report of the American Society of Echocardiography Committee on Nomenclature and Standards in Two-dimensional Echocardiography. *Circulation.* 1980;62:212-217.

8. American Institute of Ultrasound in Medicine. Transducer manipulation for echocardiography. *J Ultrasound Med.* 2005;24:733-736.

9. Lang RM, Badano LP, Mor-Avi V, Afilalo J, Armstrong A, Ernande L, Flachskampf FA, Foster E, Goldstein SA, Kuznetsova T, Lancellotti P, Muraru, D., Picard MH, Rietzschel ER, Rudski L, Spenser KT, Tsang W and Vioigt J-U. Recommendations for cardiac chamber quantification by echocardiography in adults: An update from the American Society Echocardiography and the European Association of Cardiovascular Imaging. *Am Soc Echocardiogr.* 2015; 28:1-39.

10. Rudski LG, Lai WW, Afilalo J, Hua L, Handschumacher MD, Chandrasekaran K, Solomon SD, Louie EK and Schiller NB. Guidelines for the echocardiographic assessment of the right heart in adults: a report from the American Society of Echocardiography endorsed by the European Association of Echocardiography, a registered branch of the European Society of Cardiology, and the Canadian Society of Echocardiography. *J Am Soc Echocardiogr.* 2010;23:685-713; quiz 786-788.

11. Lang RM, Badano LP, Tsang W, Adams DH, Agricola E, Buck T, Faletra FF, Franke A, Hung J, Perez de Isla L, Kamp O, Kasprzak JD, Lancellotti P, Marwick TH, McCulloch ML, Monaghan MJ, Nihoyannopoulos P, Pandian NG, Pellikka PA, Pepi M, Roberson DA, Shernan SK, Shirali GS, Sugeng L, Ten Cate FJ, Vannan MA, Zamorano JL and Zoghbi WA. EAE/ASE Recommendations for Image Acquisition and Display Using Three-Dimensional Echocardiography. *J Am Soc Echocardiogr.* 2012;25:3-46.

12. Horton KD, Meece RW and Hill JC. Assessment of the right ventricle by echocardiography: a primer for cardiac sonographers. *J Am Soc Echocardiogr.* 2009;22:776-792; quiz 861-862.

13. Zoghbi WA, Adams D, Bonow RO, Enriquez-Sarano M, Foster E, Grayburn PA, Hahn RT, Han Y, Hung J, Lang RM, Little SH, Shah DJ, Shernan S, Thavendiranathan P, Thomas JD and Weissman NJ. Recommendations for Noninvasive Evaluation of Native Valvular Regurgitation: A Report from the American Society of Echocardiography Developed in Collaboration with the Society for Cardiovascular Magnetic Resonance. *J Am Soc Echocardiogr.* 2017;30:303-371.

14. Nagueh SF, Smiseth OA, Appleton CP, Byrd BF, 3rd, Dokainish H, Edvardsen T, Flachskampf FA, Gillebert TC, Klein AL, Lancellotti P, Marino P, Oh JK, Popescu BA and Waggoner AD. Recommendations for the Evaluation of Left Ventricular Diastolic Function by Echocardiography: An Update from the American Society of Echocardiography and the European Association of Cardiovascular Imaging. *J Am Soc Echocardiogr.* 2016;29:277-314.

15. Quiñones MA, Otto CM, Stoddard M, Waggoner A, Zoghbi WA; Doppler Quantification Task Force of the Nomenclature and Standards Committee of the American Society of Echocardiography. Recommendations for quantification of Doppler echocardiography: a report from the Doppler Quantification Task Force of the Nomenclature and Standards Committee of the American Society of Echocardiography. *J Am Soc Echocardiogr.* 2002;15(2):167-184.

16. Baumgartner H, Hung J, Bermejo J, Chambers JB, Edvardsen T, Goldstein S, Lancellotti P, LeFevre M, Miller F, Jr. and Otto CM. Recommendations on the Echocardiographic Assessment of Aortic Valve Stenosis: A Focused Update from the European Association of Cardiovascular Imaging and the American Society of Echocardiography. *J Am Soc Echocardiogr.* 2017;30:372-392.

17. Baumgartner H, Hung J, Bermejo J, Chambers JB, Evangelista A, Griffin BP, Iung B, Otto CM, Pellikka PA, Quiñones M, American Society of Echocardiography; European Association of Echocardiography. Echocardiographic assessment of valve stenosis: EAE/ASE recommendations for clinical practice. *J Am Soc Echocardiogr.* 2009;22:1-23; quiz 101-102.

4

Echo Views / Comprehensive Echo Exam / Transthoracic Echocardiography Doppler Views and Measurements / Suprasternal Notch Window

Chamber and Great Vessels Evaluation and Quantification
Steve Walling, RCS, RDCS, FASE

Left Ventricle 2D Measurements

	Table 5.1: **Parasternal Long-axis** *(ASE Recommendations)* [1]		
1	**Right Ventricular Minor Axis (RVIDd)**	**The inner-edge to inner-edge:** Anterior RV wall to the IVS-aortic junction	2.0 to 3.0cm Apical 4-chamber view preferred for RV measurements
2	**IVS Diastolic Thickness (IVSd)**	**Vertical distance:** Right ventricular side of the IVS to the left ventricular side of the IVS at end-diastole	Men 0.6 to 1.0cm Women 0.6 to 0.9cm
3	**LV Minor Axis End-Diastole (LVIDd)**	**Vertical distance:** Endocardium of the IVS to the endocardium of the LVPW at end-diastole	Men 4.2 to 5.8cm Women 3.8 to 5.2cm
4	**LV Minor Axis End-Systole (LVIDs)**	**Vertical distance:** Endocardium of the IVS to the endocardium of the LVPW at end-systolex	Men 2.5 to 4.0cm Women 2.2 to 3.5cm
5	**LV Posterior Wall Diastolic Thickness (LVPWd)**	**Vertical distance:** Endocardium of the LVPW to the epicardium at end-diastole	Men 0.6 to 1.0cm Women 0.6 to 0.9cm
6	**Aorta (AoRd)**	**The leading-edge to leading-edge:** At end-diastole at the valve plane perpendicular to the walls of the aortic root	*(Table 5.5)*
7	**Left Atrium End-Systole (LAs)**	**The leading-edge to leading-edge:** At the aortic valve plane, also perpendicular to the aortic root	Men 3.0 to 4.0cm Women 2.7 to 3.8cm Volume measurement preferred

American Society of Echocardiography Recommendations include:

• 2D linear measurements of the interventricular septum, posterior wall and LV internal dimensions should be recorded from the parasternal long-axis view at the level of the LV minor axis, approximately at the mitral valve leaflet tips.

• Only the compacted portion of the IVS should be included in the IVS end diastolic measurement. Avoid including RV trabeculae, the moderator band, or the TV apparatus as septal thickness.

• If there is a septal bulge, the LV should be measured just apical from the hypertrophy in diastole and systole. One can measure the focal septal thickening as a separate basic measurement, but should not be averaged as the IVS thickening.

- Chamber dimensions and wall thicknesses can be acquired from the parasternal short-axis view of the LV using direct 2D measurements or targeted M-mode echocardiography provided that the M-mode cursor can be positioned perpendicular to the septum and LV posterior wall.
- End-diastole can be defined as the onset of the QRS complex on the ECG, the first frame after mitral valve closure or the frame in the cardiac cycle in which the cardiac chamber dimension is largest.
- End-systole is defined as the frame after aortic valve closure or the time in the cardiac cycle in which the cardiac chamber dimension is smallest. (For atria end-systole is when chamber is largest in dimension)

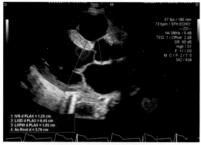

Figure 5.1: **PLAX Diastole**
(IVSd, LVIDd, LVPWd, AoRd)

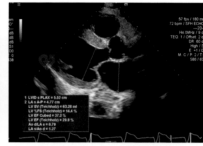

Figure 5.2: **PLAX Systole (LVIDs, LAs)**

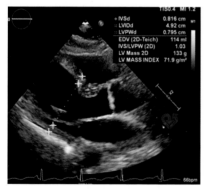

Figure 5.3: **Correct measurements of LV**

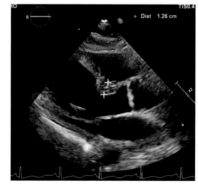

Figure 5.4: **Septal Bulge (PLAX)**

Left Ventricular Mass (Area Length and Linear Method)

- LV mass is calculated as the LV muscle volume multiplied by the specific gravity of muscle (1.04g/mL).
- M-mode and or 2D echocardiography can be used to estimate LV muscle volume and, therefore LV mass.
- LV muscle volume is the difference between the epicardial volume and the endocardial volume *(Figure 5.7)*.

Area Length Method

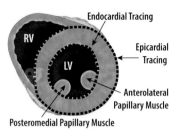

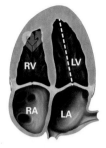

Figure 5.5: **Epicardial and endocardial tracing**

Figure 5.6: **Length of left ventricle at end-diastole**

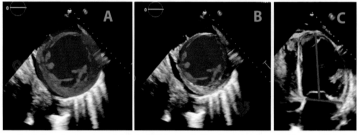

Figure 5.7: **LV Mass by Area Length Method (A) Epicardial Border, (B) Endocardial Border, (C) LV length**

Steps in Acquiring Left Ventricular Mass by Area Length Method (2D)

1. Trace the epicardial border of the left ventricle in PSAX view at the level of the papillary muscles at end-diastole (end-diastole can be defined as the onset of the QRS complex, the frame after mitral valve closure or the frame in the cardiac cycle in which the cardiac chamber dimension is largest).

2. Trace the endocardial border of the left ventricle at the level of the papillary muscles at end-diastole.

3. Measure the length of the left ventricle in the apical 4-chamber view at end-diastole from the mid mitral annulus to the cardiac apex.

4. The left ventricular mass is determined by subtracting the left ventricular volume enclosed by the endocardial surface (cavitary volume) from the volume enclosed by the epicardial surface (total volume). The specific weight of the myocardium is also considered.

5. Left ventricular mass divided by body surface area will determine left ventricular mass index.

6. Important to note that UEA's (ultrasound enhancing agents) can improve the accuracy of visualizing the myocardium and making an LV mass measurement (*Figure 5.9*).

Steps in Acquiring Left Ventricular Mass by Linear Method

1. Linear measurements of the LV are obtained in the PLAX view perpendicular to the LV long axis and measured at the level of the mitral valve leaflet tips during end-diastole (IVS, LVID, LVPW)

2. The linear method is done using the Cube formula and can be done by an M-mode tracing or 2D LV long axis view as seen 5.8.

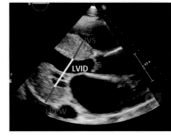

Figure 5.8: **2D Diastolic Derived Linear LV measurements**

LVM = 1.04 ([LVEDD + PW + IVS] - LVEDD³) x 0.8 + 0.6

LVM = left ventricular mass (g)
$LVEDD$ = left ventricular end-diastolic dimension(cm)
PW = left ventricular posterior wall thickness (cm)
IVS = interventricular septal thickness (cm)
1.04 = specific gravity of muscle (g/mL)

• Both M-mode and 2D formulas to calculate LV mass can be used, but should be indexed to BSA. [1]

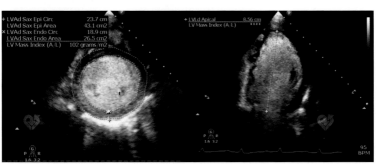

Figure 5.9: **Left Ventricular Mass by Area Length Method with an Ultrasound Enhancing Agent (UEA)**

Steps in Acquiring Relative Wall Thickness (RWT)

• RWT is calculated from the LV posterior wall thickness at end diastole and the LV end diastolic chamber diameter.

$RWT = (2\ PW)\ /\ LVEDD$
RWT = relative wall thickness
$LVEDD$ = LV end diastolic chamber diameter
PW = left ventricular end-diastolic PW thickness (cm)

Based on a combination of LVM and RWT, LV remodeling can be classified into four patterns of hypertrophy. (Tables 5.3 and 5.4)

Table 5.2: Normal Ranges and Severity Partition Cutoff Values for 2D Derived LV Size, Function and Mass *(ASE Recommendations)* [1]

	Normal range		Mildly abnormal		Moderately abnormal		Severely abnormal	
	Men	Women	Men	Women	Men	Women	Men	Women
LV dimension								
LV diastolic diameter (cm)	4.2 - 5.8	3.8 - 5.2	5.9 - 6.3	5.3 - 5.6	6.4 - 6.8	5.7 - 6.1	>6.8	>6.1
LV diastolic diameter/BSA (cm/m²)	2.2 - 3.0	2.3 - 3.1	3.1 - 3.3	3.2 - 3.4	3.4 - 3.6	3.5 - 3.7	>3.6	>3.7
LV systolic diameter (cm)	2.5 - 4.0	2.2 - 3.5	4.1 - 4.3	3.6 - 3.8	4.4 - 4.5	3.9 - 4.1	>4.5	>4.1
LV systolic diameter/BSA (cm/m²)	1.3 - 2.1	1.3 - 2.1	2.2 - 2.3	2.2 - 2.3	2.4 - 2.5	2.4 - 2.6	>2.5	>2.6
LV dimension 2D								
LV diastolic volume (mL)	62 - 150	46 - 106	151 - 174	107 - 120	175 - 200	121 - 130	>200	>130
LV diastolic volume/BSA (mL/m²)	34 - 74	29 - 61	75 - 89	62 - 70	90 - 100	71 - 80	>100	>80
LV systolic volume (mL)	21 - 61	14 - 42	62 - 73	43 - 55	74 - 85	56 - 67	>85	>67
LV systolic volume/BSA (mL/m²)	11 - 31	8 - 24	32 - 38	25 - 32	39 - 45	33 - 40	>45	>40
LV volume 3D								
LV diastolic volume/BSA (mL)/m²)	Men: >79mL/m² Women: >71mL/m²							
LV systolic volume/BSA (mL/m²)	Men: >32mL/m² Women: >28mL/m²							
LV function								
LV EF (%)	52 - 72	54 - 74	41 - 51	41 - 53	30 - 40	30 - 40	<30	<30
Septal wall thickness (cm)	0.6 - 1.0	0.6 - 0.9	1.1 - 1.3	1.0 - 1.2	1.4 - 1.6	1.3 - 1.5	>1.6	>1.5
Posterior wall thickness (cm)	0.6 - 1.0	0.6 - 0.9	1.1 - 1.3	1.0 - 1.2	1.4 - 1.6	1.3 - 1.5	>1.6	>1.5
LV mass (g)	88 - 224	67 - 162	225 - 258	163 - 186	259 - 292	187 - 210	>292	>210
LV mass/BSA (g/m²)	49 - 115	43 - 95	116 - 131	96 - 108	132 - 148	109 - 121	>148	>121
LV mass by 2D method								
LV mass (g)	96 - 200	66 - 150	201 - 227	151 - 171	228 - 254	172 - 193	>254	>193
LV mass/BSA (g/m²)	50 - 102	44 - 88	103 - 116	89 - 100	117 - 130	101 - 112	>130	>112

Table 5.3: Patterns of LV Geometry

Concentric hypertrophy	Equally distributed (uniform) increase in ventricular wall thickness with normal ventricular chamber dimensions, increased relative wall thickness (>0.42) and increased ventricular mass
Concentric remodeling	Normal chamber dimensions, elliptical ventricular chamber shape, increase in relative wall thickness (>0.42) and normal ventricular mass representing an adaptive response to an increase in afterload. Present in a subgroup of patients with high blood pressure, reduced cardiac index and the highest values of peripheral vascular resistance.
Eccentric hypertrophy	Increased ventricular dimensions, spherical ventricular chamber shape, normal wall thickness, low or normal relative wall thickness (≤0.42) and increased ventricular mass, most commonly seen in patients with significant chronic mitral regurgitation and/or aortic regurgitation
Normal geometry	Normal LV mass and normal regional wall thickness.

Table 5.4: Comparison of RWT with LV Mass Measurements Based on Linear Measurements

		Left Ventricular Mass Index (gm/m^2)		
		Women: ≤95 Men: ≤115	Women: ≤95 Men: ≤115	
Relative Wall Thickness	>0.42	**Concentric Remodeling**	**Concentric Hypertrophy**	
	≤0.42	**Normal Geometry**	**Eccentric Hypertrophy**	

Aortic Root and Ascending Aorta Measurements

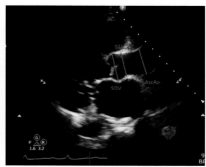

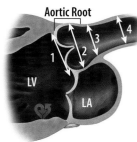

Figure 5.10: 1. Aortic Annulus, 2. Sinus of Valsalva (SOV), 3. Sinotubular Junction (STJ), 4. Ascending Aorta (Asc Ao)

Table 5.5: Aortic Root Dimensions (ASE Recommendations) [1]

	Absolute Values (cm)		Indexed Values (cm/m^2)	
Aortic Root	Men	Women	Men	Women
Annulus	2.6 ± 0.3	2.3 ± 0.2	1.3 ± 0.1	1.3 ± 0.1
Sinus of Valsalva	3.4 ± 0.3	3.0 ± .03	1.7 ± 0.2	1.8 ± 0.2
Sinotubular Junction	2.9 ± 0.3	2.6 ± 0.3	1.5 ± 0.2	1.5 ± 0.2
Proximal Ascending Aorta	3.0 ± 0.4	2.7 ± 0.4	1.5 ± 0.2	1.6 ± 0.3

Adapted from Roman et al. and Hiratzka et al.

Left Ventricular Out Flow Tract

- LVOT is measured in a zoomed parasternal long axis view in mid systole using the inner-edge to inner-edge method parallel to the aortic valve plane. Some experts prefer to measure within 0.3 to 1.0cm of the valve orifice whereas others prefer the measurement at the aortic valve annulus (hinge points) level.

Important to Note

- Measure the aortic root and ascending aorta at four levels (1 through 4) when clinically indicated. [1]

- Views used for measurements should be those that show the largest diameter of the aortic root (e.g., parasternal long-axis, right parasternal). [1]

- Measurement of the aortic diameter should be made perpendicular to the long-axis of the vessel. The inner-edge to inner-edge technique is used for the aortic annulus in mid systole. Everything past the aortic valve (aortic root, sinotubular junction and ascending aorta) are measured using the leading-edge to leading-edge technique at end diastole. [1]

- The aortic annulus should be performed between the hinge points of the aortic valve leaflets from inner edge to inner edge. Zoom mode can help with accuracy. [1]

- The ascending aorta is often best visualized from a higher intercostal space in the PLAX view closer to the sternum (left sternal border).

- If an ascending aortic aneurysm is suspected, an attempt at a right sternal border (RSB) view with the patient in the right lateral decubitus could help visualize more of the ascending aorta.

- It is important to measure 1 through 3 for homograft placement, Ross procedure, stentless valve procedure, TAVI.

Left Ventricular Systolic Function Evaluation

- Dimension(s) (end-diastolic, end-systolic)
- Volumes (end-diastolic, end-systolic)
- Wall thickness (end-diastolic, end-systolic)
- Longitudinal motion (base to apex)
- Radial motion (inward motion toward the cavity of the left ventricle)
- Circumferential (twist, torsion)
- Segmental wall motion (e.g., systolic wall thickening, systolic wall motion, diastolic wall thickness)
- Wall motion score index

M-mode/2D/3D

Determine:

- Left ventricular global systolic function with qualitative visualization of the left ventricle utilizing multiple views
- Segmental wall motion abnormalities systolic wall thickening (most important), diastolic wall thickness
- Wall motion score index
- LVIDd, LVIDs, left ventricular end-diastolic septal and posterior wall thickness, left ventricular end-systolic septal and posterior wall thickness
- Left ventricular fractional shortening *(not recommended by the ASE)*

- Left ventricular end-diastolic volume, end-systolic volume, stroke volume, cardiac output, cardiac index and ejection fraction (2D, or 3D)
- Global longitudinal strain (GLS) (normal >20%) (abnormal <15%)
- Mitral valve E point to septal separation (EPSS) of the mitral valve (>20mm indicates an ejection fraction <30%)
- Geometry (shape) of left ventricle
- Left ventricular mass index (normal LV Mass Index: men 49 to 115g/m^2; women 43 to 95g/m^2)
- Descent of the base (MAPSE) (≥10mm predicts a normal ejection fraction)

Doppler

- Evaluate aortic flow velocity tracing
- Determine:
    - Left ventricular outflow tract velocity time integral
    - Stroke volume/cardiac output/cardiac index
    - Change in pressure over time (dP/dt)
    - S' wave velocity by TDI (normal >9.5cm/s)

Left Ventricular Systolic Performance (dP/dt)

1. Optimize mitral regurgitation jet by CW Doppler.
2. On screen or paper, draw horizontal lines at 1m/s and 3m/s
3. Draw a vertical line from intercept of mitral regurgitation jet at 1m/s and 3m/s
4. Measure time (msec)
5. dP/dt = (32mmHg x 1000) ÷ change in time in msec

- The rate of pressure rise in the ventricles (dP/dt) is an index of ventricular contractility or systolic function (abnormal <400mmHg) [1]

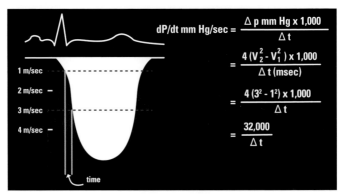

$$dP/dt \text{ mm Hg/sec} = \frac{\Delta p \text{ mm Hg} \times 1,000}{\Delta t}$$

$$= \frac{4 (V_2^2 - V_1^2) \times 1,000}{\Delta t \text{ (msec)}}$$

$$= \frac{4 (3^2 - 1^2) \times 1,000}{\Delta t}$$

$$= \frac{32,000}{\Delta t}$$

Figure 5.11: **LV dP/dt**

Biplane Simpson's Method of Discs (LV Volumes)

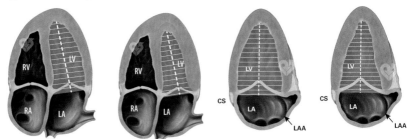

Figure 5.12: **Apical 4-chamber in end-diastole**

Figure 5.13: **Apical 4-chamber in end-systole**

Figure 5.14: **Apical 2-chamber in end-diastole**

Figure 5.15: **Apical 2-chamber in end-systole**

Steps in Acquiring Left Ventricular Volumes

1. Acquire an apical 4-chamber view, trace the left ventricular cavity at ventricular end-diastole (end-diastole can be defined as the onset of the QRS complex, the frame after mitral valve closure or the frame in the cardiac cycle in which the cardiac chamber dimension is largest). Measure the left ventricular end-diastolic length from the mid mitral annulus to the cardiac apex. This will yield the left ventricular end-diastolic volume. The same steps are repeated at end-systole (end-systole is defined as the frame after aortic valve closure or the time in the cardiac

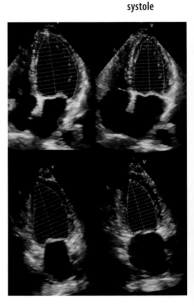

cycle in which the cardiac chamber dimension is smallest) to determine the ventricular end-systolic volume.

2. The apical 2-chamber view is then acquired and the same end-diastolic and end-systolic measurements are performed.

3. The calculation of end-diastolic volume, end-systolic volume, stroke volume, cardiac output, cardiac index and ejection fraction will be calculated from the summation of areas from the diameters of 20 cylinders or discs of equal height.

4. The percentage difference in length between the apical 4-chamber view and apical 2-chamber view should be less than 10%.

Important to Note

- When tracing the endocardial border for LV volumes it is important to be consistent in diastole and systole.

- After your diastolic area is traced, it is best practice to scroll left to right into systole. This way you can follow the diastolic traced borders into systole and be sure that the compacted myocardium and papillary muscles are included in your tracing. LV volumes are often underestimated in echocardiography due to some of these limitations

- UEA's can improve accuracy and consistency in LV volume measurements as they are much closer to MRI.

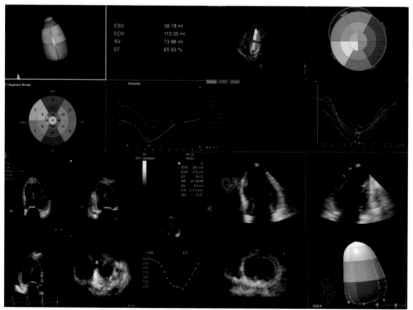

Figure 5.16: **3D LV Volume Quantification**

Evaluation of the Left Atrium

Common Causes of Left Atrial Dilatation

- Mitral valve disease (e.g., mitral stenosis, significant chronic mitral regurgitation)
- Left ventricular systolic and/or diastolic dysfunction
- Left ventricular pressure overload (e.g., systemic hypertension, aortic stenosis)
- Atrial arrhythmias (e.g., atrial fibrillation)
- Congenital heart disease (e.g., ventricular septal defect, patent ductus arteriosus)
- Cardiac transplantation

Left Atrial Linear Dimensions

M-mode

Determine left atrial linear dimension (parasternal long-axis view at end-systole) (normal: men 3.0 to 4.0cm; women 2.7 to 3.8cm)

2D

Determine:

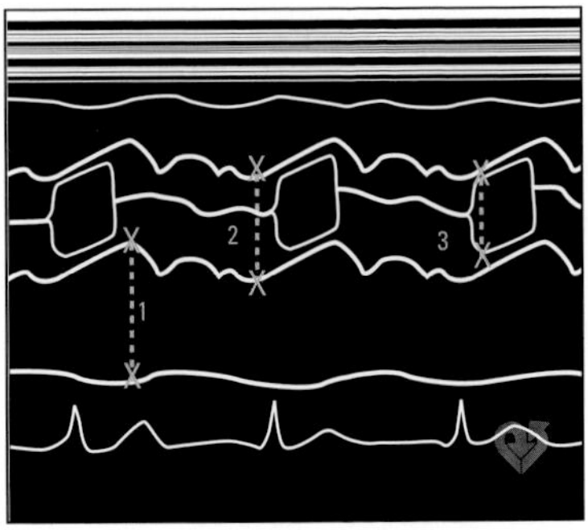

Figure 5.17: **M-mode (end-systole)**
1. LA   2. AoR   3. ACS

- Left atrial volume index (Simpson's biplane method of discs at end-systole or biplane area-length method) maximal area at end-systole (men/women normal: ≤34mL/m^2) [1]
- Left atrial linear dimension (leading-edge to leading-edge) (parasternal long-axis view at end-systole) (normal: men 3.0 to 4.0cm; women 2.7 to 3.8cm) [1]

Transesophageal Echocardiography

Possible approaches include:

- Transgastric long-axis (120°) and 2-chamber (90°) views
- Lower/Middle Esophageal at 0°, 30 to 60°, 90°, 130 to 150°
- Upper esophageal at 0 to 30°, 40 to 60°, 60 to 75°, 90 100°, 110°, 130 to 150°
- Left atrial appendage transgastric at 90°, midesophageal position with sequential steering from 0 to 135°, upper esophagus at 30 to 60°
- Pulmonary veins upper esophageal position 0 to 30° for left upper pulmonary vein with downward movement of the shaft of the probe for left lower pulmonary vein
- Right pulmonary veins upper esophageal position 0 to 110° for right upper pulmonary vein downward movement of the shaft with slight anteflexion allows visualization of the right lower pulmonary vein at 0 to 110°

Important to Note

- Left atrial volume measurements (Simpson's biplane method of discs) are preferred over linear measurements because of left atrial asymmetric remodeling.
- The maximal area imaging plane for the LA will commonly be a different imaging plane then the ideal apical window. (ensure proper angulation to bring in the maximal area for the LA with a focused imaging plane)
- The length of the LA should not change by more than 5mm between the A2C and A4C. This ensures proper imaging planes are taken and avoids foreshortening.
- Left atrial volume index of >34 mL/m^2 is an independent predictor of death, heart failure, atrial fibrillation and ischemic stroke
- Left atrial enlargement may be a marker for both the severity and chronicity of diastolic dysfunction and may indicate the magnitude of left atrial pressure elevation.
- Left atrial enlargement may be seen in patients with bradycardia, anemia, atrial flutter or fibrillation, significant mitral valve disease, and elite athletes.
- Left atrium may be compared to the aorta to determine left atrial dilatation, with the LA/Ao ratio equal to 1:1. The ratio is not valid in the presence of aortic dilatation or aortic hypoplasia.
- Bowing of the interatrial septum towards the right atrium throughout the cardiac cycle suggests left atrial dilatation and/or increased left atrial pressure. The same principle can be applied to the right atrium.
- Dilated pulmonary veins may suggest increased left atrial pressure.
- Dilated left atrial appendage may suggest increased left atrial pressure.
- The modified parasternal short-axis view of the aortic valve is used to visualize the left atrial appendage. To obtain this view, the transducer is first oriented for the standard parasternal short-axis view at the aortic valve level. The plane of the beam is then tilted superiorly with lateral angulation of the transducer, so that the pulmonary and aortic valves, but not the tricuspid, are imaged. Positioning the transducer in a high intercostal space is sometimes helpful for optimal imaging of the left atrial appendage. The left atrial appendage may also be well visualized in the apical 2-chamber view.

Biplane Simpson's Method of Discs (LA Volumes)

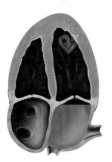
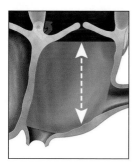
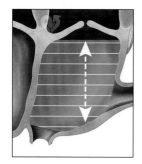

Steps in Acquiring Left Atrial Volumes

1. Acquire an apical 4-chamber view, zoom the left atrium, trace the left atrial cavity excluding the left atrial appendage and the pulmonary veins at ventricular end-systole (ventricular end-systole is defined as one frame immediately preceding mitral valve opening or when the left atrium is at its largest). Measure the left atrial end-systolic length from the mid mitral annulus to the superior portion of the left atrium. These steps will yield the left atrial end-systolic volume. The same steps are repeated at end-diastole for the left atrial end-diastolic volume.

2. The apical 2-chamber view is then acquired and the same end-systolic and end-diastolic measurements are performed (not shown).

3. The calculation of end-systolic volume, end-diastolic volume and ejection fraction will be calculated from the summation of areas from the diameters of 20 cylinders or discs of equal height.

4. The difference in left atrial lengths between the apical 4-chamber view and the apical 2-chamber view should be less than 5mm.

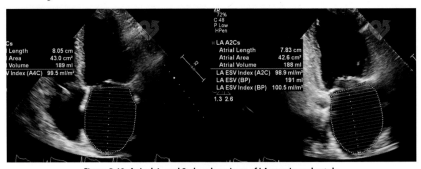

Figure 5.18: Apical 4- and 2-chamber views of LA area in end sytole

Biplane Area-Length Method (LA Volumes)

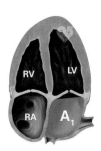 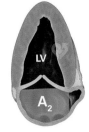 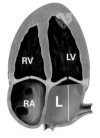 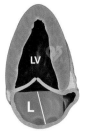

Figure 5.19: **Apical 4-chamber view LA area in end systole**

Figure 5.20: **Apical 2-chamber view LA area in end systole**

Figure 5.21: **Apical 4-chamber view LA length in end systole**

Figure 5.22: **Apical 2-chamber view LA length in end systole**

Steps in Acquiring Left Atrial Volumes

1. Acquire an apical 4-chamber view, zoom the left atrium, trace the left atrial cavity excluding the left atrial appendage and the pulmonary veins at ventricular end-systole (ventricular end-systole is defined as one frame immediately preceding mitral valve opening or when the left atrium is at its largest). Measure the length of the left atrium from the mid-annulus plane to the superior aspect of the left atrium.

2. Acquire the apical 2-chamber view and the same end-systolic measurements are performed. In the area-length formula the length is measured in both the four and 2-chamber views and the shortest of these two length measurements is used in the formula:

Left atrial volume (mL) = 8/3pi x [(A$_1$) x (A$_2$) / (L)]

3. The difference in left atrial lengths between the apical 4-chamber view and the apical 2-chamber view should be less than 5mm.

Table 5.6: Normal Ranges and Severity Partition Cutoff Values for 2D Derived LA Volume

Maximum LA volume/BSA (mL/m^2)	Normal Range	Mildly Abnormal	Moderately Abnormal	Severely Abnormal
Men	16 to 34	35 to 41	42 to 48	>48
Women	16 to 34	35 to 41	42 to 48	>48

Table 5.7: Left Atrial Dimensions and Volume Values *(ASE Recommendations)* [1]

	Men	Women
Anterior-posterior dimension (cm)	3.0 to 4.0	2.7 to 3.8
Anterior-posterior dimension index (cm/m^2)	1.5 to 2.3	1.5 to 2.3
Apical 4-chamber area index (cm^2/m^2)	8.9 ± 1.5	9.3 ± 1.7
Apical 2-chamber area index (cm^2/m^2)	9.3 ±1.6	9.6 ± 1.4
Apical 4-chamber volume index MOD (mL/m^2)	24.5 ± 6.4	25.1 ± 7.2
Apical 4-chamber volume index AL (mL/m^2)	27.0 ± 7.0	27.3 ± 7.9
Apical 2-chamber volume index MOD (mL/m^2)	27.1 ± 79	26.1 ± 6.7
Apical 2-chamber volume index AL (mL/m^2)	28.9 ± 8.5	28.0 ± 7.3

MOD = method of discs AL = area-length

5

Chamber and Great Vessels Evaluation and Quantification / Evaluation of the Left Atrium

Table 5.8: **Additional Left Atrial Dimensions and Volume Values** *(ASE Recommendations)* [1]	Reference Range	Mildly Abnormal	Moderately Abnormal	Severely Abnormal
Men				
LA diameter (cm)	3.0 to 4.0	4.1 to 4.6	4.7 to 5.2	>5.2
LA diameter/BSA (cm/m²)	1.5 to 2.3	2.4 to 2.6	2.7 to 2.9	≥3.0
LA area (cm²)	20	20 to 30	30 to 40	>40
LA volume (mL)	18 to 58	59 to 68	69 to 78	≥79
Women				
LA diameter (cm)	2.7 to 3.8	3.9 to 4.2	4.3 to 4.6	≥4.7
LA diameter/BSA (cm/m²)	1.5 to 2.3	2.4 to 2.6	2.7 to 2.9	≥3.0
LA area (cm²)	20	20 to 30	30 to 40	>40
LA volume (mL)	22 to 52	53 to 62	63 to 72	≥73

Right Ventricle Measurements

In all studies the right ventricle should be evaluated in multiple views, and the report should include:

• A measure of RV dimension

• RA dimension

• RV systolic function by a combination of the following parameters:

  - Fractional area change (FAC)

  - TDI S' peak velocity

  - Tricuspid annular plane systolic excursion (TAPSE)

  - Right Index or Myocardial Performance (RIMP or MPI)

  - SPAP using tricuspid regurgitation peak velocity with the estimate of RA pressure using the inferior vena cava dimension and degree of inspiratory collapse.

Linear Dimensions

• The right ventricle can be measured from the apical 4-chamber RV focused view at end-diastole.

• This is not to be confused with the regular apical 4-chamber view.

• The RV focused apical 4-chamber view should display the LV apex in the center of the screen with the largest basal RV diameter. Additional tilting towards the right heart or sliding laterally may be necessary to best visualize the entire RV.

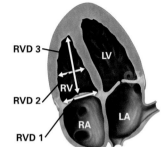

Figure 5.23: **RV focused view for linear dimensions**

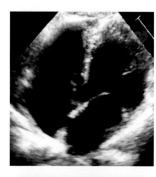

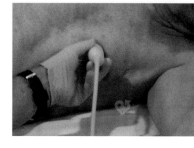

Figure 5.24: **RV modified 4-chamber view**

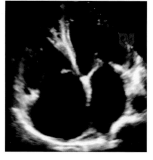

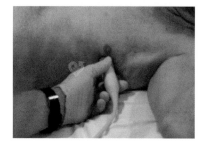

Figure 5.25: **RV focused apical 4-chamber view**

- **Basal diameter:** Maximal short axis dimension in the basal one third of the right ventricle seen in the RV focused apical 4-chamber view (RVD1) (>4.1cm abnormal)

- **Mid-cavity dimension:** Measured in the middle third of the right ventricle at the level of the left ventricular papillary muscles (RVD2) (>3.5cm abnormal)

- **Longitudinal dimension**: Measured from the mid-plane of the tricuspid annulus to the right ventricular apex (RVD3) (>8.3cm abnormal)

Wall Thickness

- RV free wall thickness can be measured at end-diastole with M-mode or 2D echocardiography from the subcostal window, preferably at the level of the tip of the anterior tricuspid valve leaflet. Left parasternal windows may be used. (normal: <0.5cm)

- It is important to note that you angle the transducer to ensure measurement of the RV free wall without including any of the tricuspid valve papillary muscle.

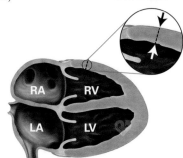

Figure 5.26: **Subcostal 4-chamber view RV free wall thickness**

Right Ventricular Outflow Tract

- The right ventricular outflow tract (RVOT) dimension should be measured using
the left parasternal or subcostal windows at end-diastole (onset of the QRS complex)
- **RVOT (proximal)** – In the parasternal long axis or short axis of the aortic valve, the proximal RVOT can be measured (>3.5cm abnormal)
- **RVOT (distal)** – In the parasternal short axis of the aortic valve, the distal RVOT diameter just proximal to the pulmonary valve annulus is the most reproducible and should be generally used (>2.7cm abnormal)

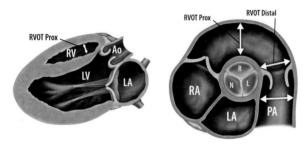

Right Ventricular Systolic Function

M-mode/2D

Determine:

- Right ventricular global systolic function with qualitative visualization of the right ventricle utilizing multiple views including the RV focused view. [1]
- All chamber measurements should be made using the inner-edge to inner-edge technique. [1]
- Segmental wall motion abnormalities systolic wall thickening (most important), diastolic wall thickness [1]
- RVIDd at end-diastole, RV end-diastolic longitudinal dimension, RV end-diastolic wall thickness [1]
- Right ventricular fractional area change (FAC) (abnormal <35%) [1]
- TAPSE (M-mode) (abnormal: <17mm) [1]
- Global longitudinal strain (GLS) (RV free wall 2D strain <20% is abnormal)
- Right ventricular end diastolic volume, end systolic volume, EF using 3D (abnormal EF <45%) [1]
- Geometry (shape) of right ventricle (e.g., D-shaped left ventricle due to right ventricular volume overload, right ventricular pressure overload) [1]

Doppler

Determine:

- Tissue Doppler S' peak velocity at the tricuspid valve lateral annulus (abnormal: <9.5cm/s) [1]

- RIMP by PW Doppler (abnormal: >0.43)
- RIMP by tissue Doppler (abnormal: >0.54) [1]
- RVOT VTI (normal: 13 to 15cm)
- RV dP/dt (<400mmHg/sec abnormal) [1]
- SPAP/MPAP/PAEDP/PVR at rest and exercise [1]

Right Ventricular Segmental Perfusion

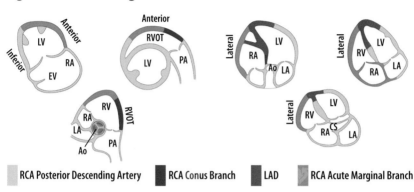

RCA Posterior Descending Artery | RCA Conus Branch | LAD | RCA Acute Marginal Branch

Right Ventricular Area and Right Ventricular Fractional Area Change

Right ventricular area may be acquired using the apical RV focused apical 4-chamber view by tracing from the tricuspid annulus along the free wall to the apex back to the annulus along the interventricular septum. Tracing at end-diastole and end-systole will allow calculation of the right ventricular area change (abnormal <35%).

Trabeculations, papillary muscles, and moderator band should be included in the RV area. The RV chamber is often difficult to view for an accurate tracing. UEA's can be used to better visualize RV volumes for FAC calculations.

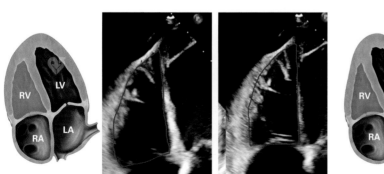

Figure 5.27: **RV FAC, (left) end diastole, (right) end systole**

Right Ventricular Ejection Fraction

The method of discs has been used to determine the right ventricular "body" volume using the apical 4-chamber view. RV volumes are underestimated because of exclusion of the right ventricular outflow tract. The lower reference value of the right ventricular ejection fraction is 44%.

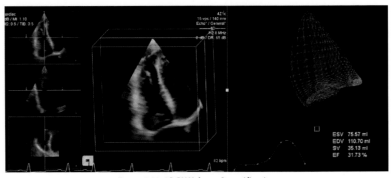

Figure 5.28: **3D RV Volume Quantification**

Tricuspid Annular Plane Systolic Excursion (TAPSE) or Tricuspid Annular Motion (TAM)

- TAPSE or TAM is a method to measure the distance of the systolic excursion of the RV annular segment along its longitudinal plane from the modified apical 4-chamber view. It is inferred that the greater the descent of the base during systole, the better the RV global systolic function. It assumes that it is representative of the entire right ventricle and may be invalid in many disease states or in the presence of RV segmental wall motion abnormalities

- TAPSE is acquired by placing an M-mode cursor through the tricuspid annulus from the modified apical 4-chamber view and measuring the amount of longitudinal motion of the tricuspid annulus at peak systole.

- The cursor should be parallel to the movement of the TV annulus towards the RV apex and Zoom mode may be helpful in proper identification and more accurate measurements.

- It is important to follow the same line from end diastole to the peak systolic measurement of the tricuspid annulus.

- The distance moved by the leading edge of the annulus from end-diastole toward the apex at end-systole is measured.

- TAPSE should be used routinely as a simple method of estimating RV global function. [1] (≥1.7cm normal)

- If the proper angulation is not acquired, TAPSE can be difficult to measure.

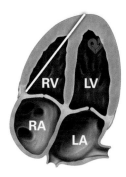

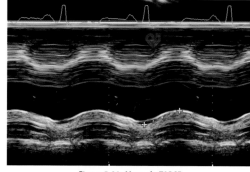

Figure 5.29: **M-mode TAPSE**

Tissue Doppler Imaging

RV S' (systolic excursion velocity)

- To obtain the RV S' velocity, an apical 4-chamber is acquired, the TDI sample volume is placed in either the tricuspid annulus or the middle of the basal segment of the RV free wall. The velocity S' is read as the highest systolic velocity without over gaining the Doppler envelope. (<9.5cm/s abnormal) [1]

- It is important to differentiate IVCT form the S' velocity. Increasing the sweep speed can help with this.

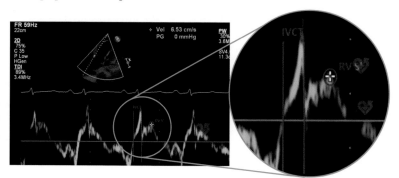

Figure 5.30: **RV free wall pulsed doppler S wave (cm/s)**

Table 5.9: **Evaluation of RV Global and Segmental Systolic Function** *(ASE Recommendations)* [1]

- Examine the right heart using multiple acoustic windows
- Report should include qualitative (e.g., evaluation of global/segmental function) and quantitative parameters including the RV focused view)

Report should include:

- A measure of right ventricular dimension at end-diastole
  (abnormal: >41mm at the base; >35mm at the mid-level in the RV focused view)
- Right atrial dimension at end-systole
  - Normal volume: Men >25mL/m^2 ± 7mL/m^2; Women: >21mL/m^2 ± 6mL/m^2
- RV systolic function (at least one of the following):
  - Fractional area change (FAC) (abnormal <35%)
  - TAPSE (abnormal <17mm)
  - TDI S' (abnormal <9.5cm/s)
  - RVSP/SPAP using tricuspid regurgitation method
  - RV index of myocardial performance (RIMP) (PW Doppler abnormal: >0.43) (TDI abnormal: >0.54)

Additional Parameters that may be determined when clinically indicated

- Pulmonary artery end-diastolic pressure using the pulmonary regurgitation method
- Assessment of RV diastolic function

Table 5.10: **Normal Values for RV Chamber Size** *(ASE Recommendations)* [1]

Parameter	Mean ± SD	Normal range
RV basal diameter (mm)	33 ± 4	25 to 41
RV mid diameter (mm)	27 ± 4	19 to 35
RV longitudinal diameter (mm)	71 ± 6	59 to 83
RVOT PLAX diameter (mm)	25 ± 2.5	20 to 30
RVOT proximal diameter (mm)	28 ± 3.5	21 to 35
RVOT distal diameter (mm)	22 ± 2.5	17 to 27
RV wall thickness (mm)	3 ± 1	1 to 5
RVOT EDA (cm^2)	Men: 17 ± 3.5 Women: 14 ± 3	Men: 10 to 24 Women: 8 to 20
RV EDA indexed to BSA (cm^2/m^2)	Men: 8.8 ± 1.9 Women: 8.0 ± 1.75	Men: 5 to 12.6 Women: 4.5 to 11.5
RV ESA (cm^2)	Men: 9 ± 3 Women: 7 ± 2	Men: 3 to 15 Women: 3 to 11
RV ESA indexed to BSA (cm^2/m^2)	Men: 4.7 ± 1.35 Women: 4.0 ± 1.2	Men: 2.0 to 7.4 Women: 1.6 to 6.4
RV EDV indexed to BSA (mL/m^2)	Men: 61 ± 13 Women: 53 ± 10.5	Men: 35 to 87 Women: 32 to 74
RV ESV indexed to BSA (mL/m^2)	Men: 27 ± 8.5 Women: 22 ± 7	Men: 10 to 44 Women: 8 to 36

EDA = end-diastolic area; ESA = end-systolic area; PLAX = parasternal long-axis view; RVOT = RV outflow tract.

Table 5.11: Normal Values for Parameters of RV Function (ASE Recommendations) [1]

Parameter	Mean ± SD	Abnormality Threshold
TAPSE (mm)	24 ± 3.5	<17
Pulsed Doppler S wave (cm/s)	14.1 ± 2.3	>9.5
Color Doppler S wave (cm/s)	9.7 ± 1.85	<6.0
RV fractional area change (%)	49 ± 7	<35
RV free wall 2D strain (%)	-29 ± 4.5	<20%
RV 3D EF (%)	58 ± 6.5	<45
Pulsed Doppler MPI	0.26 ± 0.085	>0.43
Tissue Doppler MPI	0.38 ± 0.08	>0.54
E wave deceleration time (msec)	180 ± 31	<119 or >242
E/A	1.4 ± 0.3	<0.8 or >2.0
e'/a'	1.18 ± 0.33	<0.52
e' (cm/s)	14.0 ± 0.31	>7.8
E/e'	4.0 ± 1.0	>6.0

MPI = Myocardial performance index.
*Limited data; values may vary depending on vendor and software version

Table 5.12: Additional Parameters for the Right Ventricle and Pulmonary Artery

Reference limits and partition values of right ventricular and pulmonary artery size			
RV dimensions			
Basal RV diameter (cm)	2.0 to 2.8	2.9 to 3.3	3.4 to 3.8	≥3.9
Mid-RV diameter (cm)	2.7 to 3.3	3.4 to 3.7	3.8 to 4.1	≥4.2
Base-to-apex length (cm)	7.1 to 7.9	8.0 to 8.5	8.6 to 9.1	≥9.2
RVOT diameters			
Above aortic valve (cm)	2.5 to 2.9	3.0 to 3.2	3.3 to 3.5	≥3.6
Above pulmonic valve (cm)	1.7 to 2.3	2.4 to 2.7	2.8 to 3.1	≥3.2
PA diameter			
Below pulmonic valve (cm)	1.5 to 2.1	2.2 to 2.5	2.6 to 2.9	≥3.0
Reference limits and partition values of right ventricular size and function as measured in the apical 4-chamber view			
RV diastolic area (cm²)	11 to 28	29 to 32	33 to 37	≥38
RV systolic area (cm²)	7.5 to 16	17 to 19	20 to 22	≥23
RV fractional area change (%)	32 to 60	25 to 31	18 to 24	≤17

Table 5.13: Summary of Reference Limits for Recommended Measures of Right Heart Structure and Function (*ASE Recommendations*) [1]

Variable	Abnormal
Chamber dimensions	
RV basal diameter	>4.1cm
RV mid diameter	>35mm
RV longitudinal diameter	>83mm
RVOT PLAX proximal diameter	>3.0cm
RVOT PSAX distal diameter	>2.7cm
RVOT PSAX distal diameter	>27mm
RV subcostal wall thickness	>0.5cm
RA volume	Men: 25 ± 7mL/m² Women 21 ± 6mL/m²
RA end-systolic area	>18cm²
RA major dimension	>5.3cm
RA minor dimension	>4.4cm
Systolic function	
TAPSE	<1.7cm
Pulsed Doppler peak velocity at the annulus	<9.5cm/s
Pulsed Doppler IMP	>0.43
Tissue Doppler IMP	>0.54
FAC	<35%
Diastolic function	
E/A ratio	<0.8 or >2.0
E/e' ratio	>6
Deceleration time	<119 msec

FAC, Fractional area change; MPI, myocardial performance index; PLAX, parasternal long-axis; PSAX, parasternal short-axis; RA, right atrium; RV, right ventricle; RVD, right ventricular diameter; RVOT, right ventricular outflow tract; TAPSE, tricuspid annular plane systolic excursion.

Evaluation of the Right Atrium

Common Causes of Right Atrial Dilatation

• Tricuspid valve disease (e.g., tricuspid stenosis, significant tricuspid regurgitation)
• Right ventricular systolic and/or diastolic dysfunction
• Right ventricular pressure overload (e.g., pulmonary hypertension, pulmonary stenosis)
• Atrial arrhythmias (e.g., atrial fibrillation)
• Congenital heart disease (e.g., atrial septal defect, partial anomalous pulmonary venous return)
• Cardiac transplantation

2D

Determine:

- Right atrial volume index (normal: men 25mL/m^2 ± 7; women 21mL/m^2 ± 6mL/m^2 end-systole) [1]
- Right atrial area (abnormal: >18cm^2 end-systole) [1]
- Right atrial major axis (superior to inferior) (abnormal: >5.3cm end-systole) [1]
- Right atrial minor dimension (medial to lateral) (abnormal: >4.4cm end-systole) [1]
- Right atrium larger than the left atrium suggests right atrial dilatation (apical 4-chamber view)
- 3D may be useful in the evaluation of right atrial dimension/volume

Right Atrial Pressure

- Estimated by evaluating the inferior vena cava and the presence of respiratory collapse [1]
- Interatrial septum deviated towards the left atrium throughout the cardiac cycle suggests increased right atrial pressure
- Dilated coronary sinus may suggest increased right atrial pressure (may also be dilated with persistent left superior vena cava, coronary artery AV fistula, anomalous hepatic venous drainage to the coronary sinus, total anomalous pulmonary venous return, severe tricuspid regurgitation)

Transesophageal Echocardiography

Possible approaches include:

- Mid-esophageal basal 4-chamber view (0º with posterior angulation to visualize the coronary sinus)
- Mid-esophageal right ventricular inflow-outflow tract view (60 to 90º with probe turned toward patient's right side)
- Mid-esophageal bicaval view (80 to 110º)
- Transgastric long axis view of right ventricle (0º)

Important to Note

- There is limited data available concerning right atrial dimensions and volume.
- There are several normal anatomic structures located in the right atrium including the eustachian valve, Chiari network, crista terminalis, and pectinate muscles.

Table 5.14: Normal Right Atrial Dimensions *(ASE Recommendations)* [1]

	Men	Women
2D echocardiographic right atrial volume index (mL/m^2)	25 ± 7	21 ± 6
Right atrial area (cm^2)	≤18	≤18
Right atrial major axis (cm)	≤5.3	≤5.3
Right atrial major axis dimension (cm/m^2)	2.4 ± 0.3	2.5 ± 0.3
Right atrial minor dimension (cm)	≤4.4	≤4.4
Right atrial minor axis dimension (cm/m^2)	1.9 ± 0.3	1.9 ± 0.3

Data are expressed as mean + SD. Measured at end-systole

Table 5.15: Right Atrial Pressures *(ASE Recommendations)* [1]

Variable	Normal (0 – 5 [3]mmHg)	Intermediate (5 – 10 [8]mmHg)		High (15mmHg)
IVC diameter	≤2.1cm	≤2.1cm	>2.1cm	>2.1cm
Collapse with sniff	>50%	<50%	>50%	<50%
Secondary indices of Elevated RAP		• Restrictive filling of elevated RAP • Tricuspid E/e' >6 • Diastolic flow predominance in hepatic veins (systolic filling fraction <55%)		

- A dilated IVC in a mechanically ventilated patient may not indicate an elevated RAP.
- Athletes may have dilated IVC with normal collapsibility.
- Ranges are provided for low and intermediate categories, but for simplicity, midrange values of 3mmHg for normal and 8mmHg for intermediate are suggested. Intermediate (8mmHg) RA pressures may be downgraded to normal (3mmHg) if no secondary indices of elevated RA pressure are present, upgraded to high if minimal collapse with sniff (<35%) and secondary indices of elevated RA pressures are present, or left at 8mmHg if uncertain.
- BSA, Body surface area; LA, left atrial; RA, right atrial.

Right Atrial Measurements

The primary transthoracic window for the evaluation of right atrial dimensions is the apical 4-chamber view.

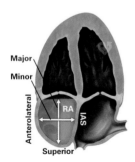

Figure 5.31: **Apical 4-chamber view of choice for evaluation of the right atrium** [1]

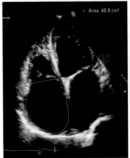

Figure 5.32: **Apical 4-chamber view of right atrial area**

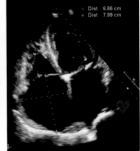

Figure 5.33: **Apical 4-chamber view – right atrial major and minor axis**

Right Atrial Volume

The recommended parameter to assess right atrial size is right atrial volume calculated using the single plane Simpson's method of discs or area-length method. (normal indexed range: men $25 \pm 7mL/m^2$; women $21 \pm 6mL/m^2$) [1]

Right Atrial Area

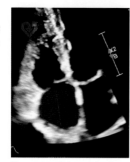

Figure 5.34: **Right atrial volume**

- Right atrial area should be obtained routinely in patients with RV and/or LV dysfunction
- Right atrial area is traced at the end of ventricular systole (largest volume) from the lateral aspect of the tricuspid annulus, following the right atrial endocardium, excluding the inferior vena cava and right atrial appendage. (>18cm² is abnormal)

Superior-Inferior (Major Dimension)

The maximal superior-inferior measurement of the right atrium is from the center of the tricuspid valve annulus to the center of the superior right atrial wall parallel to the interatrial septum at the end of ventricular systole. (>5.3cm is abnormal)

Medial-Lateral (Minor Dimension)

The mid-minor distance is measured at end ventricular systole from the mid-level of the right atrial free wall to the interatrial septum perpendicular to the long axis of the right atrium. (>4.4cm is abnormal)

Right Ventricular Diastolic Function

Determine:
- Tricuspid valve E/A ratio (normal 0.8 to 2.0) and deceleration time (normal 119 to 242 msec) [1]
- Tissue Doppler e' (abnormal <7.8cm/s) [1]
- Tissue Doppler E/e' (abnormal >6) [1]
- Tissue Doppler e'/a' (abnormal <0.52) [1]
- Hepatic vein flow (S wave dominant is normal) [1]
- Right atrial end-systolic volume index (abnormal: men >25mL/m² ± 7mL/m²; women >21 ± 6mL/m²) [1]
- Right atrial pressure [1]

Table 5.16: Evaluation of RV Diastolic Function
(ASE Recommendations) [1]

	E/A	E/e'	Additional Findings
Normal	0.8 to 2.0	<6	–
Impaired Relaxation	<0.8	<6	–
Pseudonormal	0.8 to 2.0	>6	Diastolic flow predominance in HV
Restrictive	>2.0	>6	Late diastolic antegrade flow in PA

References

1. Lang RM, Badano, LP, et al. Recommendations for chamber quantification: a report from the American Society of Echocardiography's Guidelines and Standards Committee and the Chamber Quantification. J Am Soc Echocardiogr 2015 Jan;28(1):1-39.

2. Mitchell C, Rahko PS, Blauwet LA, Canaday B, Finstuen JA, Foster MC, Horton K, Ogunyankin KO, Palma RA and Velazquez EJ. Guidelines for Performing a Comprehensive Transthoracic Echocardiographic Examination in Adults: Recommendations from the American Society of Echocardiography. J Am Soc Echocardiogr. 2019;32:1-64.

Evaluation of Diastolic Function
Jeffrey C. Hill, BS, ACS, FASE

The American Society of Echocardiography (ASE) and the European Association of Cardiovascular Imaging published guidelines and standards for the evaluation of left ventricular (LV) diastolic function by echocardiography. [1] This information included a comprehensive approach to the assessment of LV myocardial relaxation and filling pressures. The guidelines address heart failure patients with preserved LV ejection fraction (HFpEF), reduced ejection fraction (HFrEF), and in special populations. Moreover, the guidelines and standards align with the Intersocietal Accreditation Commission for adult echocardiography laboratory accreditation [2] requiring the assessment of LV diastolic function be included in the comprehensive transthoracic echocardiogram.

Key Measurements

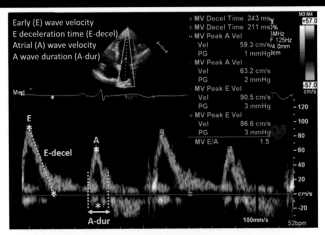

Figure 6.1: **Mitral Inflow Doppler tracings and measurements**

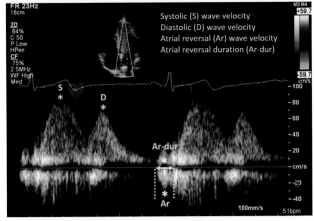

Figure 6.2: **Pulmonary vein Doppler tracings and measurements**

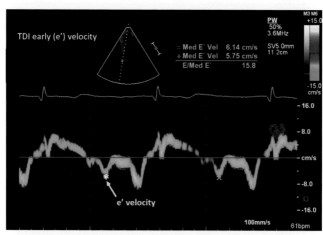

Figure 6.3: **Tissue Doppler imaging (TDI) tracings and measurements**

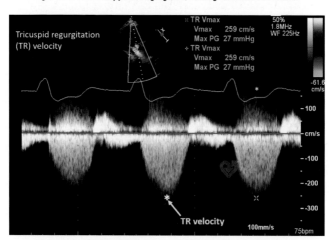

Figure 6.4: **Tricuspid regurgitation tracings and measurements**

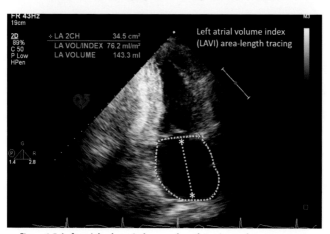

Figure 6.5: **Left atrial volume index area-length tracing and measurements**

Normal LV Diastolic Function

- Diastole involves a complex process and interaction of properties including ventricular relaxation and diastolic suction (elastic recoil) during early diastole, and atrial systolic contribution during late diastole.

- Normal diastolic function allows for adequate filling of the ventricles during rest and exercise without an abnormal increase in diastolic pressures.

- In normal, young subjects, LV untwisting is vigorous and myocardial relaxation is rapid. This results in "restrictive-like" filling with most of the ventricular filling occurring in early diastole and a small atrial systolic contribution during late diastole *(Figure 6.6)*. A normal E/A ratio is >1.

- With normal aging, there is a gradual decrease in the rate of myocardial relaxation and elastic recoil, and a slower LV pressure decline, which results in decreased early diastolic filling (reduced E-wave velocity) and a longer E-wave deceleration time. At age 65, the mitral E-wave velocity approaches the A-wave velocity. At age 70 and older, the E/A ratio is usually <1.0 *(Figure 6.7)*.

- Importantly, the accuracy in the grading of diastolic function requires the sonographer to obtain high-quality 2D and Doppler measurements as seen in all figures throughout this chapter.

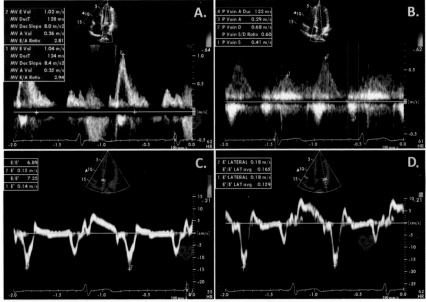

Figure 6.6: **Echocardiographic variables obtained in a normal, healthy 21-year-old female. A) The mitral inflow E-wave velocity = 100cm/sec, E-wave deceleration time = 126msec, A-wave velocity = 36cm/sec, E/A ratio = 2.9. All variables are consistent with "restrictive" filling. However, this profile is not due to high left atrial pressure, but vigorous LV untwisting and myocardial relaxation creating a "suction" effect in early diastole; B) pulmonary vein Doppler profile demonstrates S-wave <D-wave, or "D-wave dominant." This is due to the above-mentioned early diastolic filling and relaxation mechanism; tissue Doppler imaging (TDI) obtained from the septal (medial) annulus (C) and lateral annulus (D). The measured TDI e' velocities are 15cm/sec and 18cm/sec, reflecting normal LV relaxation. All findings are consistent with normal diastolic function seen in a healthy young person.**

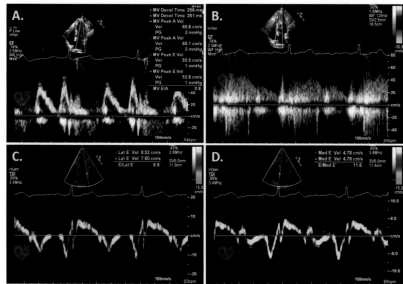

Figure 6.7: **Echocardiographic variables obtained in a normal, healthy 72-year-old male. A) mitral inflow E-wave velocity = 55cm/sec, E-wave deceleration time = 256 msec, A-wave velocity = 66cm/sec, E/A ratio = 0.8; B) pulmonary vein Doppler profile demonstrates S-wave >D-wave, or "S-wave dominant"; tissue Doppler imaging (TDI) obtained from the lateral annulus (C) and septal (medial) annulus (D). The measured e' velocities are 8cm/sec and 5cm/sec, reflecting a decrease in the rate of LV relaxation with aging. The height of the TDI e' velocities are in stark contrast to the e' velocities measured in Figure 6.6, demonstrating the effects of aging on early LV relaxation. All findings are c/w normal diastolic function and aging.**

Impact of LV Ejection Fraction on the Assessment of Diastolic Function

The ASE guidelines and standards [1] specifically focus on the assessment of diastolic function in heart failure patients with reduced ejection fraction (HFrEF), "heff-reff" and with preserved LV ejection fraction (HFpEF) "heff-peff". In patients with reduced ejection fraction, the PW Doppler mitral inflow variables correlate well with LV filling pressures and can be used to accurately estimate the various degrees of diastolic function. However, in patients with HFpEF the mitral inflow variables correlate poorly with LV filling pressures and often requires additional 2D and Doppler variables.

• One exception to consider is when the E/A ratio ≥2. This most likely indicates filling pressures are elevated in both preserved and reduced EF.

• In addition, the mitral E-wave deceleration time is usually short (<160 msec) in patients with HFrEF, however in patients with HFpEF the E-wave deceleration time can be normal despite elevate filling pressures. This is likely due to the intact EF.

Grading of Diastolic Function

Determining the absence or presence of elevated LV filling pressures is the first step when grading the severity of LV diastolic dysfunction. Grading of diastolic function, includes normal, mild, moderate and severe *(See Table 6.1 – Table 6.4)*. The most important factors to consider when assessing diastolic function is whether underlying disease is present. This includes myocardial disease, increased left atrial (LA) size/volumes, and at least mildly elevated pulmonary artery pressures. If not, the suspicion for diastolic dysfunction and elevated filling pressures is low.

Echo Variables in the Assessment of Diastolic Function

2D and Doppler echocardiographic variables for the assessment of left ventricular diastolic function include the following parameters:

PW Doppler: Mitral Inflow

- Used for estimation of LV filling pressures and myocardial relaxation.
- Obtained from the apical 4-chamber view.
- Measurements include the E-wave velocity, E-wave deceleration time, A-wave velocity, A-wave duration, and E/A ratio.

Technical Tips

- Color flow Doppler sector is placed over the mitral inflow for optimal alignment with blood flow.
- Tilt (left to right) the 2D image until the mitral valve inflow appears parallel to the Doppler sample volume (SV).
- SV positioning that is non-parallel to the flow *(Figure 6.8 A)* during normal respiration may result in inaccurate measurements of the mitral inflow velocities *(Figure 6.9 A)*.
- Position the Doppler SV at the leaflet tips during shallow breathing or apnea *(Figure 6.8 B)*.
- Optimal Doppler gain will display easily defined peaks and slopes with absence of "artifact-like" spikes and feathering of the signal *(Figure 6.9 B)*.
- When measuring A-wave duration, if not clearly visualized, position the SV at the level of the mitral annulus and decrease the wall filter setting and overall gain to better define the demarcation points of the onset and ending of the A-wave *(Figure 6.10)*.

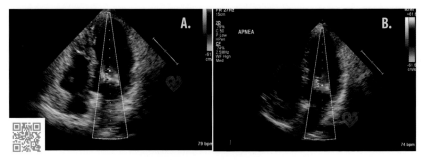

Figure 6.8: A) SV placed too far into the LV cavity non-parallel to flow during normal respiration B) Optimized SV positioning for accurate assessment of mitral inflow velocities

PW Doppler optimization of mitral Inflow

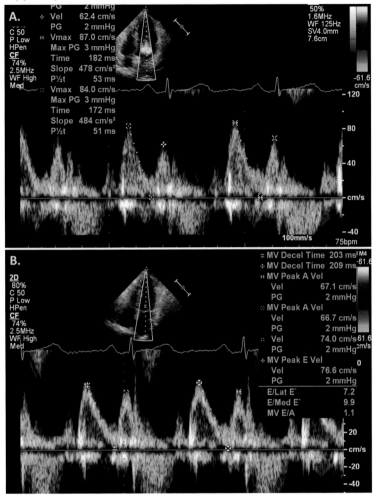

Figure 6.9: **Incorrect SV placement too far into the LV cavity during normal respiration A). Doppler waveforms are course and are poorly optimized with increased spectral broadening (i.e., area below the peak waveforms); SV placed at the leaflet tips during apnea B). Peak E-wave, E-wave deceleration time and A-wave are clearly defined and minimal spectral broadening is seen. Note the significant differences in the peak E-wave velocities (85 vs. 67cm/sec) and deceleration time (177 vs. 206 msec).**

PW Doppler optimization of mitral A-wave duration

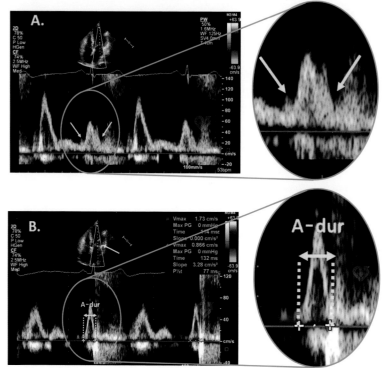

Figure 6.10: A) The sample volume (SV) was placed at the mitral leaflet tips. Although the peak E-wave, E-wave deceleration time and A-wave are clearly defined, onset and ending of the A-wave duration is difficult to visualize and measure correctly (double arrows) SV was placed towards the annulus (upper arrow), onset and ending B) of the A-wave duration at the Doppler baseline are clearly defined (vertical dotted lines) allowing for accurate measurement of A-wave duration.

2D: LA Volume Index (LAVI)

- Variable used to determine the estimation of LA pressure.
- Obtained from the apical 4-chamber and 2-chamber view.
- Measured at end-ventricular systole (when LA size is at its maximum).
- Measurements of LAVI requires tracing of the interface of the LA wall reflectors and blood pool.

Technical Tips

- In order to improve the accuracy of LAVI, the sonographer should pan or sweep through the "live" 2D image to identify the LA at its largest area *(Figure 6.11)*. The same optimization applies to the apical 2-chamber view.

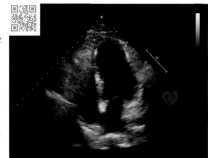

Figure 6.11: **LA optimization for volumes**

- The pulmonary vein orifice, left atrial appendage entry into the LA, and tenting area of the mitral valve should be excluded from the tracing.

- Significant far-field 2D imaging artifacts (horizontal reflectors) that appear to be part of the LA wall should be included in the tracing *(Figure 6.11, 6.12)*.

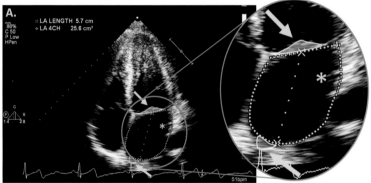

Figure 6.12: **Optimized tracings of the LA area and length measurement for LAVI calculation at end-ventricular systole in the apical 4-chamber view. The mitral valve tenting area (upper arrow) and the pulmonary vein orifice (lower arrow) were excluded from the area tracing. In addition, the 2D far-field lateral resolution artifacts (horizontal reflectors) were included in the area tracing (asterisk)**

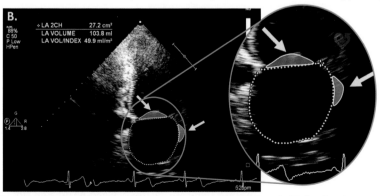

Figure 6.13: **Tracing of the LA for LAVI at end-ventricular systole in the apical 2-chamber view. Like the apical 4-chamber view, the tenting area highlighted in red, "upper arrow" and the left atrial appendage "right arrow" were excluded from the area tracing.**

PW Tissue Doppler Imaging (TDI) of the Mitral Valve Annulus

- Used to estimate LV relaxation (e' velocity); when combined with the mitral E-wave velocity (E/e' ratio), used to estimate LV filling pressures.
- Obtained from the apical 4-chamber view.
- Measurements include the peak e' velocities of the septal (medial) and the lateral mitral annulus.

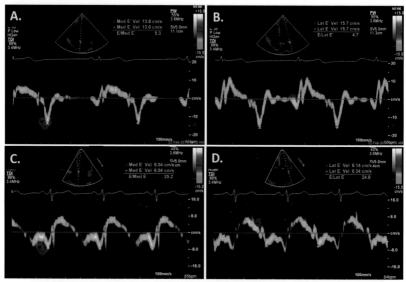

Figure 6.14: **TDI waveforms obtained from the septal (A) and lateral (B) annulus in a 25-year-old male from the apical 4-chamber view. The SV was positioned at the annuli during apnea. The Doppler gain was optimized demonstrating minimal background noise and the peak TDI velocities are clearly defined. The peak septal e' velocities measure 14cm/sec and the lateral e' velocity measures 16cm/sec; the averaged E/e' ratio is 5. Findings consistent with normal diastolic function. Note the lateral e' velocity is almost always higher than the septal e' velocity in normal patients. This is in stark contrast to Figures C and D where the TDI was obtained in a patient with HFpEF. The peak TDI e' velocity measures 6cm/sec at the septal annulus and 6cm/sec at the lateral annulus; the averaged E/e' ratio = 25. Findings consistent with abnormal relaxation (low e' velocities) and highly elevated filling pressures.**

Technical Tips

- Tilt the 2D image until the mitral valve annulus is as parallel as possible to the SV.
- Position the SV at the mitral valve annulus (leaflet insertion point) and activate color TDI.
- TDI obtained during normal respiration can result in poor quality recordings *(Figure 6.17 A)*.
- To reduce error in measurements, TDI should be obtained during shallow breathing or apnea *(Figure 6.17 B)*. [3]
- Optimize the Doppler gain until there are clearly defined peaks and slopes *(Figure 6.17 B)*.
- Avoid measuring artifact or incorrect waveforms that do not represent the peak e' velocities. *(Figure 6.16, 6.24 F)*.

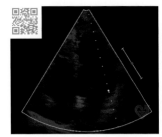

Figure 6.15: TDI SV placed at the lateral annulus during respiration

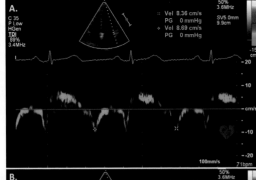

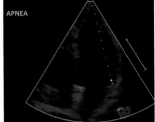

Figure 6.16: Lateral annulus during apnea during apnea

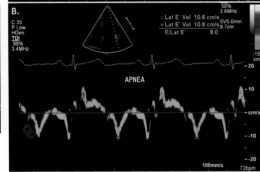

Figure 6.17: Example of a TDI obtained from the lateral annulus during respiration (A). The TDI signals are of poor quality with the ave. peak e' velocities measuring 8.5cm/sec; TDI obtained during apnea in the same patient (B). The TDI signals are of high quality and clearly defined with the average peak e' velocities measuring 10.6cm/sec. There is a >25% difference in the peak e' velocities compared to example A, representing the true peak myocardial velocities.

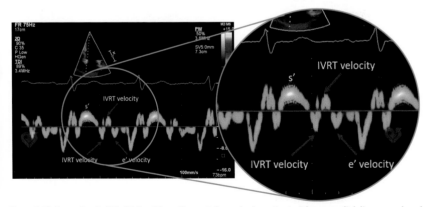

Figure 6.18: Example of a TDI obtained from the septal annulus in patient with myocardial disease, reduced EF and left bundle branch block. The first waveform below the Doppler baseline after the s' velocity is the isovolumic relaxation time (IVRT) velocity. Because of the myocardial disease, the IVRT is prolonged resulting in biphasic IVRT waveforms. The TDI e' velocity is the second negative waveform. An additional observation are the biphasic waveforms displayed below the QRS complex due to the prolongation of the isovolumic contraction time.

6

Evaluation of Diastolic Function / Echo Variables in the Assessment of Diastolic Function

6

Evaluation of Diastolic Function / Echo Variables in the Assessment of Diastolic Function

PW Doppler: Pulmonary Vein Flow

- Variable used to estimate LA and LV filling pressures.
- Typically obtained in the apical 4-chamber view (may require slight angulation towards the apical 5-chamber view).
- Measurements include the peak systolic (S) wave, diastolic (D) wave, atrial reversal (Ar) velocity and its duration (Ar-dur). *(Figure 6.19)*

Technical Tips

- Activate color Doppler over the entry of the pulmonary vein into the LA to identify blood flow.
- Decreasing the color scale or increasing the color gain may improve visualization of the blood flow.
- Position the Doppler SV an estimated 1cm into the pulmonary vein.
- Optimize the Doppler signals whereby minimizing the Doppler gain and clearly defining the peaks velocities.
- Avoid measuring artifact that does not represent the true peak velocities.
- If significant variation in the peak S, D and Ar velocities are seen, obtain during apnea or shallow breathing.

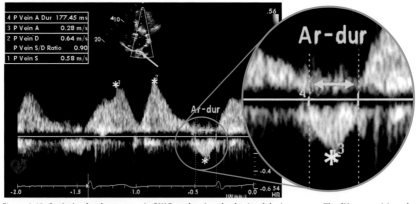

Figure 6.19: **Optimized pulmonary vein PW Doppler signals obtained during apnea. The SV was positioned approximately 1cm into the right upper pulmonary vein in the apical 4-chamber view (arrow). Note the peak S-wave, D-wave and A-wave reversal velocities, and A-wave duration are clearly defined (arrows).**

CW Doppler: Tricuspid Valve Regurgitation Peak Velocity

- Variable used as a surrogate measurement to predict LA pressure (in the absence of pulmonary disease).
- Obtained from the echocardiographic view that most accurately displays the peak velocity.
- Measurement includes the peak regurgitation velocity reflecting the right ventricular systolic pressure (RVSP).

Technical Tips

- Activate color Doppler to identify the extent of the tricuspid valve regurgitation.
- Align the 2D image so the color jet is as parallel as possible to the CW Doppler cursor. *(Figure 6.20 C)*
- Optimize the Doppler signals whereby minimizing the Doppler gain and clearly defining the peaks velocities. *(Figure 6.20 D)*
- Avoid measuring artifact that does not represent the true peak velocities.

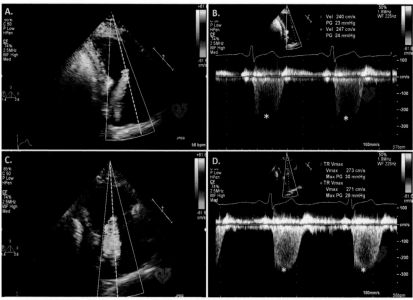

Figure 6.20: **Optimization of the CW Doppler peak tricuspid regurgitation (TR) signal to improve accuracy in reporting of the right pulmonary artery systolic pressure. A)** CW Doppler cursor non-parallel to the direction of the color Doppler jet; **B)** Peak TR velocity was measured = 2.45 m/sec. Note the degree of TR is significant by Color Doppler display, however the density of the TR jet is faint likely underestimating the true peak velocities; **C)** The sonographer repositioned the probe so the color Doppler jet is more parallel to the CW Doppler cursor; **D)** Peak TR velocity was re-measured = 2.72 m/sec. There is increased density of the TR jet representing increased TR increasing the accuracy in obtaining the peak velocities.

Table 6.1: **Normal Diastolic Function** *(ASE Recommendations)*[1]	
LV relaxation	Normal
LA pressure	Normal
Mitral E/A ratio	≥0.8
Averaged E/e' ratio (septal and lateral annulus)	<10
Peak TR velocity (m/s)	<2.8
LA volume index (mL/m^2)	≤34

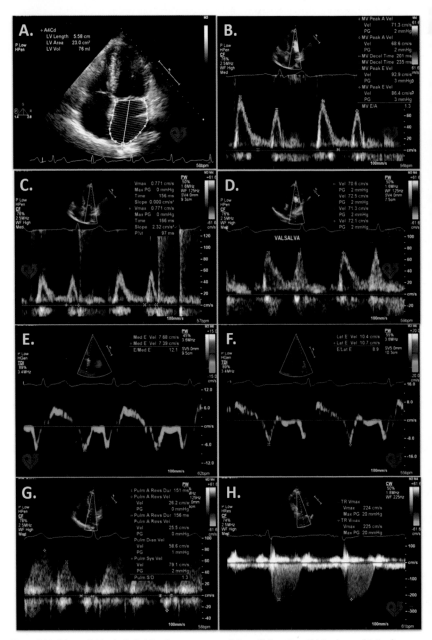

Figure 6.21: **Echo variables included for the assessment of diastolic function.** A) LA volume obtained from the apical 4-chamber view; B) mitral Inflow Doppler with the SV placed at the leaflet tips for the measurement of the peak E-wave, E-wave deceleration time, A-wave from the apical 4-chamber view; C) mitral inflow with SV placed at the MV annulus to measure the A-wave duration; D) mitral inflow obtained during the Valsalva maneuver; E) TDI e' velocity obtained from the septal (medial) mitral valve annulus in the apical 4-chamber view; F) TDI e' velocity obtained from the lateral mitral valve annulus; G) Pulmonary vein Doppler obtained from the right upper pulmonary vein in the apical 4-chamber view; H) Peak TR jet obtain from the RV inflow view. All echo variables are consistent with normal diastolic function.

Assessing Abnormal Diastolic Function Grades (I – III)

- In patients with myocardial disease, an increase in ventricular volume may lead to an abnormal increase in LV filling pressures. Abnormal increase in LV filling pressures at rest is consistent with abnormal diastolic function (i.e., moderate or severe diastolic dysfunction); on the other hand, abnormal diastolic function can be associated with abnormal or slowed LV relaxation, but normal filling pressures (i.e., mild diastolic dysfunction).

- As the myocardium becomes diseased, changes in relaxation and/or compliance occur. In the earliest stage of diastolic dysfunction, the LV relaxation becomes abnormal or prolonged, without an abnormal increase in LA pressure (Grade I).

- The patient with abnormal relaxation may at some point, transition to a more advanced state of diastolic dysfunction including not only abnormal relaxation, but increased LV filling pressures. Patients with moderate diastolic dysfunction have abnormal filling pressures (Grade II).

- Further increase in LV filling pressures and exacerbation of myocardial disease can result in the patient developing significantly increased filling pressures consistent with severe diastolic dysfunction (Grade III).

- Remember, all patients with diastolic dysfunction have some form of abnormal relaxation. However, filling pressures are only elevated in Grades II and III. *(Table 6.6)*

Grade I: Mild Diastolic Dysfunction

(Abnormal relaxation, normal LA pressure)

- **Significance:** The first abnormality in diastolic function. Impaired (slowed) LV relaxation reduces the rate of filling in early diastole.

- **Signs and symptoms:** None at rest, may develop with moderate to extreme exertion.

- **Functional status:** Mild impairment with moderate to extreme exertion.

- **Left atrium:** Normal dimension/dilated (may be hypercontractile).

- **LV filling pressures:** Normal. *(Figure 6.22)*

- **Treatment:** Beta-adrenergic or calcium channel blocking agents to increase diastolic filling period and allow relaxation to be completed before atrial contraction. If abnormal relaxation is caused by left ventricular hypertrophy, drugs which aid in regression of hypertrophy may be indicated (e.g., angiotensin converting inhibitors) and maintaining normal sinus rhythm is essential in these patients.

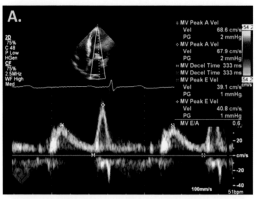

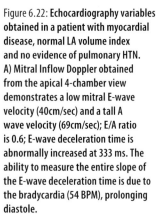

Figure 6.22: **Echocardiography variables obtained in a patient with myocardial disease, normal LA volume index and no evidence of pulmonary HTN.** A) Mitral Inflow Doppler obtained from the apical 4-chamber view demonstrates a low mitral E-wave velocity (40cm/sec) and a tall A wave velocity (69cm/sec); E/A ratio is 0.6; E-wave deceleration time is abnormally increased at 333 ms. The ability to measure the entire slope of the E-wave deceleration time is due to the bradycardia (54 BPM), prolonging diastole.

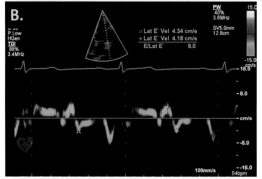

B) TDI obtained from the lateral annulus demonstrates a low (<10cm/sec) e' velocity measuring 4.2cm/sec, which is consistent with abnormal relaxation. The E/e' ratio = 9.5.

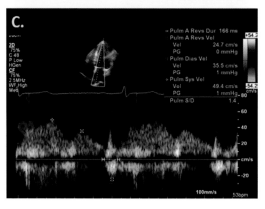

C) Pulmonary vein Doppler profile demonstrating an S-wave >D-wave. The A-wave reversal velocity = 25cm/sec and the A-wave duration is 166 msec. Note the low D-wave of 36cm/sec coincides with a low mitral E-wave, as the height of the D and E wave go hand-in-hand. In other words, the smaller the E the smaller the D, and vice versa. All echocardiographic findings in this patient are consistent with Grade I, mild diastolic dysfunction. *(Table 6.2)*

Table 6.2: **Grade I Diastolic Dysfunction** *(ASE Recommendations)* [1]	
LV relaxation	Impaired (slowed)
LAP	Normal or low
Mitral E/A ratio	≤0.8
Averaged E/e' ratio (septal and lateral annulus)	<10
Peak TR velocity (m/s)	<2.8
LA volume index (mL/m²)*	Normal or can be increased
* note: increased LA volumes would indicate the LA pressure was most likely elevated at some point in time	

Table 6.2: Grade I filling pattern in a patient with impaired (slowed) early LV relaxation usually demonstrates a low E-wave velocity. At this point, the patient is usually asymptomatic with normal filling pressures. Patients with Grade I diastolic dysfunction may develop symptoms of heart failure with moderate to extreme exertion or may develop heart failure symptoms if the atrial contribution to diastolic filling is lost such as in atrial fibrillation.

Special considerations in a patient with Grade I diastolic dysfunction

A Grade IA should be considered if the pulmonary vein A wave velocity is >35cm/s, the pulmonary vein A wave duration is ≥30 msec compared to the mitral valve A wave duration, if the mitral valve A wave velocity increases during the Valsalva maneuver and/or if the E/e' is >15. These findings suggest impaired relaxation with a mild reduction in left ventricular compliance resulting in an elevation of the left ventricular end-diastolic pressure.

Grade II: Moderate Diastolic Dysfunction

(Abnormal relaxation + at least mildly elevated filling pressures)

- **Significance** — Suggests impaired (slow) early left ventricular relaxation with moderately decreased left ventricular compliance and increased LA pressure.

- **Signs and symptoms** — Dyspnea with mild to moderate exertion

- **Functional status** — Mild to moderate impairment

- **Left atrium** — Enlarged and hypocontractile

- **Filling pressures** — Increased *(Figure 6.23)*

- **Treatment** — May include vasodilator, diuretic therapy and afterload reduction

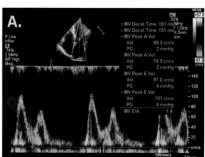 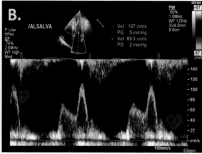

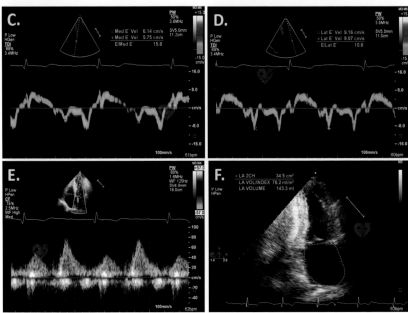

Figure 6.23: **Echo variables obtained in a patient with myocardial disease, increased LA volume index and evidence of increased TR velocity = 3.47 m/sec (48mmHg). A) Mitral Inflow Doppler demonstrates a tall mitral E-wave velocity (99cm/sec), A wave velocity (72cm/sec); E/A ratio is 1.4; E-wave deceleration time = 156 msec. All findings consistent with "normal appearing" mitral inflow A-wave duration could not be measured. B) Valsalva maneuver performed during the recording of mitral inflow demonstrating a significant reduction in the E-wave velocity and significant increase in the A-wave velocity. E/A ratio is now 0.6; C) TDI obtained from the septal annulus = 6cm/sec; D) TDI obtained from the lateral annulus = 9cm/sec; averaged e' velocities = 7.5 and the E/e' ratio = 14. E) Pulmonary vein Doppler profile demonstrating an S-wave <D-wave. A-wave reversal velocity and duration could not be measured. Note the tall D-wave of 81cm/sec coincides with a tall mitral E-wave. F) LA volume index = 76.2mL/m². All echo findings this patient are consistent with Grade II, moderate diastolic dysfunction.** *(Table 6.3).*

Table 6.3: **Grade II Diastolic Dysfunction** *(ASE Recommendations)* [1]	
LV relaxation	Impaired
LAP	Elevated
Mitral E/A ratio	>0.8 to <2
Averaged E/e' ratio (septal and lateral annulus)	10 to 14
Peak TR velocity (m/s)	>2.8
LA volume index (mL/m²)	Increased (>34)

Table 6.3: With Grade II, the effects of impaired (slow) early left ventricular relaxation on early diastolic filling become opposed by the elevated left atrial pressure and the early diastolic transmitral pressure gradient and mitral valve flow velocity pattern return to normal. This phenomenon is called pseudonormalization (historically has been referred to as pseudonormalization although the term does not appear in the 2016 guidelines) to indicate that although left ventricular filling appears normal, significant abnormalities of diastolic function are present. In most patients with Grade II, left atrial and

left ventricular end-diastolic filling pressures are elevated, the left atrium is increased in size and patients often complain of exertional dyspnea. Grade II suggests impaired relaxation, a mild to moderate decrease in left ventricular compliance, a mild to moderate increase in filling pressures which will produce symptoms of heart failure with mild to moderate exertion.

Grade III: Diastolic Dysfunction

(Abnormal relaxation + highly elevated filling pressures)

- **Significance:** Severe decrease in left ventricular compliance and impaired (slow) early left ventricular relaxation with a significant increase in filling pressures which may be altered with preload reduction maneuvers
- **Signs and symptoms:** Dyspnea with minimal exertion
- **Functional status:** Marked impairment
- **Left atrium:** Enlarged and hypocontractile
- **Filling pressures:** Markedly increased
- **Treatment:** Cautious use of venodilators, diuretics, afterload reduction or inotropic agents

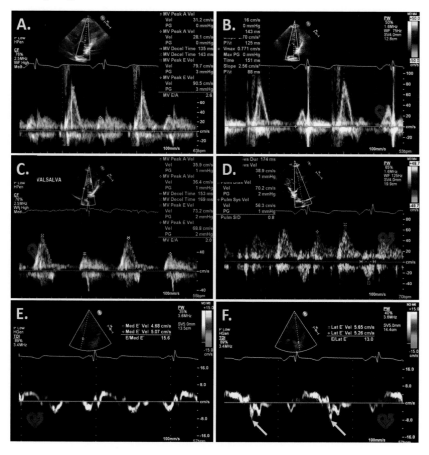

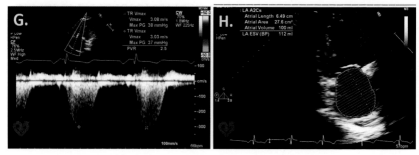

Figure 6.24: **Echocardiography variables obtained in a patient with myocardial disease, increased LA volume index and evidence of increased TR velocity = 3.1 m/sec (38.44mmHg). A) Mitral inflow Doppler demonstrates a tall mitral E-wave velocity (86cm/sec), A wave velocity (36cm/sec); E/A ratio is 2.6; E-wave deceleration time = 139 msec. All findings are consistent with a restrictive filling pattern; B) Sample volume was placed at the mitral annulus and the A-wave duration = 134 msec; C) Adequate Valsalva maneuver was performed during the recording of mitral inflow demonstrating a slight reduction in the E-wave velocity from 86cm/sec to 71cm/sec. No significant change was observed in the A-wave velocity. E/A ratio is now 2.0. Findings consistent with Stage III b irreversible restrictive. D) Pulmonary vein Doppler profile demonstrating an S-wave <D-wave. A-wave reversal velocity = 39cm/sec and the duration = 174 msec; the mitral A-wave duration (134 msec) was then compared to the pulmonary vein A-wave duration (174 msec), demonstrating a 40 msec difference. Note the tall D-wave coincides with a tall mitral E-wave; F) TDI obtained from the septal annulus = 5cm/sec; E) TDI obtained from the lateral annulus = 5.4cm/sec, averaged e' velocities = 5 and the E/e' ratio = 15; G) Not the TDI isovolumic velocity is higher than the e' velocity (Arrows). As mentioned above, the TR velocity is elevated; H) LA volume index = 62.2mL/m².** All echocardiographic findings in this patient are consistent with Grade III, severe diastolic dysfunction.*(Table 6.4)*.

Table 6.4: **Grade III Diastolic Dysfunction** *(ASE Recommendations)*[1]	
LV relaxation	Impaired
LAP	Elevated
Mitral E/A ratio	>2
Averaged E/e' ratio (septal and lateral annulus)	>14
Peak TR velocity (m/s)	>2.8
LA volume index	Increased (>34)

Table 6.4: Grade III represents a severe decrease in LV chamber compliance. Diastolic filling pressures are elevated. The LA is dilated and hypocontractile. Despite the presence of impaired left ventricular relaxation, the markedly elevated LA pressure results in a high velocity of early diastolic filling, which stops abruptly because of an abnormally rapid rise in ventricular pressure and atrial dysfunction. The patient is typically symptomatic at rest or with minimal exertion, and demonstrates a severely reduced functional capacity.

Table 6.5: **Sonographer's Check List Evaluation of Diastolic Function**
1. Patient information (e.g., age, cardiac history, blood pressure)
2. Evaluation of structural abnormalities/ventricular systolic function
3. Measurement of LA volume index
4. Measurements of mitral valve PW Doppler E/A ratio, TDI E/e', pulmonary veins
5. Measurement of CW Doppler tricuspid regurgitation peak velocity for RVSP

Table 6.6: **Evaluation of Diastolic Function** *(ASE Recommendations)*[1]				
	Normal	**Grade I**	**Grade II**	**Grade III**
LV relaxation	Normal	Impaired	Impaired	Impaired
LAP	Normal	Low or normal	Elevated	Elevated
Mitral E/A ratio	≥0.8	≤0.8	>0.8 to <2	>2
Average E/e' ratio	<10	<10	10 to 14	>14
Peak TR velocity (m/s)	<2.8	<2.8	>2.8	>2.8
LA volume index	Normal	Normal or increased	Increased	Increased

Table 6.7: **Examples of Conclusions for Reporting LV Diastolic Function** *(ASE Recommendations)* [1]

Example 1 Conclusion would contain an item from each of 1, 2, and 3	1. LV relaxation impaired or normal 2. LV filling pressures normal, elevated or borderline elevated 3. Grade I diastolic dysfunction or grade II diastolic dysfunction or grade III diastolic dysfunction
Example 2 Conclusion would contain one of the six options shown to the right	1. Normal diastolic function 2. Impaired LV relaxation, normal LAP 3. Impaired LV relaxation, mildly elevated LAP 4. Impaired LV relaxation, elevated LAP 5. Restrictive LV filling pattern, indicating markedly elevated LAP 6. Indeterminate
Example 3 Conclusion would contain one of the six options shown to the right	1. Normal diastolic function 2. Impaired LV relaxation, normal LAP 3. Impaired LV relaxation, increased LVEDP 4. Impaired LV relaxation, elevated LAP 5. Restrictive LV filling pattern, indicating markedly elevated LAP 6. Indeterminate
Example 4 Conclusion would contain one of the four options shown to the right	1. Normal diastolic function and filling pressure 2. Grade 1 (impaired relaxation with low to normal filling pressure) 3. Grade 2 (moderate increase in filling pressure) 4. Grade 3 (marked elevation in filling pressure)
Example 5 Conclusion would contain one of the three options shown to the right	1. Increased filling pressure 2. Normal filling pressure 3. Constrictive pericarditis
Example 6 Conclusion would contain one of the three options shown to the right	1. Findings consistent with diastolic dysfunction 2. Findings suggestive of probable diastolic dysfunction 3. Findings raise the possibility of diastolic dysfunction.

6

Evaluation of Diastolic Function / Assessing Abnormal Diastolic Function Grades (I – III)

Table 6.8: Assessment of LV Filling Pressures in Special Populations *(ASE Recommendations)*[1]

Disease	Echocardiographic measurements and cutoff values
Atrial fibrillation	• Peak acceleration rate of mitral E velocity (≥1,900cm/s2) • DT of pulmonary venous diastolic velocity (≤220msec) • Septal or lateral E/e' ratio (≥11)
Sinus tachycardia	• Mitral inflow pattern with predominant early LV filling in patients with EFs <50% • Pulmonary vein systolic filling fraction ≤40% is specific (88%) • Average E/e' >14 (this cutoff has highest specificity but low sensitivity) • When E and A velocities are partially or completely fused, the presence of a compensatory period after premature beats often leads to separation of E and A velocities which can be used for assessment of diastolic function
Hypertrophic cardiomyopathy	• Average E/e' (>14) • Ar-A (≥30 msec) • TR peak velocity (>2.8m/s) • LA volume index (>34mL/m²)
Noncardiac pulmonary hypertension	• Lateral E/e' can be applied to determine whether a cardiac etiology is the underlying reason for the increased pulmonary artery pressures • When cardiac etiology is present, lateral E/e' is >13, whereas in patients with pulmonary hypertension due to a noncardiac etiology, lateral E/e' is <8
Mitral stenosis	• Mitral A velocity (>1.5 m/s)
Mitral regurgitation	• Ar-A (≥30 msec) • Average E/e' (>14) may be considered only in patients with depressed EFs

A comprehensive approach is recommended in all of the above settings, which includes estimation of systolic pulmonary artery pressure using peak velocity of TR jet (>2.8 m/s) and LA maximum volume index (abnormal: >34mL/m²). Conclusions should not be based on single measurements. Specificity comments refer to predicting filling pressure >15mmHg. Note that the role of LA maximum volume index to draw inferences on left atrial pressure is limited in athletes, patients with atrial fibrillation, and/or those with mitral valve disease.

LV Diastolic Function in Patients with Normal LVEF

(ASE Recommendations) [1]

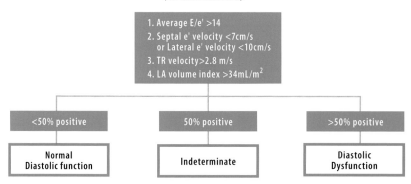

Estimation of Filling Pressures and Grading Diastolic Function in Patients with Depressed LVEF

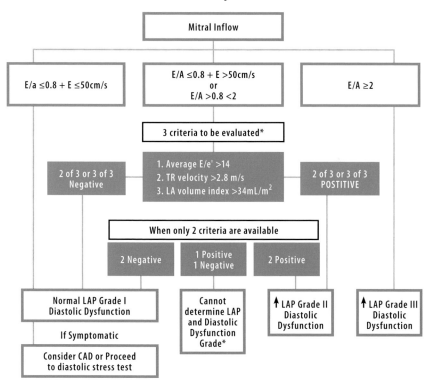

*LAP indeterminate if only 1 of 3 parameters available.
Pulmonary vein S/D ratio <1 applicable to conclude elevated LAP in patients with depressed LV EF

Patterns of Diastolic Function

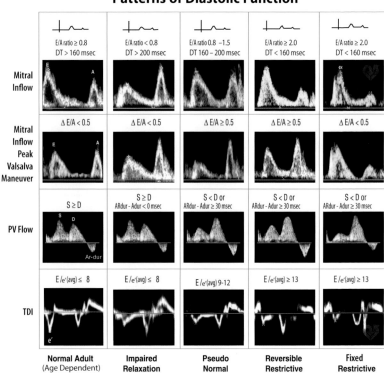

	35-44	45-54	55-64	65-75	P-value
MITRAL VALVE					
E (cm/s)	75.0 ± 15.3	72.5 ± 14.7	74.1 + 16.7	64.7 ± 14.8	0.01
A (cm/s)	57.5 ± 12.4	63.1 ± 13.9	72.0 ± 17.9	71.8 ± 16.7	<0.001
E/Λ ratio	1.3 ± 0.3	1.2 ± - 0.4	1.1 + 0.2	0.9 ± 0.2	<0.001
SEPTAL ANNULUS					
s'$_{septal}$ (cm/s) (Range)	8.2 ± 1.4 (6.4-10.9)	8.2 ± 1.6 (5.9-11.0)	8.2 ± 1.6 (6.0-10.9)	7.6 ± 1.2 (5.2-9 .8)	0.20
e'$_{septal}$ (cm/s) (Range)	9.5 ± 2.1 (6.1-13.3)	8.7 ± 1.7 (6.0-11.7)	8.1 ± 1.8 (5.4-11.4)	7.5 ± 1.4 (4.9-9.9)	<0.001
E/e'$_{septum}$ (Range)	8.2 ± 2.1 (5.5 -12.0)	8.5 ± 1.9 (5.9-12.2)	9.5 ± 2.6 (6.3-14.3)	8.9 ± 2.3 (6.1-13.3)	<0.001
LATERAL ANNULUS					
s'$_{lateral}$ (cm/s) (Range)	10.6 ± 2.4 (7.3-15.9)	10.3 ± 2.4 (6.7-14.7)	9.6 ± 2.3 (6.3-13.9)	9.9 ± 2.3 (5.9-14.5)	0.006
e'$_{lateral}$ (Range)	14.0 ± 3.0 (9.6-19 .2)	12.3 ± 2.8 (8.2-17.5)	10.7 ± 2.5 (6.9-14.7)	1 0.5 ± 1 .9 (7. 3 -1 3 .6)	<0.001
E/e'$_{lateral}$ (Range)	5.5 ± 1.4 (3.2-8.3)	6.1 ± 1.6 (3.9-9.2)	7.3 ± 2.4 (4.3-11.0)	6.3 ± 1.8 (3.9-11.4)	<0.001

Table 6.9: Normal Mitral Valve and TDI Values with Aging

P-value <0.05 indicates significant differences in mean values. Note: the mitral valve E wave and TDI septal s' do not demonstrate changes with normal aging.

Adapted from Normative reference values for the mitral valve and tissue Doppler imaging parameters of left ventricular function: a population-based study; Navtej S. Chahal, Tiong K. Lim, Piyush Jain, John C. Chambers, Jaspal S. Kooner, and Roxy Senior.

Important to Note

- The sonographer's ability to obtain high-quality 2D and Doppler tracings is critical to the success of the evaluation of diastolic function. It must be emphasized that the mitral valve anterior leaflet is longer and larger than the posterior mitral valve leaflet, which means the left ventricle fills laterally and posteriorly. The sonographer should move off of the cardiac apex and tilt posteriorly when obtaining the mitral valve flow velocities *(Figure 6.8 B)*.

- Age is a primary consideration when defining normal mitral inflow and TDI velocities. *(Table 6.9)*

- In general, the higher the mitral valve E-wave velocity, the higher the left atrial pressure in patients with reduced ejection fraction and global left ventricular systolic function.

- The shorter the mitral valve deceleration time, the greater the reduction in ventricular compliance in patients with significantly reduced ejection fraction and global left ventricular systolic function.

- A mid-diastolic wave (L-wave) seen on the mitral inflow suggests increased LV filling pressures in the absence of myocardial disease and bradycardia. *(Figure 6.10)*

- In patients with atrial fibrillation, the peak E-wave velocity and deceleration time (the deceleration time should only be measured if the E velocity ends by the onset of the QRS complex) should be measured. A consistent increased E-wave velocity of >1.0 m/s and/or a shortened deceleration time (<130 msec) may indicate increased LV filling pressures.

- An E/e' ratio of ≥11 predicts elevated left ventricular filling pressures (≥15mmHg) in patients with atrial fibrillation.

- In patients with fusion of the mitral valve E wave and A wave velocities (e.g., sinus tachycardia), an E/e' septal ratio of >14 may indicate elevated LV filling pressure (≥15mmHg).

- The inclusion of peak TR velocities are important to obtain and document, especially in symptomatic patients with diastolic dysfunction. *(Figure 6.20)*

- Use caution on measuring the correct TDI e' velocity. Note the first deflection below the baseline just after the end of the s' velocity is most likely the isovolumic relaxation waveform. A longer isovolumic period may result in more than one isovolumic waveform *(Figure 6.18, 6.24 F)*.

- If there is reduced left ventricular systolic function there is diastolic dysfunction.

- Importantly, normal left atrial volume virtually excludes significant diastolic dysfunction and elevated filling pressures.

Acknowledgment I would like to thank Marie Ficociello, RDCS, MA for her helpful review of this chapter.

References

1. Nagueh SF, Smiseth OA, Appleton CP, et al. Recommendations for the Evaluation of Left Ventricular Diastolic Function by Echocardiography: An Update from the American Society of Echocardiography and the European Association of Cardiovascular Imaging. J Am Soc Echocardiogr. 2016;29(4):277-314. doi:10.1016/j.echo.2016.01.011

2. Intersocietal Accreditation Commission Standards and Guidelines for Adult Echocardiography Accreditation. 2018. Available at: https://www.intersocietal.org/echo/standards/IACAdultEchocardiographyStandards2017.pdf. Accessed December 5, 2019.

3. Hill JC, Palma RA. Doppler tissue imaging for the assessment of left ventricular diastolic function: a systematic approach for the sonographer. J Am Soc Echocardiogr. 2005;18(1):80-89. doi:10.1016/j.echo.2004.09.007

4. Chahal NS, Lim TK, Jain P, Chambers JC, Kooner JS, Senior R. Normative reference values for the tissue Doppler imaging parameters of left ventricular function: a population-based study. Eur J Echocardiogr. 2010;11(1):51-56. doi:10.1093/ejechocard/jep164

6

Evaluation of Diastolic Function / Assessing Abnormal Diastolic Function Grades (I – III)

Hypertension
Margaret M. Park, BS, ACS, RDCS, RVT, FSDMS, FASE

Systemic Hypertension

Definition

- Hypertension (high blood pressure) begins at 130/80
- Systolic blood pressure above 130mmHg, diastolic blood pressure above 80mmHg or both based on the mean of two or more readings on two separate office visits.

Classification

- Hypertension or high blood pressure is classified as either essential or secondary.
- Essential hypertension also known as primary or idiopathic hypertension has no identifiable cause and is assigned to approximately 90 to 95% of patients with systemic hypertension.
- Secondary hypertension is caused by an identifiable underlying mechanism such as arterial renal disease, renal parenchymal disease, aortic coarctation, endocrine diseases, neurogenic diseases, drugs, chemical, food ingestion, or as a complication from certain medical therapies.

Table 7.1: 2017 ACC/AHA High Blood Pressure Guidelines for Adults		
BP Category	**Systolic (mmHg)**	**Diastolic (mmHg)**
Normal	<120	<80
Elevated	120 to 129	<80
Stage 1 hypertension	130 to 139	80 to 89
Stage 2 hypertension	≥140	>90
Hypertensive urgency/emergency**	≥180	>120

ACC, American College of Cardiology, AHA, American Heart Association,
BP indicates blood pressure (based on an average of ≥2 careful readings obtained on ≥2 occasions

**Hypertensive urgency definition: Systolic pressure over 180mmHg and/or diastolic pressure over 120mmHg, with patients needing prompt changes in medication if there are no other indications of problems, or immediate hospitalization if there are signs of organ damage.

Important to Note

The previously used term "hypertensive crisis" has been replaced by "hypertensive urgency" or "hypertensive emergency." Hypertensive urgency and emergency are differentiated by the absence or presence of new or worsening target organ damage, respectively. For both conditions, the classification is based on the blood pressure of a systolic blood pressure >180mmHg and/or a diastolic blood pressure >120mmHg.

Table 7.2: Blood Pressure Measurement Definitions	
BP Component	Definition
Systolic Blood Pressure (SBP)	First Korotkoff* sound
Diastolic Blood Pressure (DBP)	Fifth Korotkoff* sound
Pulse pressure	SBP minus DBP
Mean arterial pressure	DBP plus 1/3 the pulse pressure
Mid BP	Sum SBP + DBP divided by 2

Korotkoff arterial sounds are what is heard through a stethoscope when applied on the brachial artery and change with varying reduction of cuff pressure. These sounds are used to determine the systolic (first sound) and diastolic (last sound) blood pressure. There are 5 phases:

- **Phase 1:** Sharp thuds, begin at systolic blood pressure
- **Phase 2:** Blowing sound; may disappear entirely (the auscultatory gap)
- **Phase 3:** Crisp thud, a bit quieter than phase 1
- **Phase 4:** Sounds become muffled
- **Phase 5:** End of sounds, end at diastolic blood pressure

Accurate blood pressure readings require the correct cuff size to avoid over or underestimation of blood pressure.

Table 7.3: Blood Pressure Cuff Size	
Arm Circumference (cm)	BP Cuff Size
22 to 26	Small Adult
27 to 34	Adult
35 to 44	Large Adult
45 to 52	Adult Thigh

Risk Factors of Elevated Blood Pressure

Modifiable Risk Factors

When changed may reduce the risk of cardiovascular disease (CVD) as a result of hypertension and include:

- Smoking and/or exposure to secondhand smoke
- Diabetes mellitus
- Obesity (especially abdomen obesity)
- Dyslipidemia/hypercholesterolemia (independent of obesity)
- Physical inactivity
- Low physical fitness
- Unhealthy diet
- Inadequate intake of potassium and calcium
- Sodium intake
- Alcohol consumption
- Emotional and work-related stress

Fixed Risk Factors

Those risk factors which are difficult to change, may not be altered or even when changed may not reduce CVD risk:

• Chronic kidney disease

• Family history

• Increased age

• Male sex

• Race (higher incidence in African Americans)

• Low socioeconomic/educational status

• Obstructive sleep apnea

• Psychosocial stress

Patient Complaints

• May be asymptomatic

• Headaches (common complaint)

• Dyspnea (suggests heart failure)

• Palpitations

• Anxiety

• Tinnitus

• Blurred vision

• Dizziness

• Sweats

• Pallor

• Orthostatic hypotension (suggests pheochromocytoma)

Identifiable Causes of Secondary Hypertension

• Endocrine, hormonal Changes

• Acromegaly

• Congenital adrenal hyperplasia

• Cushing Syndrome

• Exogenous hormones (corticosteroids, estrogen)

• Hypothyroidism, hyperthyroidism

• Pheochromocytoma

• Primary hyperaldosteronism

• Sympathomimetic drugs

• Renal causes

  - Chronic renal disease and failure

  - Intrarenal vasculitis

  - Polycystic kidney disease

  - Renal parenchymal disease

  - Renal artery stenosis

• Vascular causes

  - Aortic coarctation

  - Collagen vascular disease

  - Renovascular disease

  - Intracranial hypertension

  - Vasculitis

• Other causes

  - Pregnancy induced

  - Obstructive sleep apnea

  - Hyperdynamic circulation issues resulting in increased cardiac output

  - Aortic insufficiency

  - Patent ductus arteriosus

  - Atrioventricular fistulas

Complications

- Complications associated with hypertension can affect multiple systems including the brain, eye, heart, kidney and vascular tree.
- Atherosclerotic complications, coronary artery disease (angina, myocardial ischemia, acute myocardial infarction)
- Left ventricular hypertrophy
- Heart failure (dyspnea, orthopnea, paroxysmal nocturnal dyspnea, fatigue, cough, weight gain)
- Transient ischemic attacks/stroke
- Hypertensive encephalopathy, intracerebral hemorrhage, dementia
- Hypertensive renal disease (nephrosclerosis, renal failure, glomerulosclerosis)
- Hypertensive retinopathy, optic neuropathy, choroidopathy
- Aortic aneurysm (ascending aorta, abdominal aorta)
- Aortic dissection
- Arteriosclerosis

Cardiac Auscultation

- Early systolic ejection murmur (aortic valve sclerosis/dilated ascending aorta)
- Ejection sound (dilated ascending aorta)
- S4 (decreased left ventricular compliance)
- S3 (heart failure or mitral regurgitation)
- Murmur of aortic regurgitation secondary to aortic root dilatation
- Murmur of mitral regurgitation (mitral annular calcification/dilated left ventricle)

Electrocardiogram

- Left ventricular hypertrophy (predictor of poor outcome)
- Left atrial enlargement
- Atrial fibrillation
- Ventricular arrhythmias
- Evidence of myocardial ischemia/infarction

Chest X-ray

- Cardiomegaly due to left ventricular enlargement
- Pulmonary congestion (suggests heart failure)
- Aortic aneurysm/dissection

Medical Treatment

- - Non-pharmacologic therapy
- - Weight loss
- - Heart healthy diet (reduction in sodium, cholesterol, saturated fats, coffee
- - Increased physical activity (aerobic exercise 90 to 150 min./week)
- - Reduce alcohol consumption (moderate intake)
- - Cessation of tobacco consumption
- - Stress reduction via psychotherapy, relaxation methods, biofeedback, environmental modification
- Pharmacologic therapy:
  - - Diuretics (first drug of choice) (e.g., hydrochlorothiazide)
  - - Beta blockers (e.g., metoprolol)
  - - Central acting anti-adrenergic agents (e.g., clonidine)
  - - Alpha-beta blockers (e.g., labetalol)
  - - ACE inhibitors (e.g., captopril)
  - - ARB's (e.g., losartan)
  - - Calcium channel blockers (e.g., nifedipine)
  - - Direct vasodilators (e.g., minoxidil)
  - - Treatment of hypertensive emergency (e.g., sodium nitroprusside)

Surgical Treatment

Treat cause of secondary systemic hypertension (e.g., reconstruction of stenotic renal artery, excision of aortic coarctation)

Role of Echocardiography

The role of echocardiography is to evaluate secondary complications of hypertension (HTN) to the heart:

- The presence of and degree of left ventricular hypertrophy and/or increased mass
- Assessment of left ventricular systolic function
- Assessment of left ventricular diastolic function
- Identify associated cardiac abnormalities associated with HTN
- Exclude any identifiable causes

Left Ventricular hypertrophy (LVH) is an adaptive response of the heart to the increased afterload caused by a chronic increase in blood pressure. An increase in left ventricular (LV) wall thickness and regional wall thickness (RWT) is known as concentric remodeling. Eventually the increased wall stress leads to concentric hypertrophy and reduced cavity size which leads to increased LV mass. LV mass is calculated as the LV muscle volume multiplied by the specific gravity of muscle (1.04g/mL). M-mode and or 2D echocardiography can be used to estimate LV muscle volume and, therefore LV mass. LV muscle volume is the difference between the epicardial volume and the endocardial volume *(Figure 7.6)*. The presence of and the degree of LVH can be determined by wall thickness measurements derived either by M-mode *(Figure 7.1)* or 2D echocardiography *(Figure 7.2)*. Care should be taken to assure the parasternal long axis view is obtained perpendicular to the LV long axis and measured at the level of the mitral valve leaflet tips during end-diastole (onset of the QRS).

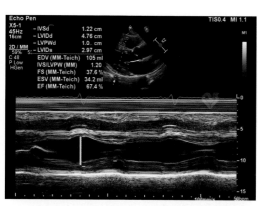

Figure 7.1: **M-mode derived linear LV internal measurements acquired in the parasternal long-axis view. Wall thickness is measured at end-diastole at the onset of the QRS complex. Measurements are performed at the blood tissue interface of the interventricular septum, LV internal dimension, and LV posterior wall. LV = left ventricle**

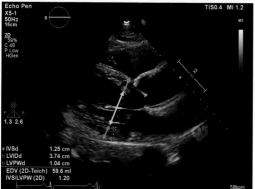

Figure 7.2: **2D derived linear LV internal measurements acquired in the parasternal long-axis view. Image should be obtained perpendicular to the LV long axis at end-diastole. Electronic calipers are used to measure the interface between the myocardial wall and cavity and the interface between the wall and the pericardium at the level of the mitral valve leaflet tips. (Blood tissue interface) 2D = two-dimensional, LV = left ventricle**

In addition, these same dimensions may be measured from the parasternal short-axis view. The use of the short axis derived linear dimensions overcomes the common problem of oblique parasternal images resulting in overestimation of cavity and wall dimensions from M-mode *(Figure 7.3)*.

7

Hypertension / Systemic Hypertension

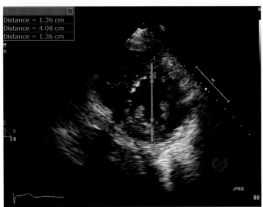

Figure 7.3: **2D-derived diastolic linear LV dimensions measured from the parasternal short-axis view papillary muscle level, left ventricular end-diastolic dimension (LVEDD) represented by green arrow, Interventricular septal (IVS) and posterior wall (PW) in blue.**

Using linear dimensions of the IVS, PW and LVEDD derived by either method LV mass (LVM) can be estimated as:

LVM = 1.04 ([LVEDD + PW + IVS] - LVEDD³) x 0.8 + 0.6

> *LVM = left ventricular mass (g)*
> *LVEDD = left ventricular end-diastolic dimension(cm)*
> *PW = left ventricular posterior wall thickness (cm)*
> *IVS = interventricular septal thickness (cm)*
> *1.04 = specific gravity of muscle (g/mL)*

In this LVM formula the specific gravity of muscle is a constant and 0.8 and 0.6 are correction factors. The (LVEDD + IVS + PW) determines the LV epicardial volume while the LVEDD determines the endocardial volume. *(Figure 7.3)*.

The 2D area length method and the truncated ellipsoid method can also be used to calculate LV mass. Measurements of the total cavity area, total epicardial area and total LV length are required. The total epicardial and endocardial area are traced in the parasternal short axis view at the level of the papillary muscles in end-diastole. The LV length is measured from the LV apical 4-chamber view from the apex to the mitral valve (MV) annulus. Calculate LV mass using the 2D Area-Length Method. *(Figures 7.4, 7.5)*

2D Area-Length Method

LVM = 1.05 [5/6 A1 (L + t)] – 5/6 A2 L]

> *LVM = left ventricular mass (g)*
> *A1 = epicardial area at end diastole (cm²)*
> *A2 = endocardial area at end diastole (cm³)*
> *L = LV length at end diastole*
> *t = average wall thickness*
> *1.05 = specific gravity of muscle (g/mL)*

Truncated Ellipse Method

$$LVM = \frac{1{:}05 \; \Pi \, b + t) \, [2/3 \, (a + t) + d^3 \,/3 \, (a + t)^2] - b^2}{[\, 2/3 \, a + d - d^3 / 3a^2]}$$

LVM = left ventricular mass (g)
a = semi-major axis length (cm)
b = short axis radius (cm)
d = truncated semi-major axis length (cm)
t = average wall thickness
1.05 = specific gravity of muscle (g/mL)
LV mass value is then indexed or normalized to body surface area (BSA)

LVMi = LVM / BSA

LVMi = left ventricular mass index (g/m^2)
LV Mass = left ventricular mass (g)
BSA = body surface area (m^2)

Important to Note

Indexing by BSA in obesity will underestimate the degree of LVH, it is recommended indexing by height in the presence of obesity.

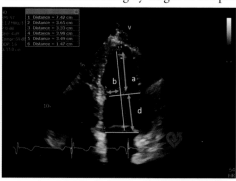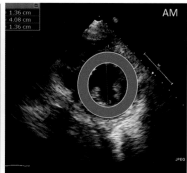

Figure 7.4: **Left and right panel: Demonstrated measurements used for the 2D based formulas to calculate LV mass**

a = distance from the minor axis to the endocardium at the LV apex;
b = LV minor radius
d = distance from the minor axis to the mitral valve plane
t = mean wall thickness.
Solid yellow line = LV length (long axis) measured from the apex to the MV annulus.
Am = mean wall thickness as t in formula

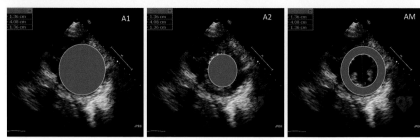

Figure 7.5: (A1) LV Epicardial Volume; (A2) LV Endocardial Volume = (AM) LV Muscle Volume

From the parasternal short axis view traced at the level of the papillary muscles at end-diastole, LV muscle volume (AM) is determined by subtracting the total endocardial volume (A2) from the total epicardial volume (A1).

Relative wall thickness (RWT) is calculated from the LV posterior wall thickness at end diastole and the LV end diastolic chamber diameter.

RWT = (2 PW) / LVEDD

RWT = relative wall thickness
LVEDD = LV end diastolic chamber diameter (cm)
PW = left ventricular end-diastolic PW thickness (cm)

Based on a combination of LVM and RWT the resulting LV remodeling can be classified into four groups: normal LV geometry, concentric hypertrophy, concentric remodeling, eccentric hypertrophy. The typical hypertensive concentric remodeling pattern is concentric hypertrophy, a combination of increased mass and increased relative wall thickness.

Table 7.4: **Patterns of LV Geometry**	
Concentric hypertrophy	Equally distributed (uniform) increase in ventricular wall thickness with normal ventricular chamber dimensions, increased relative wall thickness (>0.42) and increased ventricular mass
Concentric remodeling	Normal chamber dimensions, elliptical ventricular chamber shape, increase in relative wall thickness (>0.42) and normal ventricular mass representing an adaptive response to an increase in afterload. Present in a subgroup of patients with high blood pressure, reduced cardiac index and the highest values of peripheral vascular resistance.
Eccentric hypertrophy	Increased ventricular dimensions, spherical ventricular chamber shape, normal wall thickness, low or normal relative wall thickness (≤0.42) and increased ventricular mass. Most commonly seen in patients with significant chronic mitral regurgitation and/or aortic regurgitation.
Normal geometry	Normal LV mass and normal regional wall thickness

Table 7.5: Classical Description of LV Geometry *(ASE Recommendations)* [3]			
LV Geometry	**LVM (men)**	**LVM (women)**	**RWT**
Normal	≤115g/m²	≤95g/m²	<0.42
Concentric hypertrophy	>115g/m²	>95g/m²	>0.42
Eccentric Hypertrophy	>115g/m²	>95g/m²	<0.42
Concentric Remodelling	≤115g/m²	≤95g/m²	>0.42
Measurements performed using 2D -direct M-mode			

The LV geometry changes that occur in hypertensive heart disease usually have effects on the LV systolic and diastolic performance. Chronic hypertension often develops into heart failure therefore LV systolic function should be evaluated along with a complete LV diastolic function examination. LV systolic function may present with increased wall thickness and hyperdynamic contractility, consequently careful interrogation for a dynamic LVOT obstruction is warranted. Look for the typical systolic late-peaking dagger shaped Doppler profile. MV inflow signals will commonly display impaired relaxation patterns; E/A ratio >1 and prolongation of the deceleration time are common in hypertensive individuals as is the presence of an L-wave with early diastolic E and late diastolic A MV filling waves indicating a pseudonormal filling pattern. *(Figure 7.6)*

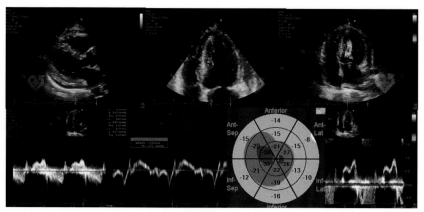

Figure 7.6: **Hypertensive patient with concentric LVH, pericardial effusion, normal systolic function and abnormal diastolic dysfunction**

The aorta and aortic valve should be carefully evaluated using 2D imaging including suprasternal notch and subcostal Doppler imaging to r/o the presence of color flow turbulence as seen in aortic coarctation. Aortic coarctation is a secondary sign of hypertension *(Figure 7.7)* which can be diagnosed with echo/Doppler echocardiography. Other cardiac lesions associated with systemic hypertension include aortic valve sclerosis, mild aortic insufficiency, dilated ascending aortic root, aortic atheroma or atherosclerosis.

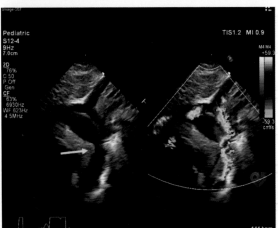

Figure 7.7: Suprasternal arch image of the aorta with a coarctation at the onset of the descending aorta (arrow) with turbulent color flow Doppler. Aortic coarctation, an identifiable cause of secondary systemic hypertension is a vascular complication that often causes LVH secondary to the chronic LV pressure overload. Interrogation of the aorta should be performed on all subjects presenting with systemic hypertension and LVH (left ventricular hypertrophy).

Table 7.6: Degrees of Abnormality of Left Ventricular Mass (LVM) Men *(ASE Recommendations)*[3]

Men	Reference range	Mildly abnormal	Moderately abnormal	Severely Abnormal
Linear method				
LVM (g)	88 to 224	225 to 258	259 to 292	≥293
LVM/BSA (g/m²)	49 to 115	116 to 131	132 to 148	≥149
LVM/height (g/m)	52 to 126	127 to 144	145 to 162	≥163
Relative wall thickness (cm)	0.24 to 0.42	0.43 to 0.46	0.47 to 0.51	≥0.52
Septal thickness (cm)	0.6 to 1.0	1.1 to 1.3	1.4 to 1.6	≥1.7
Posterior wall thickness (cm)	0.6 to 1.0	1.1 to 1.3	1.4 to 1.6	≥1.7
2D method				
LVM (g)	96 to 200	201 to 227	228 to 254	≥255
LVM/BSA (g/m²)	50 to 102	103 to 116	117 to 130	≥131

BSA = body surface area; LV = left ventricular; 2D = two-dimensional; Bold values = recommended and best validated.

Table 7.7: Degrees of Abnormality of Left Ventricular Mass (LVM) Women *(ASE Recommendations)* [3]

Women	Reference range	Mildly abnormal	Moderately abnormal	Severely Abnormal
Linear method				
LVM (g)	67 to 162	163 to 186	187 to 210	≥211
LVM/BSA (g/m^2)	43 to 95	96 to 108	109 to 121	≥122
LVM/height (g/m)	41 to 99	100 to 115	116 to 128	≥129
Relative wall thickness (cm)	0.22 to 0.42	0.43 to 0.47	0.48 to 0.52	≥0.53
Septal thickness (cm)	0.6 to 0.9	1.0 to 1.2	1.3 to 1.5	≥1.6
Posterior wall thickness (cm)	0.6 to 0.9	1.0 to 1.2	1.3 to 1.5	≥1.6
2D method				
LVM (g)	66 to 150	151 to 171	172 to 182	>193
LVM/BSA (g/m^2)	44 to 88	89 to 100	101 to 112	≥113

BSA = body surface area; LV = left ventricular; 2D = two-dimensional; Bold values = recommended and best validated.

7

Hypertension / Systemic Hypertension

- There are other disorders and diseases that can cause increased LV wall thickness on echocardiography and therefore left ventricular hypertrophy or LVH should not be used in the echo report unless LVH has been previously diagnosed and/or associated ECG findings are present.

- ECG evidence of left ventricular hypertrophy include deep S waves in V1, and tall R waves in V5 and V6. When the sum of the tallest R wave of either V5 or V6 and the S wave is greater than 35mm the ECG is positive for LVH. If associated inverted T waves are present in leads V5 and V6 significant LV strain is indicated.

- Other disorders which may present with increased wall thickness on echocardiography include:

  - **Hemochromatosis** – A hereditary disease in which excess iron from the digestive system accumulate in the myocardium

  - **Anderson-Fabry Disease** – A rare disorder with intracellular accumulation of glycolipids in the heart muscle

  - **Amyloidosis (cardiac)** – An infiltrative systemic disorder in which amyloid proteins depositions build within the cardiac myocytes

  - **Oxalosis** – An infiltrative rare hereditary disorder in which calcium oxalate crystals accumulate in the myocardial fibers

  - **Myocarditis** – Inflammation of the myocardium as seen in acute myocardial disease secondary to viral infections, toxins, drugs, and autoimmune reactions.

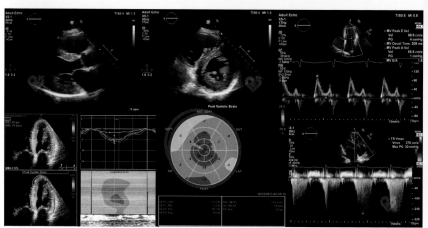

Figure 7.8: **Echo and Doppler and speckle tracking strain images of a patient with cardiac amyloidosis, an infiltrative systemic disorder in which amyloid protein depositions build within the cardiac myocytes causing increased wall thickness, low preserved systolic function, diastolic dysfunction, pulmonary hypertension and valve thickening as shown. Longitudinal strain imaging is key in identification of this pathology, apical sparing nicknamed "cherry on top" as shown on the bull's eye plot and individual wall segment strain values.**

Pulmonary Hypertension

Pulmonary hypertension (PH): A progressive and often fatal disease resulting from an increase in pulmonary artery pressures related to multiple causes. Overtime sustained increased pressure in the arterial bed leads to increased right ventricular (RV) afterload and eventually RV failure.

• Pulmonary artery pressures normally are much lower than systemic pressures due to the vast cross-sectional area of the pulmonary circulation and the resulting low resistance to blood flow. Complicated mechanisms in pulmonary vascular disease can cause plaque formation, fibrosis, vasoconstriction, and resultant luminal narrowing and pruning of the pulmonary vascular tree which in turn increases pulmonary vascular resistance (PVR).

• Pulmonary changes that occur on the arterial side of the pulmonary circulation are classified as pre-capillary PH and changes occurring on the venous side of the pulmonary circulation are classified as post-capillary PH.

• A formal diagnosis of PH is made by right heart cardiac catheterization as a mean pulmonary artery pressure >20mmHg accompanied by a pulmonary vascular resistance (PVR) ≥3 wood units (WU). Pulmonary arterial hypertension (PAH) or pre-capillary PH is further characterized as a pulmonary artery wedge pressure ≤15mmHg. Post-capillary PH has a pulmonary artery wedge pressure >15mmHg. Some patients may be further classified with combined pre-capillary PH and post-capillary PH. Additional testing during right heart catheterization of pulmonary artery pressure and cardiac output response to exercise, oxygen, vasodilators and/or nitric oxide aid in the classification and disease severity.

Table 7.8: Hemodynamic definitions of pulmonary hypertension (PH)				
Definition	**Cath Lab Hemodynamics**			**WHO Clinical Group Classification**
	mPAP	**PAWP**	**PVR**	
Pre-capillary PH	>20mmHg	≤15mmHg	≥3 WU	1, 3, 4, and some 5
Post-capillary PH	>20mmHg	>15mmHg	<3 WU	2 and 5
Combined pre-capillary and post-capillary (CpcPH)	>20mmHg	>15mmHg	>3 WU	2 and 5

mPAP: mean pulmonary arterial pressure; PAWP: pulmonary arterial wedge pressure; PVR: pulmonary vascular resistance; WU: Wood Units.
#: group 1: PAH; group 2: PH due to left heart disease; group 3: PH due to lung diseases and/or hypoxia; group 4: PH due to pulmonary artery obstructions; group 5: PH with unclear and/or multifactorial mechanisms.

Adapted from: Hemodynamic definitions and updated clinical classification of pulmonary hypertension. Eur Respir J. 2019;53(1):1801913. Published 2019 Jan 24. doi:10.1183/13993003.01913-2018

The earliest classification of pulmonary hypertension (PH) from the World Health Organization (WHO) included Primary PH and Secondary PH. In Primary PH no identifiable risk factors or cause could be determined. Primary PH was frequently interchanged with idiopathic PH. By contrast secondary PH was based on the ability to identify risk factors and causes of PH. The WHO classification of pulmonary hypertension over the last decade has been based on the similarities in pathophysiology, clinical presentation, mechanisms, and effective treatment therapies. The current WHO classification for PH *(Table 7.9),* includes 5 major categories encompassing 1) Pulmonary Arterial Hypertension (PAH) 2) PH due to left heart disease 3) PH due to lung diseases and/or hypoxia 4) PH due to pulmonary artery obstructions and 5) PH with unclear and/or multifactorial mechanisms.

Important to Note

Pulmonary arterial hypertension (PAH) is characterized by structural changes to the pulmonary artery tree, specifically pruning of the small pulmonary arteries. A multitude of pathological changes cause constriction, thickening, fibrosis, prolific over growth and hypertrophy to the vessel lumen which restricts flow throughout the pulmonary arterial circulation increasing right sided pressures and pulmonary vascular resistance. The definition of PAH by cardiac catheterization is a mPAP >20mmHg (previously 25mmHg) with a PA wedge pressure ≤15mmHg and a PVR ≥3 WU. PAH is also identified and referenced as pre-capillary PH.

Classification WHO group 2, is the largest group in the US population with post-capillary PH due mainly to left sided heart disease as a result of ventricular dysfunction (systolic and/or diastolic) and/or valvular heart diseases. The definition of PH is a mPAP >20mmHg, PA wedge pressure >15mmHg and a PVR <3 WU. These individuals should be carefully evaluated with Doppler echocardiography for estimation of LV filling pressures.

7

Hypertension / Pulmonary Hypertension

Table 7.9: 6th World Health Organization (WHO) Classification of Pulmonary Hypertension *(Nice, France 2018)*	

Pulmonary Arterial Hypertension (PAH)	• Idiopathic PAH
	• Heritable PAH
	• Drug- and toxin-induced PAH (table 3)
	• PAH associated with:
	  - Connective tissue disease
	  - HIV infection
	  - Portal hypertension
	  - Congenital heart disease
	  - Schistosomiasis
	• PAH long-term responders to calcium channel blockers
	• PAH with overt features of venous/capillaries (PVOD/PCH) involvement
	• Persistent PH of the newborn syndrome

PH due to left heart disease	• PH due to heart failure with preserved LVEF • PH due to heart failure with reduced LVEF • Valvular heart disease • Congenital/acquired cardiovascular conditions leading to post-capillary PH
PH due to lung diseases and/or hypoxia	• Obstructive lung disease • Restrictive lung disease • Other lung disease with mixed restrictive/obstructive pattern • Hypoxia without lung disease • Developmental lung disorders
PH due to pulmonary artery obstructions	• Chronic thromboembolic PH • Other pulmonary artery obstructions
PH with unclear and/or multifactorial mechanisms	• Hematological disorders • Systemic and metabolic disorders • Others • Complex congenital heart disease

The general purpose of classification of PH is to categorize clinical conditions associated with PH based on similar pathophysiological mechanisms, clinical presentation, hemodynamic characteristics, and therapeutic management. Pulmonary hypertension (PH), PAH pulmonary arterial hypertension, pulmonary vascular occlusive disease (PVOD), pulmonary capillary hemangiomatosis (PCH), left ventricular ejection fraction (LVEF).

Role of Echocardiography in PH/PAH

Echocardiography is a vital tool in the screening of patients with symptoms and/or suspicion of PH, for those at risk for developing PH or those already diagnosed and on medical therapy as a mechanism to evaluate treatment response. The goals of the echo exam should include:

• Identify potential causes of PH
• Identify important functional and morphological changes of PH
• Estimation of pulmonary artery pressures
• Evaluation of pulmonary vascular resistance
• Estimation of right atrial size/pressure

- Indirect information on right ventricular structure and function (important prognostic implications)
- Observation of shunts and/or other hemodynamic flow abnormalities
- Identification of increased RV wall thickness (chronic)

Key identifying Signs Suggestive of PH and PAH

M-mode
- Absent or decreased "a" dip (<2mm) of the pulmonary valve cusp suggest increased pulmonary artery end-diastolic pressure
- Mid-systolic notching (flying W) of pulmonary valve cusp
- Reduced tricuspid annular excursion

2D
- Right ventricular dilatation
- Prominent RV moderator band and trabeculations
- Apex forming right ventricle
- Right ventricular dysfunction
- D-shaped left ventricle
- Pulmonary artery dilatation
- Tricuspid valve annular dilatation
- Diminished RVOT TVI, reduced acceleration time, RVOT mid systolic notching
- Coronary sinus dilatation
- Right atrial dilatation
- Deviation of the interatrial septum towards the left atrium
- Right ventricular hypertrophy
- Pericardial effusion
- Patent foramen ovale
- Dilated inferior vena cava (≥2.1cm)
- Hepatic vein systolic reversal

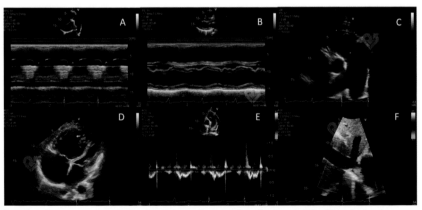

Figure 7.9: Some common signs seen in pulmonary hypertension: a) pulmonic valve M-mode showing reduced "a" wave depth and mid systolic notching often named "flying w" b) M-mode PLAX view demonstrating a dilated RV, prominent moderator band and abnormal septal motion c) PSAX view of a dilated main and branch pulmonary arteries d) A4C view with dilated right heart chambers bowing of IVS towards the LV from high RV volume/pressure e)Pulsed wave Doppler of RVOT with low flow and mid systolic notching f) dilated IVC and hepatic vein as seen with increased RA pressure.

Estimation of Pulmonary Artery Pressure from the TR Peak Velocity Profile

- Interrogation of the TR peak velocity by continuous wave (CW) Doppler reflects the right ventricular (RV) to right atrial (RA) pressure gradient.

- Using the modified Bernoulli equation, the peak TR velocity with combined right atrial pressure (RAP) estimation from the IVC collapsibility index allows for pulmonary artery systolic pressure (PASP) estimation.

- In the absence of pulmonary stenosis and/or RVOT obstruction PASP = RVSP

$$RVSP = 4V^2 + RAP \text{ (expressed as mmHg)}$$

- Careful alignment of the Doppler cursor within the direction of flow should be acquired from multiple windows using color flow Doppler.

- Assessment may require off axis imaging for eccentric jets, reversed apical 4-chamber RV window or subcostal 4C alignment to assure the highest peak is achieved.

- If the TR velocity is acquired with the aid of an ultrasound (US) enhancing agent some washout should occur before capture to avoid over estimation of noise vs the true Doppler profile signal.

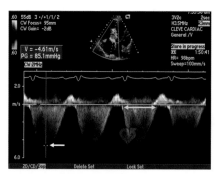

Figure 7.10: Measurement of the continuous wave Doppler peak tricuspid regurgitation velocity (white arrow) used to calculate RVSP using the modified Bernoulli equation and adding RAP. This patient has a prolonged systolic flow (yellow arrow) to diastolic flow (green arrow) duration ratio suggesting severe impairment in global RV function. V = peak velocity; PG = pressure gradient; RAP = right atrial pressure; PASP = pulmonary artery systolic pressure.

Important to Note

- Due to respiratory variation three peak velocity jets should be averaged. In severe TR there is a rapid pressure equalization between the RV and RA that blunts the peak velocity profile.

- To calculate pulmonary vascular resistance (PVR) we divide the transpulmonary pressure gradient by cardiac output therefore, in severe RV systolic function or low cardiac output states the estimated pressure may not appear elevated regardless of the presence of high vascular resistance.

Right Atrial Pressure (RAP) Estimation from IVC Collapsibility Index

RAP may be estimated using the inferior Vena Cava (IVC), hepatic veins or Doppler tissue imaging of the TV lateral annulus. The most common method involves imaging the IVC in the long axis from the subcostal window with the aid of the "inspiratory sniff." The largest(max) and smallest(min) IVC diameter (IVCd) is then measured and the **IVC collapsibility index (CI)** is calculated as:

IVC CI = ICVd max - IVCd min ÷ IVCd max x 100

The IVC should be measured perpendicular to its long axis approximately 0.5 to 2.0cm from the RA junction at end inspiration and end expiration, or pre and post respiratory sniff.

7

Hypertension / Pulmonary Hypertension

Table 7.10: Estimation of RAP Based on IVC Diameter		
IVC Diameter (cm)	**% Diameter Decrease with Sniff**	**Estimated RAP (mmHg) Normal Range**
≤2.1	>50	3 (range 0 to 5)
≤2.1	<50	8 (range 5 to 10)
≥2.1	>50	8 (range 5 to 10)
≥2.1	<50	15 (high)
Secondary indices of RAP		
Restrictive filling; Tricuspid E/e' >6; Diastolic flow predominance in HV (systolic filling fraction <55%)		

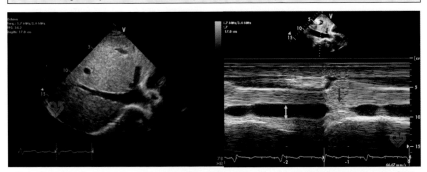

Figure 7.11: 2D subcostal image of the IVC and medial hepatic vein, M-mode of adjacent 2D image of IVC showing maximal diameter (yellow arrow) and near full collapse with brief sniff (red arrow)

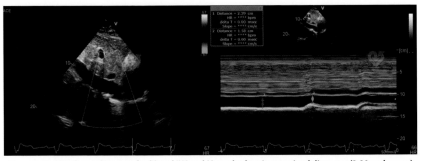

Figure 7.12: 2D subcostal image of a dilated IVC and M-mode showing maximal diameter (2.39, red arrow) and minimal diameter with brief sniff (1.58, green arrow). RAP estimation 15mmHg. Central venous pressure and right atrial pressure are the same if no vena cava obstruction is present.
IVC collapsibility index = 2.39 -1.58 ÷ 2.39 x 100 = 34%.

Right Atrial Pressure Estimation Using Hepatic Vein Doppler Profile

The hepatic veins may be used in a similar fashion to measure the systolic filling fraction (SFF). The Doppler sample volume should be placed within the medial hepatic vein and optimized. From the Doppler trace the peak systolic and diastolic Doppler velocities or the velocity time integral trace is measured and the systolic filling fraction (SFF) can be calculated as:

SFF = Systolic V ÷ (Systolic V + Diastolic V) x 100

SFF <55% suggests a RAP >8mmHg

Pulmonary Regurgitation Doppler for Estimation of Mean Pulmonary Artery pressure

- The pulmonary regurgitant (PR) velocity (V) reflects the pressure gradient between the PA and the RV during diastole.

- Using the modified Bernoulli equation, the PR early peak velocity can be converted to a pressure gradient and when the RAP is added the mean pulmonary artery pressure gradient(mPAP) is the result:

mPAP = 4V² PR early + RAP

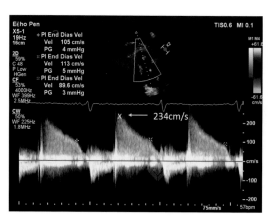

Figure 7.13: **CW Doppler across the PV, PR early peak velocity measurement** as shown used to calculate mean pulmonary artery pressure gradient.

Peak V = 234cm/s
mPAP = 4V2 PR early + RAP

Pulmonary Regurgitation Doppler for Estimation of Pulmonary Artery End Diastolic Pressure

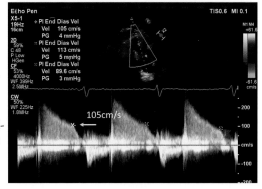

Similarly, in the absence of TV stenosis it can be assumed that RVEDP is equal to RAP and therefore pulmonary artery end-diastolic pressure (PAEDP) can be calculated using the PR end diastolic peak velocity as:

$$PAEDP = 4V^2 \text{ PR late} + RAP$$

Figure 7.14: **Calculation of PAEDP using late PR peak V. PAEDP, pulmonary artery end-diastolic pressure, PR, pulmonary regurgitation, V, peak velocity.**

RV Acceleration Time for Estimation of Mean Pulmonary Artery Pressure

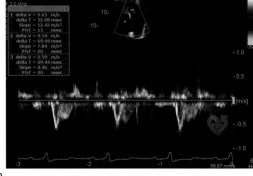

Using the RV outflow tract (RVOT) pulsed wave (PW) Doppler waveform the RV acceleration time (RVAT) can be used to estimate mean pulmonary artery pressure(mPAP).

Formulas are only accurate when heart rates fall between 60 to 100 bpm, either equation may be used:

Figure 7.15: **RVAT is measured as the time from the beginning of the RVOT signal at zero baseline to the peak of the signal.**

$$mPAP = 79 - (0.45 \times RVAT)$$
$$mPAP = 90 - (0.62 \times RVAT)$$

A RVAT greater than 120ms is associated with a normal mPAP.

TR Doppler for Estimation of Mean Pulmonary Artery Pressure (mPAP)

mPAP may also be calculated from the TR CW Doppler signal. The TR Doppler envelope is traced from its beginning to end to derive the RV to RA gradient and adding the RAP the mPAP is estimated as:

mPAP = mean RV - RA PG + RAP

Estimation of Pulmonary Vascular Resistance (PVR)

- Pulmonary vascular resistance (PVR) is directly proportional to the pressure gradient across the entire lungs from the PAP to the LA pressure.

- A normal value range for PVR is 0.25 to 1.6 wood units (WU).

- PVR can be calculated as:

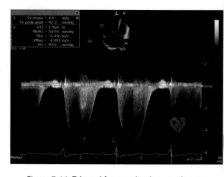

Figure 7.16: **Tricuspid regurgitation continuous wave Doppler trace to determine right ventricle to right atrial gradient (55mmHg in this example) to which RAP pressure is added to determine mean pulmonary artery pressure.**

PVR = TRV (m/s) / RVOT TVI (cm) x 10 + 0.16
or
as a direct ratio of the TRV to RVOT VTI:

TRV/RVOT VTI

A value of <0.2 equates to normal PVR, a value >0.2 equates to a PVR >2 WU

Important to Note

The first hemodynamic change in patients with PAH that respond to vasodilator pharmacology is a decrease in PVR and an increase in cardiac output (CO); Pulmonary artery pressure does not change significantly.

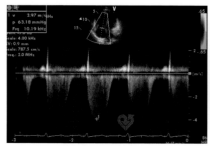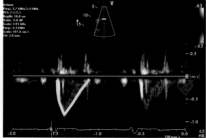

Figure 7.17: **Left panel, demonstration of Peak TR velocity (TRV = 3.97 m/s, 63mmHg), right panel tracing of RVOT time velocity integral (RVOT VTI = 15.91cm.) the necessary components for Pulmonary Vascular Resistance(PVR) calculation by echocardiography.**

- The highest Doppler signal will be parallel to the jet direction.
- In the absence of pulmonic stenosis, RVSP and PASP are equal.
- When RV outflow obstruction is present, PASP is calculated by subtracting the RV to PA gradient from the estimated RVSP.
- RA pressure is estimated from the IVC size and amount of collapse during respiratory changes and/or HV flow patterns.
- Increased RV wall thickness indicates chronic increased RV pressures.
- Increased PA pressures do not always mean vessel narrowing, increased pressures can also result from high PA flow (increased cardiac output).

Evaluation of Right Atrial Chamber Size

- Right atrial pressure is a manifestation of RV failure caused by high RV diastolic pressure and linked to outcomes in PAH. Therefore, careful interrogation of RA size is important.
- RA area >27cm^2 predictive of increased risk of mortality or transplantation
- RA size has also been shown to respond to PAH therapy
- Capture a A4C dedicated right heart view — avoid RA foreshortening
- Maximize RA length ensuring alignment along the true long axis of the RA
- The base of the RA should be at its largest size indicating that the imaging plane passes through the maximal short-axis area.
- The RA should be measured at end-ventricular systole when the RA chamber is at its greatest dimension, prior to TV opening.

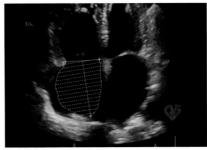

Figure 7.18: RA measurement for volume (mL). Generally indexed by BSA, or in some instances height.

- RA volumes recommended over areas
- Method of disc or single-plane area-length method
- When performing planimetry of the RA, trace the RA inner border excluding the area under the TV annulus and the confluences of the RA appendage.
- Area-length method: the length should be performed at the center of the area under the TV annulus to the superior RA wall.
- Values in men > women

Rv Free Wall Thickness

- RV free wall thickness is a useful measurement for RVH and usually a resultant of increased chronic RV systolic pressure overload.
- RV increased thickness can be seen in infiltrative and hypertrophic cardiomyopathies and in significant left ventricular hypertrophy independent of PH.

- Measured in end diastole from the subcostal window at approximately the tip of the TV leaflets. Normal values are 0.5cm or less.
- Zoom view may be helpful but be careful to avoid adjacent liver fat in the wall thickness.

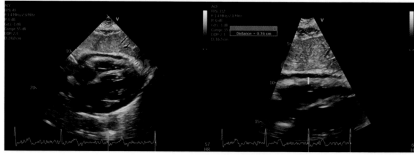

Figure 7.19: Subcostal 4-C view image for analysis of RV free wall thickness. Right panel is zoom of original image with focus on RV wall for accuracy in measurement. RVH is present in this image at 0.76cm, normal values >0.5cm.

Imaging views for RV assessment

- Left parasternal long-axis view (PLAX)
- Left parasternal short-axis view (PSAX)
- Left parasternal RV inflow view
- Apical 4-chamber view
- Focused apical 4-chamber RV view
- Modified apical 4-chamber view
- Subcostal views

Evaluation of RV chamber size

- RV size should be assessed using multiple acoustic windows, PLAX, PSAX, Apical 4-chamber dedicated RV view, modified RV view, off axis imaging as necessary and subcostal 4-chamber view. All chamber measurements should be made inner-edge to inner-edge.
- Optimize the RV image to a focused RV view. The RV focused apical 4-chamber view is a dedicated view which keeps the LV apex in the center and displays the largest basal RV diameter. This view should be attempted to for the most accurate 2D areas and linear measures. Since RV linear dimensions are dependent on probe rotation and different RV views, the echocardiographic report should indicate if an alternate view was used.
- Slide laterally and below the apex from a conventional 4-chamber view and slightly rotate the transducer until the maximum plane is obtained without foreshortening the LV.
- RV apex shape changes indicate enlargement
- Report qualitative and quantitative analysis

- RV volumes and RVEF with 3D can complement 2D derived linear and area measurements

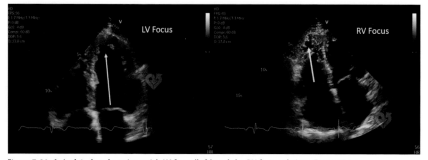

Figure 7.20: Apical 4-chamber view with LV focus(left) and the RV focused view. From a true non-foreshortened apical view rotate the transducer counter clockwise to maximize the RV area.

Evaluation of LV Shape in the PSAX

Evaluation of LV shape in the PSAX view should be carefully evaluated for any signs of septal flattening and or abnormal motion indicative of pressure/volume changes. This requires scanning carefully and slowly from the base to the apex, capture images at base, mid and apical levels.

- **RV Volume Overload** – RV is enlarged and septal motion is flat in diastole. In systole the chamber is circular, and the contour of the septum is normal.

- **RV Pressure Overload** – RV is enlarged and increased pressure results in septal flattening in both diastole and systole, creating the "D" shape

- Septal flattening or "D" shape may be subtle and only seen in mid or late systole

- Septal flattening or "D" shape may also be isolated to only one level, sweeping the probe from base to apex may tease out this finding.

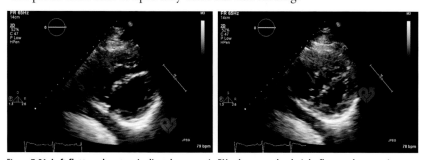

Figure 7.21: Left flattened septum in diastole as seen in RV volume overload, right flattened septum in systole from pressure overload. It is not unusual for both diastolic and systolic flattening to be present in PH.

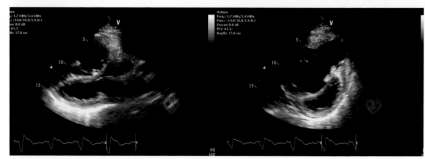

Figure 7.22: Parasternal long (left) and parasternal short axis images(right) of LV shape changes seen in increased volume and pressure overload in this patient with severe pulmonary arterial hypertension.

Evaluation of RV Systolic Function

RV systolic function should be assessed by a combination of recommended parameters including:

- FAC (fractional area change)
- TAPSE (Tricuspid Annular Plane Systolic Excursion)
- DTI-Derived Tricuspid Lateral Annular Systolic Velocity S'
- RV longitudinal strain
- Right Index of Myocardial Performance (RIMP or MPI)
- 3D EF

RV Fractional Area Change (FAC)

Because the RV is not seen in its entirety in any one view volumes from 2D imaging are not recommended. RV fractional area change utilizes the largest RV end diastolic area (RVEDA) and the smallest RV end systolic area (RVESA) and is expressed as a percentage. Cut off value for abnormal <35%.

- Acquire Focused apical 4-chamber RV view
- Trace the inner edge of the RV chamber from the base of the TV lateral to medial annulus.
- Trabeculations, papillary muscles and moderator band should be included in the cavity area.
- Multiple measures should be performed and averaged if not in normal sinus rhythm
- Careful to measure the largest and smallest dimensions from the same beat
- FAC reflects both longitudinal and radial components of RV contraction. It does not include the contribution of the RV outflow tract to overall systolic function.
- Correlates with PAP, TAPSE, cardiac MRI
- Independent predictor of HF, sudden death and stroke post PE and MI
- Fractional Area Change is calculated as:

$$FAC = RVEDA - RVESA \div RVEDA \times 100 \ (\%)$$

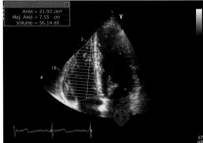

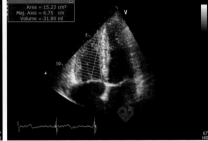

Figure 7.23: **Area trace of largest diastolic cavity**

Figure 7.24: **Area trace area of smallest systolic cavity**

In this example RV fractional area change is calculated at 32%:

RVEDA = 22cm²
RVESA = 15cm²
22 -15 = 7
7 ÷ 22 = 0.318
0.32 x 100 = 32%

Possible RV FAC Pitfalls

• Because RV FAC assess the ventricle in only one plane other means of RV assessment should be performed.

• The correct RV view must be used for analysis, if other than the RV focused view is used documented on the report for serial follow-up analysis to be performed likewise.

• Often the RV chamber is difficult to view the entire wall in diastole and traced areas may be under or overestimated, look at the RV size in other views (except subcostal) it should all correlate.

• Saline contrast or a commercial ultrasound enhancing agent (UEA) can be beneficial in RV wall border delineation.

• Caution in interpreting severity of area size (cm²) when using an UEA as the areas may be larger than unenhanced images in which normal values have derived from. **For FAC the percent change result will be unaffected with an UEA on board.

Tricuspid Annular Plane Systolic Excursion (TAPSE)

Tricuspid Annular Plane Systolic Excursion (TAPSE or TAM) is a measure of longitudinal performance, it measures the displacement from diastole to systole relative to the transducer. An M-mode cursor should be aligned along the RV free wall as perpendicular to the TV annulus as possible and parallel to movement of the TV annulus towards the apex. Use of the Zoom mode or color Doppler M-mode may help in proper identification.

• Movement of TVA from end-diastole to end-systole towards the apex

• Surrogate for global RV longitudinal function

• Correlates with MRI derived RVEF

- Predictor of prognosis
- RV Systolic dysfunction is likely impaired <1.6cm
- TAPSE may over- or underestimate RV function because of cardiac translation and angle dependency

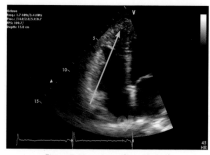

Figure 7.25: **proper alignment of M-mode cursor for TAPSE**

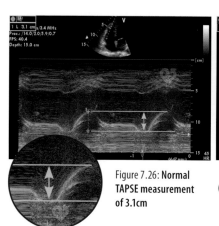

Figure 7.26: **Normal TAPSE measurement of 3.1cm**

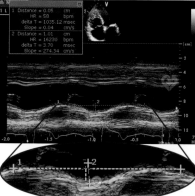

Figure 7.27: **Abnormal TAPSE measurement of 1.1cm**

Careful of TAPSE Pitfalls

- Inaccurate with elevated RAP
- Assumes basal segment is representative of entire RV lateral wall
- The measurement of displacement relative to the transducer makes this parameter susceptible to angle dependence, translational motion, and changes in LV systolic function
- Does not correlate well with severe RV dysfunction
- Can be difficult to measure

Tissue Doppler Imaging of the TV Lateral Annulus: Estimation of Systolic "S" Wave, RV Diastolic Function

- Tissue Doppler imaging (TDI) of the lateral TV annulus is used to estimate peak systolic lateral TV annular motion towards the apex as a measure of RV performance. Performed in the RV focused 4-chamber view using pulsed wave color tissue Doppler and a sample volume (SV) size of 4 to 6mm.

- The SV should be placed on the basal portion of the RV free wall near the annulus but not encroaching on the right atrium and in parallel with the RV basal wall to avoid overestimation.

- The systolic (s'), early diastolic (e') and (a') waves should be clearly recognized when the TDI Doppler is properly optimized, isovolumic contraction and isovolumic relaxation waves should also be distinguishable. *(Figures 7.28 and 7.29)*

   - An (s') value <10 is suggestive of impaired RV systolic performance

   - When paired with TV inflow Doppler (E) TDI can be used to speculate on RV diastolic dysfunction.

   - E/e'<0.8 suggest impaired RV relaxation

   - TV E/A ratio >2.1 with DT <120ms suggest restrictive filling pattern

   - E/e' ≥4 suggest increased right atrial pressure

   - Dominant diastolic flow predominance in the hepatic veins suggests RV diastolic dysfunction

   - Emphasis is on clarity for valued analysis so Doppler optimization is key

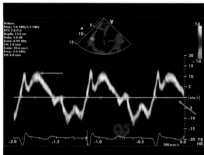 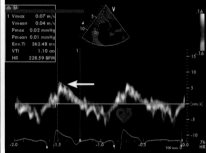

Figure 7.28: **Pulsed wave (PW) Tissue Doppler Imaging (TDI) of the TV annulus for RV systolic performance, "S" peak velocity (green arrow) >10 suggest normal RV function.**

Figure 7.29: **In comparison to Figure 7.28, PW TDI tracing with "S" peak velocity <10 suggesting abnormal RV systolic performance.**

- Record tricuspid valve (TV) inflow at the TV leaflet tips with a sample volume size of 1.5 to 2.0mm. Normal TV inflow will have some inspiratory E&A respiratory changes while DT and E/A ratio should show no change. For optimal recording acquire on held expiration and average over three cycles.

7

Hypertension / Pulmonary Hypertension

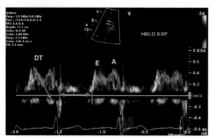

Figure 7.30: **Pulsed wave Doppler TV inflow diastolic early (E)wave, (A)wave and deceleration time (DT) as labelled. Time of TV closure to opening (green arrow).**

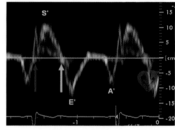

Figure 7.31: **Optimized TDI Doppler tracing with systolic (s'), early diastolic (e') and (a') waves as labeled. Isovolumetric contraction time (yellow arrow) and isovolumetric relaxation time (orange arrow) components.**

TDI Systolic S wave pitfalls:

• RV TDI (S') like TAPSE is angle dependent and may lead to underestimation, and susceptibility to translational motion, which may cause overestimation.

• Is not typically reliable in PAH subjects with moderately severe RV dysfunction

Echocardiographic Pulmonary to Left Atrial Ratio (ePLAR)

Echocardiographic pulmonary to left atrial ratio (ePLAR) is calculated form the maximum TV regurgitation velocity (m/s) divided by the transmitral E-wave (septal or lateral)mitral annular Doppler tissue imaging e' ratio (E/e'). This parameter utilizes the TR maximum velocity (m/sec) as an indicator of pulmonary artery pressure and E/e' as a surrogate for left atrial pressure to differentiate pre-capillary from post-capillary PH. In pre capillary PH the PAP and TRV will increase without significant elevation in LAP, therefore patients with post capillary hypertension will have lower values.

ePLAR = TRV max ÷ mitral E/e'

TRV = peak TR velocity (m/s)
E/e' = mitral E to septal e' ratio

Important to Note

In pre capillary PH the PAP and TRV will increase without significant elevation in LAP, therefore patients with post capillary hypertension will have lower values. The normal cut off value for ePLAR is 0.28 m/s. Patients with post-capillary PH tend to have values of 0.25 m/s or lower and those with pre-capillary PH have values over 0.40 m/s. (Scalia et al)

Myocardial Performance Index (MPI or TEI Index)

Myocardial Performance Index (MPI) or (TEI Index) is the ratio between the sum of isovolumetric contraction time (ICT) and isovolumetric relaxation time (IRT) divided by the RV ejection time (ET). It can be measured from the pulsed (PW) TDI of the RV lateral annulus. Alternatively, it can be measured from PW Doppler of the RVOT outflow track and TV inflow waveforms. It is best measured with TDI as all timing can be measured from the same Doppler waveform(beat). For analysis with (PW) TDI method, abnormal values >0.54. MPI is a prognostic marker and measures >0.98(TDI) have been associated with mortality in PAH.

Myocardial Performance Index (MPI) =

$$\frac{\text{isovolumetric contraction time (ICT) + isovolumetric relaxation time (IRT)}}{\text{ejection time (ET)}}$$

MPI = ICT + IRT ÷ ET *as simplified as: a − b ÷ b*

a = tricuspid valve closure to opening time
b = right ventricular ejection time

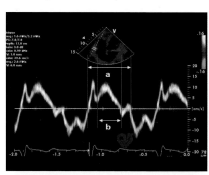

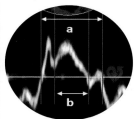

Figure 7.32: **TV PW annular TDI with systolic component (b) and time from TV closure to opening (a) as labeled.**

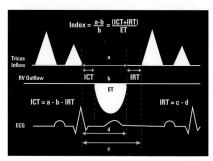

Figure 7.33: **Top section PW Doppler of TV inflow showing TV closure to opening time (a), middle line and labelled as RV outflow demonstrating isovolumetric contraction time (ICT) and isovolumetric relaxation time (IRT) and ejection time (ET) as (b), bottom section showing ECG with timing events from peak R wave to end of isovolumetric relaxation time (IRT) labeled as (c) peak R wave to end of isovolumetric contraction time (ICT). Labeled as (d). ICT = a − b and IRT = c − d.**

- The same MPI formula can be applied using pulsed wave (PW) Doppler of the RVOT and TV inflow however, two separate tracings must be analyzed so care should be taken that the Doppler samples are collected sequentially assuring the same heart rate and/or R-R interval is represented.

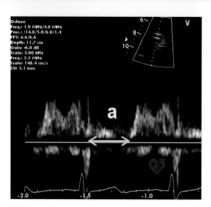

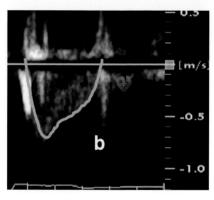

Figure 7.34: **TV pulsed wave Doppler inflow with closure to opening time shown (yellow arrow) labeled as (a)**

Figure 7.35: **RVOT pulsed wave Doppler tracing with RV ejection time (ET) orange arrow labeled as (b)**

Refer to figure 7.32 demonstrating graphic cartoon of formula for calculating MPI from both tracings,
$$MPI = a - b \div b = IVC + IRT \div ET$$

MPI pitfalls
• Not valid with irregular heart rates
• MPI is load-dependent
• MPI may underestimate the severity of RV dysfunction, as in early equalization of pressures when an elevated RAP causes a shortening of isovolumetric relaxation time

RV Systolic Strain for Assessment of Myocardial Function

RV assessment of Myocardial Function with 2D strain imaging allows evaluation of ventricular global and regional function, using standard B-mode images for speckle tracking analysis [Tissue Tracking (TT) and/ or Vector Velocity Imaging (VVI)]. Method based on reflection, interference and scattering of the ultrasound beam in myocardial tissue, "speckles." The speckles represent tissue markers that can be tracked from frame to frame within the myocardium.

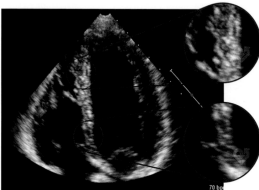

Figure 7.36: **Representative of how echo speckles represent tissue markers that can be tracked from frame to frame within the myocardium.**

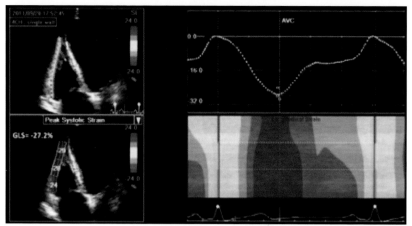

Figure 7.37: **Longitudinal 3 segment free wall RV longitudinal speckle tracking strain. Each wall segment is color coded and the segmental strain deformation value is represented on the segment and coordinated graph. Peak systolic strain occurring at pulmonic valve closure line (marked AVC). The white dotted line is the average of all segmental values or global strain. As the values fall below the zero baseline the strain is "negative". Color M-mode representation bottom right.**

Global Longitudinal Strain (GLS)

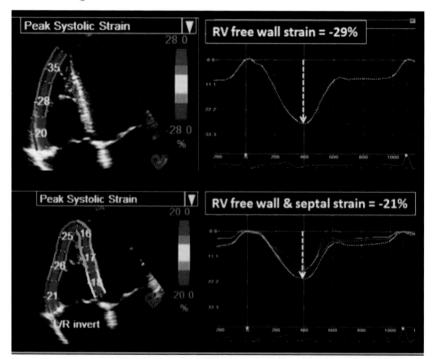

Figure 7.38: **Top panel: Global longitudinal strain (GLS) averaged over three segments of the RV free wall in the RV-focused apical 4-chamber view, lower panel GLS averaged over 6 segments. RV longitudinal strain averaged from the 3 free wall segments is significantly higher (as an absolute value) than the strain averaged from both septal and RV free wall segments (6 wall strain) as in the lower panel.**

Strain performance tips:
- Optimize ECG signal
- Acquire a focused RV image
- Frame rates between 50 to 70 fps
- Capture on held expiration
- Identify pulmonic valve closure time
- Avoid image translation

3D Volumetric Assessment of the Right Ventricle

- 3D Volumetric assessment of the right ventricle using either summation of disc or surface remodeling methods is the most accurate echocardiographic measure of RV volumes to determine RV systolic function precisely as RV ejection fraction.

- Patients with advanced chronic disease often have exceptionally large RV chambers and/or technically poor windows providing 3D challenges.

- Newer ultrasound systems have overcome the need for reduced sector capture size and are showing significant promise with 3D software algorithms dedicated for RV analysis *(Figure 7.39)*. These newer systems allow for ease of collection and analysis for accurate RVEF analysis. Current normal RV ejection fraction values ≥45% with ≤35% indicative of impaired RV systolic function.

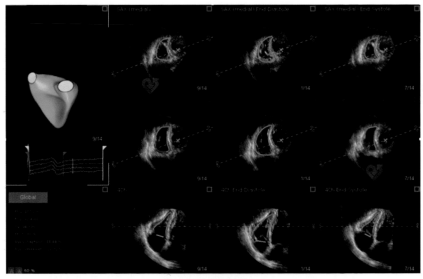

Figure 7.39: **RV 3D volume**

Important to Note

- More than one parameter of systolic function should always be evaluated to accurately determine normal from abnormal and to best assess the degree of dysfunction.

- Pulmonary hypertension is an increase in pulmonary arterial pressures (MPAP ≥20mmHg) which results in a pressure overload of the right heart. The right ventricle first responds with hypertrophy followed by right ventricular dilatation, tricuspid regurgitation, pulmonary regurgitation and right atrial dilatation.

- Right ventricular dilatation occurs early in pulmonary hypertension and dilatation occurs more in the short-axis rather than in the long-axis.

- Cor pulmonale is pulmonary hypertension due to diseases of the lung parenchyma and/or pulmonary vasculature unrelated to the left side of the heart. It may be acute (e.g., pulmonary embolism) or chronic (e.g., COPD).

- Eisenmenger's syndrome is a term which refers to patients with a congenital heart lesions and severe pulmonary hypertension in whom reversal of a left to right shunt has occurred.

7

Hypertension / Pulmonary Hypertension

Table 7.11: Pulmonary Hypertension Severity Scales	
Systolic Pulmonary Artery Pressure (SPAP)	
Normal	18 to 25mmHg
Mild	35 to 45mmHg
Moderate	45 to 60mmHg
Severe	>60mmHg
Eisenmenger's physiology	≥120mmHg and/or ≥ systemic pressure
RVOT Acceleration Time	
Normal	≥120 msec
Mild	80 to 100 msec
Moderate	60 to 80 msec
Severe	<60 msec
Mean Pulmonary Artery Pressure (MPAP)	
Normal	9 to 18mmHg
Pulmonary Artery End-Diastolic Pressure (PAEDP)	
Normal	4 to 12mmHg
Pulmonary Vascular Resistance (PVR)	
Total pulmonary resistance	100 to 300 dyne-sec-cm^{-5} (1.16 to 3 Wood's units)
Pulmonary vascular resistance	20 to 130 dyne-sec-cm^{-5} (0.7 to 1.1 Wood's units)

Adapted from: Haemodynamic definitions and updated clinical classification of pulmonary hypertension. Eur Respir J. 2019;53(1):1801913. Published 2019 Jan 24. doi:10.1183/13993003.01913-2018

Table 7.12: **Normal Values for Parameters of RV Function** (*ASE Recommendations*) [3]		
Parameter	Mean ± SD	Abnormality Threshold
TAPSE (mm)	24 ± 3.5	<17
Pulsed Doppler S wave (cm/s)	14.1 ± 2.3	>9.5
Color Doppler S wave (cm/s)	9.7 ± 1.85	<6.0
RV fractional area change (%)	49 ± 7	<35
RV free wall 2D strain (%)	-29 ± 4.5	<20%
RV 3D EF (%)	58 ± 6.5	<45
Pulsed Doppler MPI	0.26 ± 0.085	>0.43
Tissue Doppler MPI	0.38 ± 0.08	>0.54
E wave deceleration time (msec)	180 ± 31	<119 or >242
E/A	1.4 ± 0.3	<0.8 or >2.0
e'/a'	1.18 ± 0.33	<0.52
e' (cm/s)	14.0 ± 0.31	>7.8
E/e'	4.0 ± 1.0	>6.0

MPI = Myocardial performance index.
*Limited data; values may vary depending on vendor and software version

Table 7.13: **Additional Parameters for the Right Ventricle and Pulmonary Artery**			
Reference limits and partition values of right ventricular and pulmonary artery size			
RV dimensions			
Basal RV diameter (cm)	2.0 to 2.8	2.9 to 3.3	3.4 to 3.8	≥3.9
Mid-RV diameter (cm)	2.7 to 3.3	3.4 to 3.7	3.8 to 4.1	≥4.2
Base-to-apex length (cm)	7.1 to 7.9	8.0 to 8.5	8.6 to 9.1	≥9.2
RVOT diameters			
Above aortic valve (cm)	2.5 to 2.9	3.0 to 3.2	3.3 to 3.5	≥3.6
Above pulmonic valve (cm)	1.7 to 2.3	2.4 to 2.7	2.8 to 3.1	≥3.2
PA diameter			
Below pulmonic valve (cm)	1.5 to 2.1	2.2 to 2.5	2.6 to 2.9	≥3.0
Reference limits and partition values of right ventricular size and function as measured in the apical 4-chamber view			
RV diastolic area (cm²)	11 to 28	29 to 32	33 to 37	≥38
RV systolic area (cm²)	7.5 to 16	17 to 19	20 to 22	≥23
RV fractional area change (%)	32 to 60	25 to 31	18 to 24	≤17

Table 7.14: Summary of Reference Limits for Recommended Measures of Right Heart Structure and Function (ASE Recommendations)[3]

Variable	Abnormal
Chamber dimensions	
RV basal diameter	>4.1cm
RV mid diameter	>35mm
RV longitudinal diameter	>83mm
RVOT PLAX proximal diameter	>3.0cm
RVOT PSAX distal diameter	>2.7cm
RVOT PSAX distal diameter	>27mm
RV subcostal wall thickness	>0.5cm
RA volume	Men: 25 ± 7mL/m^2 Women 21 ± 6mL/m^2
RA end-systolic area	>18cm^2
RA major dimension	>5.3cm
RA minor dimension	>4.4cm
Systolic function	
TAPSE	<1.7cm
Pulsed Doppler peak velocity at the annulus	<9.5cm/s
Pulsed Doppler IMP	>0.43
Tissue Doppler IMP	>0.54
FAC	<35%
Diastolic function	
E/A ratio	<0.8 or >2.0
E/e' ratio	>6
Deceleration time	<119 msec

FAC, Fractional area change; MPI, myocardial performance index; PLAX, parasternal long-axis; PSAX, parasternal short-axis; RA, right atrium; RV, right ventricle; RVD, right ventricular diameter; RVOT, right ventricular outflow tract; TAPSE, tricuspid annular plane systolic excursion.

References

1. Abbas AA, Franey LM, Marwick T, Maeder MT, Kaye DM, Vlahos,AP et al. Noninvasive Assessment of Pulmonary Vascular Resistance by Doppler Echocardiography. J Am Soc Echocardiogr 2013; 26(10) 1170 – 1177

2. Cordina RL, Playford D, Lang,I, Celermajor DS. State of the Art Review: Echocardiography in Pulmonary Hypertension. Heart, Lung and Circulation (2019) 28,1351-1364

3. Lang RM, Badano LP, Mor-Avi V, et al. Recommendations for cardiac chamber quantification by echocardiography in adults: an update from the American Society of Echocardiography and the European Association of Cardiovascular Imaging. J Am Soc Echocardiogr 2015;28:727-54.

4. Lee J-H, MD and Park J-H, Strain Analysis of the Right Ventricle Using Two-dimensional Echocardiography. J Cardiovasc Imaging. 2018 Sep; 26(3): 111–124. Published online 2018 Aug 29. doi: 10.4250/jcvi.2018.26.e11

5. Levy D, Garrison RJ, Savage DD, et al. Left ventricular mass and incidence of coronary heart disease in an elderly cohort. The Framingham Heart Study. Ann Intern Med 1989;110:101

6. Liu D, Hu K, Nordbeck P, Ertl G, Störk S, Weidemann F. Longitudi¬nal strain bull's eye plot patterns in patients with cardiomyopa¬thy and concentric left ventricular hypertrophy. Eur J Med Res. 2016;21(1):21.

7. Marwick TH, Gillebert TC, Aurigemma G, et al. Recommendations on the Use of Echocardiography in Adult Hypertension: A Report from the European Association of Cardiovascular Imaging (EACVI) and the American Society of Echocardiography (ASE). Echocardiogr 2015;28(7):727-754.

8. Rudski LG, Lai WW, Afilalo J, Hua L, Handschumacher, Chandrasekaran K, Solomon SD, Louie EK, Schiller NB. Guidelines for the Echocardiographic Assessment of the Right Heart in Adults. J Am Soc Echocardiogr 2010;23:685-713.

9. Scalia, GM, Scalia IG, Kierle R, Beaumont R, Cross DB, Fennstra, J, Burstow DJ, Fitzgerald BT, Platts D. The Echocardiographic Pulmonary to Left Atrial Ratio- A Novel non-invasive parameter to differentiate pre-capillary and post capillary pulmonary hypertension. International Journal of Cardiology 212 (2016) 379-386.

10. Simonneau G, Montani D, Celermajer DS, et al. Haemodynamic definitions and updated clinical classification of pulmonary hypertension. Eur Respir J. 2019;53(1):1801913. Published 2019 Jan 24.

11. Vonk MC, Sander MH, van den Hogen FHJ, van Reil PLCM, Verheugt FWA, van Dijk APJ. Right ventricle Tei-index: A tool to increase the accuracy of non-invasive detection of pulmonary arterial hypertension in connective tissue diseases. European Journal of Echocardiography, Volume 8, Issue 5, October 2007, Pages 317–321, https://doi.org/10.1016/j.euje.2006.06.002

12. Williams, Mancia et al. 2018 ESC/ESH Guidelines for the management of arterial hypertension. J Hypertens 2018;36:1953-2041 and Eur Heart J 2018;39:3021-3104 Soc Echocardiogr 2015; 28:1-39.

Ischemic Heart Disease
Sally J. Miller, BS, RDCS, RT(R), FASE

Definition

A narrowing or obstruction of the coronary artery(s) sufficient to prevent adequate blood and oxygen supply to the myocardium (ischemia). This narrowing may progress to the point that heart muscle is damaged (infarction).

Etiology

• Atherosclerosis
• Non-Atherosclerotic Causes
  - Congenital coronary artery anomalies
  - Coronary artery spasm
  - Coronary embolus
  - Decreased coronary perfusion
  - Inflamation
  - Radiation induced
  - Spontaneous coronary artery dissection (SCAD)

Risk Factors

Major

• Advancing age
  (men ≥45; women ≥55)
• Tobacco smoking
• Diabetes mellitus
• Elevated total and low density lipoprotein cholesterol
• Low high-density lipoprotein cholesterol
• Hypertension (HTN)

Predisposing

• Abdominal obesity
  (e.g., metabolic syndrome)
• Ethnic characteristics
• Family history
  (males first degree relative <55, females first degree relative <65)
• Obesity (>20% over ideal weight)
• Physical inactivity
• Psychosocial factors

Conditional

• Elevated serum homocystine, serum lipoprotein (a), serum triglycerides
• Inflammatory markers
  (e.g., C-reactive protein)
• Prothrombic factors (e.g., fibrinogen)
• Abnormal ankle-brachial index (ABI)
• Abnormal calcium score
• Abnormal carotid intima-media (CIMT)
• Left ventricular hypertrophy (LVH)
• Medical conditions (e.g., Takotsubo cardiomyopathy, HIV, end-stage renal disease, inflammatory connective tissue disease)

History/Physical Examination

- Angina pectoris (stable, unstable, Prinzmetal's)
- Microvascular angina (syndrome X: anginal chest pain with a normal coronary arteriogram)
- Heart failure (dyspnea, orthopnea, paroxysmal nocturnal dyspnea, fatigue, cough, weight gain)
- Myocardial infarction
- Sudden cardiac death (SCD)
- Elevated cardiac enzymes (e.g., troponin, CK-MB)

Cardiac Auscultation

- S4
- Murmur of mitral regurgitation up to 60% will have some degree of mitral regurgitation follow an acute myocardial infarction (AMI)
- Murmur of tricuspid regurgitation has increased pulmonary artery pressures, right ventricular infarction
- Systolic murmur of ventricular septal rupture
- Soft S1
- Paradoxical S2
- S3
- Pericardial friction rub

Electrocardiogram

- May be normal at rest even in patients with significant coronary artery disease
- T wave inversion may suggest cardiac ischemia
- ST segment changes (depressed ST segments suggest cardiac ischemia, while elevated ST segments may represent injury and acute myocardial infarction)
- Prominent peaked T waves (acute myocardial infarction)
- Pathologic Q waves indicate "old" myocardial infarction
- Ventricular arrhythmias
- Conduction defects (e.g., first degree AV block, LBBB)

Chest X-ray/CMR/CT

- May be normal
- Pulmonary vascular redistribution/pulmonary edema
- Cardiomegaly
- CT provides information concerning the complications of myocardial infarction (e.g., left ventricular aneurysm), ventricular function and perfusion and may provide early detection of coronary artery disease (e.g., coronary artery calcification)
- CMR provides information concerning ventricular global function segmental function, ventricular volumes, ventricular mass, plaque characterization, myocardial perfusion and myocardial viability

8

Ischemic Heart Disease

Cardiac Catheterization

- Coronary arteriogram is the gold standard for determining the presence and severity of CAD
- Segmental wall motion abnormalities
- Identification of the complications of myocardial infarction (e.g., left ventricular aneurysm, ventricular septal rupture, mitral regurgitation)
- Intravascular ultrasound may supplement coronary arteriography

Treatment

Lifestyle

- Reduce risk factors
- Exercise

Medical

- Antianginal treatment
- Nitrates (e.g., sublingual nitroglycerin)
- Beta blockers (e.g., propranolol, nadolol)
- Calcium channel blockers (e.g., diltiazem, verapamil)
- ACE inhibitors (e.g., vasotec, captopril)
- ARNI / ARB (e.g., valsartan)
- Thrombolysis (e.g., streptokinase, alteplase tPA, reteplase rPA)
- Antiplatelet therapy (e.g., aspirin, plavix)
- Anticoagulation (e.g., heparin, aspirin)
- Antiarrhythmic (e.g., amiodarone)
- Cholesterol lowering drugs (statins) (e.g., mevacor, pravachol)
- Analgesics (e.g., morphine)
- Sedation (e.g., flurazepam)
- Laxatives (e.g., dioctyl sodium sulfosuccinate)
- Diuretics (e.g., furosemide)
- Digitalis
- Volume therapy
- Oxygen therapy

Procedural

- Pacemakers
- Implantable cardiac defibrillator (ICD)
- Cardioversion
- Percutaneous transluminal coronary angioplasty (PTCA)
- Atherectomy
- Coronary stent
- Coronary laser
- Myoblast transplantation

Surgical

- Coronary artery bypass graft
- Intra-aortic balloon counterpulsation
- Left/Right ventricular assist device
- Transmyocardial revascularization (percutaneous or open heart)
- Ventricular remodeling (Batista procedure)
- Heart transplantation
- Impella device
- Extracorporeal membrane oxygenation (ECMO)
- Total artificial heart

M-mode/2D/3D

- Multiple views should be utilized
- Ejection fraction; 2D linear, M-mode, 2D volumetric, 3D volumetric (volumetric measurement recommended) (EF <52% for males and <54% for females would suggest decreased function)
- Segmental wall motion abnormality(s)
- Evaluate systolic wall thickening (most important), systolic wall motion and diastolic wall thickness (a wall thickness <7mm or 30% less than adjacent myocardium may indicate ischemia/infarction)
- Opposing wall of involved region may be hyperkinetic
- Thin, bright (scarred), akinetic muscle section suggests old infarction
- Spontaneous echo contrast may be visualized in the infarcted area (assess for possible thrombus)
- Serial echocardiograms may be useful to evaluate infarct extension (progressive increase in the necrosis within the same vascular area as the myocardial infarction). Evaluate for expansion (a thinning of the muscle mass at the site of infarction)
- In the parasternal short-axis view of the aortic valve, the left main coronary artery, proximal left anterior descending, proximal left circumflex may be visualized at the four o'clock position and the proximal right coronary artery maybe visualized at the eleven o'clock position

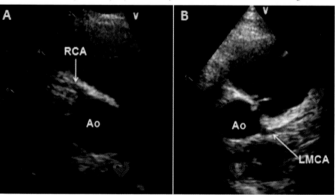

Figure 8.1: **Parasternal short axis view slightly superior to the aortic valve at the level of the sinus of Valsalva. A: Demonstrates the proximal portion of the right coronary artery (RCA) with the origin at approximately 11 o'clock. B: Demonstrates the origin of the left main coronary artery (LMCA) at approximately 4 o'clock.**

- The left main coronary artery is approximately 1 to 1.5cm in length and is then shown bifurcating into the proximal portions of the left anterior descending artery and the left circumflex artery.
- The coronary origins may sometimes be visualized in one image, but often will need a slight rotation or angulation of the imaging transducer to adequately visualize the true location of the origin and may need to be perform in two separate images as demonstrated in figure 8.1.

8

Ischemic Heart Disease

- Describe wall motion abnormality: hypokinesis is a decrease in systolic wall thickening of <40%; akinesis is systolic wall thickening of <10%, dyskinesis is present when the wall moves outward during ventricular systole with wall thinning, aneurysm is a fixed outward defect
- Determine:
  - Wall motion score index
  - Left and right ventricular size; M-mode, 2D, 3D (volumetric measurement recommended)
  - Left and right ventricular ejection fraction(EF) (volumetric measurement recommended) (LV EF <52% males and <54% females suggests decreased systolic function. RV EF <45% is considered abnormal.)
  - Global longitudinal strain (GLS) (normal strain values are more negative than -20%, values vary by vendor)
  - Which segments and coronary artery(s) are involved using the ASE wall segment and coronary distribution models shown below: (When assessing for segmental wall motion abnormalities, the 17th segment, apical cap, should not be used. 17th segment should be used in the assessment of perfusion and strain)
- The addition of ultrasound enhancing agent may be beneficial in the assessment of segmental wall motion abnormalities and for identification of thrombus

Wall Motion Score Index

1 = Normal wall motion   3 = Akinesis

2 = Hypokinesis   4 = Dyskinesis / Aneurysmal

- All segments are assigned a value. The sum of the segments is divided by the total number of segments visualized. (typically 16 segments)

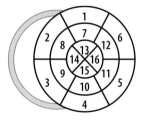 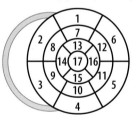 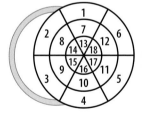

all models

1. basal anterior
2. basal anteroseptal
3. basal inferoseptal
4. basal inferior
5. basal inferolateral
6. basal anterolateral
7. mid anterior
8. mid anteroseptal
9. mid inferoseptal
10. mid inferior
11. mid inferolateral
12. mid anterolateral

16 and 17 segment model

13. apical anterior
14. apical septal
15. apical inferior
16. apical lateral

17 segment model only

17. apex

18 segment model only

13. apical anterior
14. apical anteroseptal
15. apical inferoseptal
16. apical inferior
17. apical inferolateral
18. apical anterolateral

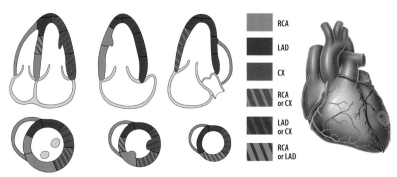

Figure 8.2: **Left ventricle segmentation** *(ASE recomendations)* [5]

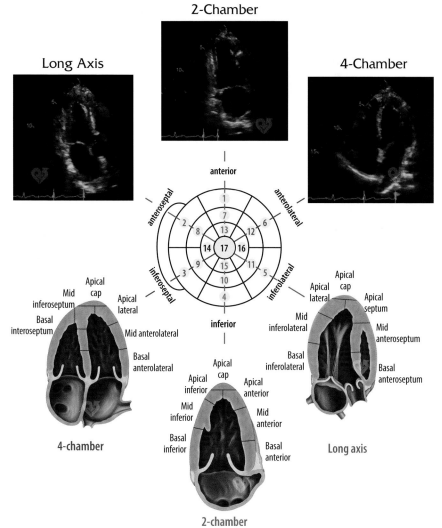

Figure 8.3: **Bull's eye diagram of 17 segments**

8

Ischemic Heart Disease / Complications of Myocardial Infarction / Post-infarction (Early) Pericarditis/Pericardial Effusion

Cardiac Doppler

Determine:

- Severity of coexisting valvular regurgitation
- Stroke volume, cardiac output, cardiac index
- SPAP/MPAP/PAEDP/PVR at rest and exercise
- Left ventricular dP/dt
- Index of myocardial performance index (IMP)
- Tissue Doppler imaging of LV and RV systolic annular velocity (S')
- Grade of diastolic dysfunction (restrictive filling pattern after acute myocardial infarction represents an increase risk of cardiac death)

Important to Note

- Myocardial infarction may be classified as a Q wave infarction (STEMI) (usually implies a transmural infarction) and non-Q wave (non-STEMI) infarction (non-transmural).
- The general echocardiographic manifestations of myocardial infarction are hypokinesis/akinesis/dyskinesis of the affected wall segment, thinning of the affected wall segment, increased echogenicity of the affected segment (old infarction) and hyperkinesis of the opposing wall segments.
- Stunned myocardium is viable myocardium salvaged by coronary reperfusion that exhibits prolonged post-ischemic dysfunction after reperfusion.
- Hibernating myocardium is ischemic myocardium supplied by a narrowed coronary artery in which ischemic cells remain viable but contraction is chronically depressed.
- Routine echocardiography tends to overlook CAD because the examination is performed while the patient is at rest, when the narrowed coronary arteries may still be able to provide adequate blood supply to the heart muscle. To better evaluate the presence and severity of CAD, a stress echocardiogram should be performed.

Complications of Myocardial Infarction

Post-infarction (Early) Pericarditis/Pericardial Effusion
Definition

Pericarditis is the inflammation of the pericardium. Irritation of the pericardium may sometimes lead to fluid within the pericardial sac, known as pericardial effusion.

History/Physical Examination

- A common acute (1 to 4 days) response to acute myocardial infarction (25%)
- Greater incidence in transmural Q wave and STEMI infractions as compared to non-transmural -Q wave and non- STEMI infratctions
- Associated with larger infarctions, anterior infarctions
- Relative contraindication for anticoagulation
- May be an absolute contraindication for thrombolysis
- May predict a more complex course (increased risk of heart failure, atrial/ventricular arrhythmias, higher 12 month mortality)
- Patient may be asymptomatic or may present with severe chest pain which may radiate to the upper abdomen, upper arms or back and increases in severity with inspiration and decreases in severity by patient leaning forward
- May have pericardial friction rub upon auscultation
- Cardiac tamponade is rare

2D

- Echolucent space within pericardial sac
- Typically no signs of tamponade, but must rule out (no chamber collapse or septal shift)
- Rule out free wall rupture if effusion is >1cm

Doppler

- Typically no signs of tamponade, but must rule out (signs of enhanced ventricular interdependence)

Dressler's Syndrome (Post-Myocardial Infarction)

Definition

- Delayed form of pericarditis with or without an effusion: an immunologic reaction occurring 1 to 8 weeks after myocardial infarction(1 to 3%)

History/Physical Examination

- Symptoms include fever, polyserositis, pleuropericardial pain, malaise, pericarditis and pleuritis
- May have pericardial friction rub upon auscultation
- Recurrences are common in setting of viral infections, greater myocardial damage, younger age, or prior history
- Treatment is aspirin (650 mg) every four hours

2D/Doppler

- Evaluate for pericardial effusion, new and old segmental wall motion abnormalities and constrictive pericarditis
- Cardiac tamponade is rare, but must rule out

Left Ventricular True Aneurysm

Definition

A thin, dyskinetic area of myocardium composed of muscle fibers and scar tissue recognized as a bulge distorting the normal contour of the left ventricular cavity in systole and diastole. Left ventricular aneurysm contains all layers of the myocardium (not a rupture) and is the final result of infarct expansion and ventricular remodeling.

Differential Diagnosis

- Left ventricular diverticulum (usually small as compared to the large, globular, saccular true aneurysm)
- Herniation of the ventricle with a partial defect of the pericardium
- Noncompaction of the left ventricle
- Takotsubo cardiomyopathy ("apical ballooning")
- Pseudoaneurysm/false aneurysm (contained rupture)

History/Physical Examination

- Palpation of the apical impulse medial to the cardiac apex
- Continuing angina pectoris
- Refractory heart failure
- Systemic emboli (due to thrombus located within aneurysm; thrombus occurs in 7 to 46%, systemic emboli occurs in ~10% post acute myocardial infarction)
- Ventricular arrhythmias

Electrocardiogram

- Evidence of myocardial infarction (usually anterior)
- Persistent ST-T wave elevation (suggests large infarction with segmental wall motion abnormality)

Chest X-ray/CMR/CT

- Aneurysmal dilatation of left heart border
- Calcification of aneurysm

Medical/Surgical Treatment

- ACE inhibitor (may inhibit post-myocardial infarction cardiac remodeling)
- Reperfusion (e.g., thrombolysis; PTCA) (may inhibit post-myocardial infarction cardiac remodeling)
- Anticoagulation
- Electrophysiology mapping for cardiac arrhythmia
- Aneurysmectomy (operative mortality 7 to 15%, varies in relation to preoperative CHF classification)

- Dor myoplasty / Endoventricular circular patch plasty (EVCPP) (intraventricular patch to exclude aneurysmal cavity)
- Coronary artery bypass graft

2D

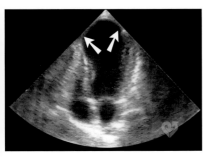

Figure 8.4: **Apical left ventricular true aneurysm**

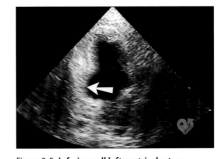

Figure 8.5: **Inferior wall left ventricular true aneurysm**

- Utilize apical/subcostal axis views and modified views. Most aneurysms are located at the cardiac apex (70 to 85%) but may be isolated to the interventricular septum, inferior wall, or lateral wall.
- Thin walls (<5mm) with distorted shape which demonstrate akinesis/dyskinesis/paradoxical motion
- "Hinge" point where "good" left ventricular myocardium meets "bad"
- Spontaneous echo contrast within aneurysm may be visualized
- Sessile or pedunculated thrombus within the aneurysm possible
- Early or late rupture is rare
- Transpulmonary ultrasound enhancing agent may be useful to identify aneurysm and assess for thrombus (e.g., Definity, Optison, Lumason)
- 3D may provide supportive information (e.g., location, size, type, ventricular volumes)
- Evaluate right ventricle for aneurysm post right ventricular infarction
- Determine:
  - Ratio of the neck diameter to the maximum body diameter of the aneurysm (>0.5 indicates a true aneurysm vs. a pseudoaneurysm)
  - Left ventricular fractional shortening of the uninvolved portion (≥17% predicts improved survival of aneurysmectomy)
  - Amount of functional residual myocardium (42% is good)
  - Left ventricular EF (volumetric measurement recommended)

8

Ischemic Heart Disease / Complications of Myocardial Infarction / Left Ventricular True Aneurysm

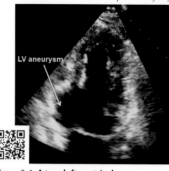

Figure 8.6: **A true left ventricular aneurysm of the basal inferior wall demonstrating a wide neck with an aneurysmal neck to body ratio >0.5. There is clear visualization of the "hinge-point" between normal and abnormal myocardium.**

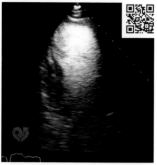

Figure 8.7: **Ultrasound enhancing agent has been used in this apical 2-chamber view with enhancing agent demonstrating swirling in the left ventricular apical aneurysm.**

Doppler

- Swirling blood flow pattern may be visualized especially when color velocity scale and wall filter is decreased
- Mitral regurgitation
- Determine grade of diastolic dysfunction

Important to Note

- Swirling of enhancing agent (or spontaneous echo contrast in a non-enhanced image) in a left ventricular aneurysm could indicate an increased likelihood of future thrombus formation.
- Incidence of aneurysm formation in patients with first anterior infarction is 22%.
- Occurs most often in Q wave (STEMI, transmural) infarction than in non-Q wave (non-STEMI, non-transmural) infarction.
- May be detected as early as five days post-myocardial infarction with development of a left ventricular aneurysm within the first five days post-myocardial infarction associated with an 80% 1-year mortality rate as compared to 25% with gradual aneurysm formation.
- Aneurysm usually occurs within 2 to 4 weeks post acute myocardial infarction (AMI); formation beyond three months is rare.
- Higher mortality rate approaching 60% in three years.
- Increased risk of thrombus formation/systemic embolization.
- Associated with ventricular arrhythmias.
- 2D/3D echocardiography aids in determining the amount of viable myocardium when aneurysmectomy is being considered.
- A true aneurysm may affect the left ventricular apex, interventricular septum, or inferior wall of the left ventricle; most commonly seen following anterior myocardial infarction with the aneurysm affecting the apex and septum.

- The difference between a dyskinetic segment and an aneurysm is that an aneurysm causes a deformity of the left ventricle during ventricular systole and diastole while a dyskinetic segment deforms only during ventricular systole.

Pseudoaneurysm/False Aneurysm/Free Wall Rupture

Definition

The free wall of the left ventricle ruptures and a hemopericardium is confined by the pericardium. A pseudoaneurysm does not contain all layers of myocardium.

Etiology

- Usually myocardial infarction (1 to 3% of all acute myocardial infarctions)
- May also be caused by cardiac surgery, blunt trauma or endocarditis

History/Physical Examination

- Myocardial infarction (free wall rupture is often associated with small infarct)
- Severe, prolonged, recurrent chest pain
- Hypotension
- Cardiac decompensation
- Apical systolic murmur
- Mass on chest x-ray (50%)
- Bifid precordial impulse

Cardiac Auscultation

- Low pitched diastolic/systolic to and fro type murmur

Surgical Treatment

- Surgical resection of necrotic/ruptured myocardium with primary reconstruction

2D

- A narrow perforation with sharp edges of the left ventricular free wall with a saccular/globular contour of the false chamber
- Systolic expansion of the pseudoaneurysm
- Thrombus may line the aneurysm
- Extension of the aneurysmal space behind the left ventricular wall (vs true aneurysm which does not)
- Displacement/compression of surrounding cardiac chambers (e.g., right ventricle against the chest wall)
- Determine "neck" diameter/true diameter ratio (<0.5 suggests pseudoaneurysm) TEE and transpulmonary ultrasound enhancing agent may be useful

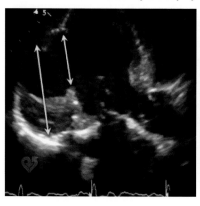

Figure 8.8: **Apical long axis image demonstrates a pseudoaneurysm in the mid inferolateral wall demonstrating a narrow neck in comparison to the widest dimension of the aneurysm. A pseudoaneurysm has an aneurysmal neck to body ratio of <0.5. The pseudoaneurysm is partially filled with thrombus. (Many pseudoaneurysms have a much smaller neck than demonstrated on this image.)**

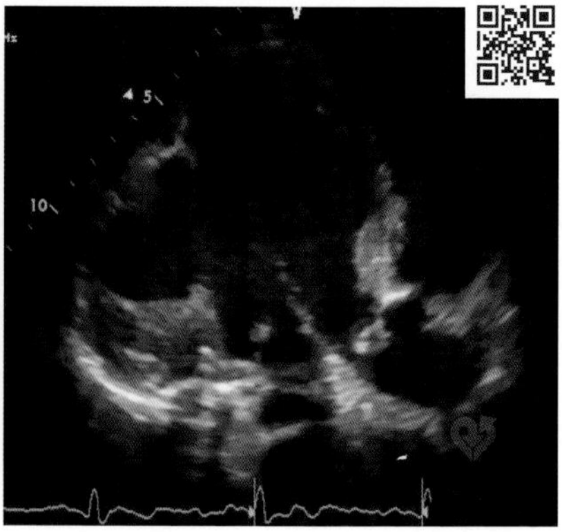

Figure 8.9: **Apical long axis image demonstrates a pseudoaneurysm in the mid inferolateral wall demonstrating a narrow neck with an aneurysmal neck to body ratio of <0.5. The pseudoaneurysm is partially filled with thrombus.**

Doppler

- Pulsed wave Doppler demonstrates characteristic to and fro waveform at the mouth of the pseudoaneurysm consisting of two peaks: atrial systolic and ventricular systolic
- Color flow Doppler demonstrates a to and fro turbulent flow pattern at the orifice of the pseudoaneurysm (flow from the left ventricle to the pseudoaneurysm occurs during systole, flow out of the pseudoaneurysm into the left ventricle occurs from end-systole to early to mid diastole) (decrease velocity scale/wall filter)
- Abnormal flow within the pseudoaneurysm may be visualized by color flow Doppler (decrease color velocity scale/wall filter)
- Respiratory variation of peak systolic velocity may be present

Important to Note

- Increased incidence in patients with pre-existing systemic hypertension, older female patients after first anterior Q wave MI, patients receiving anti-inflammatory drugs (e.g., steroids)
- Significantly increases risk of sudden death due to early/late rupture
- Free wall rupture is most likely to occur within the first 2 weeks post AMI (90%), with 50% occurring within the first 5 days
- Common cause of death within the first two weeks of acute myocardial infarction (-7% of infarct related deaths)

- Increased risk of thromboembolism
- Associated with heart failure
- May lead to cardiac tamponade
- Most common locations for pseudoaneurysm are posterior (43%), lateral (28%), apical (24%), inferior (19%), anterior (18%), basal (14%)

Left Ventricular Thrombus

Definition

Coagulation of blood appearing as an echodense mass with defined margins due to decrease movement of blood flow typically adjacent to asynergic myocardium and associated with aneurysms. Thrombus may begin to form within 24 hours post AMI.

Medical Treatment

- Thrombolytic therapy and IV heparin (during hospitalization)
- Warfarin (mural thrombus forms in 20% of AMI not treated with anticoagulation)

2D

- Utilize multiple on-axis views and modified views with special emphasis on the cardiac apex (confirm presence of thrombus in at least two orthogonal views) (apical views are best for demonstrating apical thrombus)
- Thrombus will be located adjacent to segmental wall motion abnormality (usually akinesis, dyskinesia, or aneurysmal)
- Thrombus echo density is generally greater than the adjacent endocardium and myocardium
- Thrombus margin may disrupt the continuity of the endocardial echo

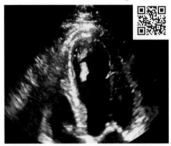

Figure 8.10: **Apical 4-chamber view demonstrating thrombus in the left ventricular apex near the septum following myocardial infarction. Notice there is also a smaller thrombus located more distally into the apex.**

- Mural thrombi demonstrate motion that is similar to the adjacent wall vs, reverberations which remain relatively stationary and do not move with the adjacent muscle and reverberations move when the transducer is moved
- Clearly identifiable throughout the cardiac cycle
- An apical thrombus is suggested present if the apical wall thickness is greater than the interventricular septal thickness (assuming there is abnormal apical wall motion)
- Describe the location (e.g., apex) type (e.g., mural/non-protruding/ sessile or protruding/pedunculated/mobile), echodensity (e.g., hypoechoic, echodense) and dimensions of the thrombus

- Pedunculated thrombus generally represent thrombus in the early stages while mural thrombi are older thrombi (embolization is more likely with pedunculated thrombus)
- New thrombi are generally hypoechoic while older clots are hyperechoic, more homogeneous
- Transpulmonary ultrasound enhancing agent may be useful (e.g., Definity, Optison, Lumason)
- Serial echocardiograms may be useful to evaluate anatomical changes of the thrombus

Doppler

- Color flow Doppler may demonstrate "filling defect" in the area of the thrombus (utilize low-velocity scale and wall filter)
- Color flow Doppler within the suspected thrombus could be suggestive of vascularity, indicating mass rather than thrombus
- Accurate display of color flow imaging is angle dependent and could be limited in some imaging planes

Important to Note

- The incidence of left ventricular thrombus formation is decreasing post-myocardial infarction due to the use of antithrombotic agents.
- Most often associated with anterior myocardial infarction followed by inferior infarctions
- Systemic embolization occurs in 10% of patients with echocardiographically detected thrombi with incidence of embolism highest within the first 3 month post-myocardial infarction.
- Factors which suggest an increased risk of embolization include, large size, protrusion into the left ventricular cavity, mobile, adjacent to a hyperkinetic segment and/or sonolucent area
- Early (<48 to 72 hours) thrombus formation may predict a poorer prognosis post-myocardial infarction.
- Spin the probe 360° when investigating the cardiac apex.
- Use a black-on-white display.
- Utilize transpulmonary ultrasound enhancing agent (e.g., Definity, Optison, Lumason).
- Prove the presence of the thrombus in at least two orthogonal views (distinguish from artifact)
- Vast majority occur in the region of the cardiac apex and/or the anterior wall, adherent to asynergic/aneurysmal areas.
- May be as small as 2mm.
- Thin (<0.6cm), layered thrombus may not be detected.
- Proposed timing of the echocardiographic evaluation of left ventricular thrombus is: 1) within 24 to 48 hours post myocardial infarction; 2) 10 to 15 days after infarction and 3) 1 to 3 months after infarction.

- Thrombus may also be seen in patients with dilated cardiomyopathy, left ventricular true and false aneurysms, endocardial fibroelastosis, hypereosinophilic syndrome or Chagas disease.
- Differential diagnosis includes near field artifact, thickened papillary muscle, hypertrophied trabeculations, ectopic chordae.
- Poor transthoracic image quality could interfere with accurate visualization of thrombus. Image optimization including optimal gain settings, zoom/res, B-Mode color, proper focal placement, and the use of high frequency and harmonic imaging are essential.
- TEE may be useful in patients with suboptimal transthoracic images or in the setting of very small thrombus (TEE provides better axial resolution).

Ventricular Septal Rupture

Definition

An acute ventricular septal defect due to rupture of the interventricular septum.

History/Physical Examination

- Occurs within the first week following AMI (1 to 3% of AMI patients), (rare after 2 weeks)
- Risk factors include first infarction, advanced age (>65), systemic hypertension, female gender, single vessel occlusion, large infarctions, infarct expansion
- Chest pain
- Acute hypotension
- Pulmonary edema
- Severe left and right heart failure/Cardiogenic shock

Cardiac Auscultation

New, loud, harsh holosystolic (crescendo-decrescendo) murmur heard best at the left sternal border and often associated with a thrill

Electrocardiogram

- Myocardial infarction
- Bradycardia
- Heart block
- Atrial fibrillation
- Electromechanical dissociation

Chest X-ray/CMR/CT

- Pulmonary congestion

Cardiac Catheterization

- Demonstrates an increase in oxygen saturation in the right ventricle due to left-to-right shunting
- Large v waves
- May demonstrate left to right shunt during left ventriculography
- Placement of umbrella device (may stabilize patient)

Medical Treatment

- Vasodilators
- Inotropic support
- Intra-aortic balloon counterpulsation

Surgical Treatment

- Urgent surgical closure in patients with unstable hemodynamics and/or end-organ damage
- Delayed surgical closure (≥3 weeks) in stable patients

2D

- Allows direct visualization of the defect (disrupted, "spliced" IVS) (off-axis views/unconventional views may be required)
- Inferoapical, anteroapical location is most common site (use parasternal short-axis view of left ventricle and apical/subcostal 4-chamber views) usually occurring at hinge point of infarcted and non-infarcted myocardium
- May be in multiple locations and have serpiginous course, making it more difficult to visualize exact location (usually when located in basal segment)
- Right ventricular volume overload (right ventricular dilatation with paradoxical septal motion)
- Decreased left ventricular/right ventricular systolic function

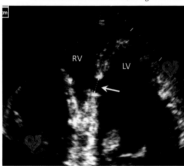

Figure 8.11: **Apical 4-chamber view demonstrating a 0.78cm ventricular septal defect resulting from ventricular septal rupture following acute myocardial infarction (AMI).**

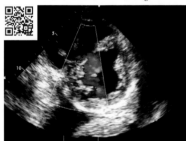

Figure 8.12: **Parasternal short axis view demonstrating high velocity, left to right shunting across a ventricular septal rupture following AMI. Notice the thinning of the myocardium adjacent to the defect.**

- Right atrial dilatation (upper limits of normal RA values: major dimension <53mm, minor dimension <44mm, end-systolic area <18cm^2)
- Bowing of the interatrial septum towards left atrium
- Inferior vena cava plethora
- 3D may provide information concerning location and size

Doppler
- A systolic high-velocity, turbulent jet with left-to-right shunting
- Increased RVOT/pulmonary artery flow
- Determine:
  - Location and width of jet
  - Right ventricular systolic function (important determinant of survival) PAP/MPAP/PAEDP/PVR
  - Shunt ratio (Qp:Qs) (may demonstrate increased RVOT/pulmonary artery flow with decreased LVOT/aortic flow)

Important to Note
- Associated with a 41 to 80% mortality (almost always fatal if not repaired).
- Rupture will most likely be located apical in the setting of anterior infarcts, and basal with inferior infarcts
- Infarction involving the right ventricle in the setting of ventricular septal rupture indicates a poor prognosis
- Identified by transthoracic imaging 90% of the time

Papillary Muscle Dysfunction
Definition
Disruption of the mitral valve support structures which produces mitral regurgitation due to improper spatial orientation of the papillary muscle due to left ventricular dilatation, papillary muscle fibrosis and/or calcification, improper contraction of the papillary muscle associated with ischemia/infarction of the papillary muscle or subjacent myocardium, rupture of the papillary muscle head(s) or trunk or improper timing of contraction such as in left bundle branch block or other types of conduction disturbances.

History/Physical Examination
- Myocardial infarction, cardiomyopathy
- Angina
- Pulmonary edema
- New, loud systolic murmur
- Heart failure (dyspnea, orthopnea, paroxysmal nocturnal dyspnea, fatigue, cough, weight gain)

2D
- An area of wall motion abnormality around either papillary muscle implies dysfunction

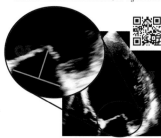

Figure 8.13: **Incomplete closure of the mitral valve leaflets failing to coapt to the level of the mitral annulus ("tenting") (best seen in the parasternal long-axis view or apical 4-chamber view with the anterior mitral valve leaflet more often involved)**

- Fibrosis/calcification (papillary muscle is denser than adjacent myocardium) of the papillary muscle implies papillary muscle dysfunction (best seen in the parasternal short-axis view of the left ventricle at the level of the papillary muscles)
- Left ventricular dilatation interrupts the spatial orientation of the papillary muscles to the rest of the mitral valve apparatus, thus inducing papillary muscle dysfunction
- Mitral valve prolapse due to inadequate contraction of the papillary muscle
- Flail mitral valve

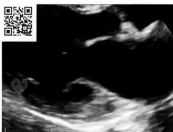

- Partial papillary muscle rupture, defined as rupture of one of the several heads of the papillary muscle, will present with the head being visualized moving within the left atrium and left ventricle and is associated with flail mitral valve
- The most severe form of papillary muscle dysfunction is the complete (frank) rupture of a papillary muscle trunk resulting in flail mitral valve with severe mitral regurgitation

Figure 8.14: Parasternal long axis view of the mitral valve demonstrating a partially torn posteromedial papillary muscle resulting in flail segments of the mitral valve.

- Mobile mass representing the papillary muscle may be seen moving between the left ventricle and left atrium during the cardiac cycle (in the left atrium during systole, in the left ventricle during diastole)

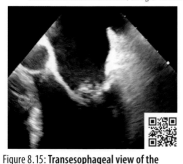

- Left atrial dilatation (normal LA volume: ≤34mL/m²)
- Left ventricular volume overload pattern (left ventricular dilatation with hyperkinesis)

Doppler

- Determine:
  - Presence and severity of the mitral regurgitation

Figure 8.15: Transesophageal view of the mitral valve demonstrating a partially torn posteromedial papillary muscle resulting in flail segments of the mitral valve.

  - Direction of the mitral regurgitation jet (anterior direction suggests posterior mitral valve leaflet involvement, posterior direction suggests anterior mitral valve leaflet involvement)
- In flail mitral valve leaflet, the severity of the mitral regurgitation may be underestimated by color flow Doppler due to the coanda effect as well as the reduced left ventricle-left atrial pressure gradient
- Increased stroke volume across the mitral valve in the setting of significant mitral regurgitation
- In the setting of acute mitral regurgitation, there may be a reduction in left ventricular stroke volume

Transesophageal Echocardiography

- TEE may be helpful especially in the evaluation of papillary muscle rupture and the severity of the mitral regurgitation
- May be useful in differentiating between ruptured papillary muscle versus ventricular septal rupture

Important to Note

- Rupture of the papillary muscle occurs in approximately 1% of patients with acute myocardial infarction.
- Papillary muscle rupture usually develops 2 to 7 days post infarction with a median survival of only three days.
- Complete papillary muscle rupture is associated with death within one hour.
- Mitral valve replacement the most common surgical treatment.
- Papillary muscle rupture most commonly occurs with inferior infarctions involving the posteromedial papillary muscle and presents as acute pulmonary edema.
- Rupture of one of the smaller heads (partial rupture) of the papillary muscle occurs more frequently than does rupture of the main trunk (complete rupture).
- Papillary muscle dysfunction is more common after an inferior infarction while annular dilatation is more common following an anterior infarction.
- Anterolateral papillary muscle most commonly becomes fibrocalcific due to the direction of left ventricular inflow.

Right Ventricular Infarction

Definition

Myocardial infarction involving the right ventricle; may be isolated to the right ventricle only, but more often associated with an inferior or inferolateral infarction.

Etiology

- Associated most often with inferior infarction (up to 1/3 of patients with inferior wall infarctions, and hemodynamically significant in 10% of inferior infarctions)
- Isolated right ventricular infarction is rare with necropsy proven myocardial infarction

History/Physical Examination

- Inferior or inferolateral MI
- Systemic hypotension
- Jugular venous distention
- Kussmaul's sign (inspiratory increase in jugular venous pressure)
- Normal to low pulmonary artery pressures
- Clear lungs
- Hypoxemia (in the setting of PFO with right to left shunt)

8

Ischemic Heart Disease / Complications of Myocardial Infarction / Right Ventricular Infarction

Cardiac Auscultation
- Murmur of tricuspid regurgitation
- Right sided S3, S4

Electrocardiogram
- Inferior myocardial infarction
- ST segment elevation in $V_4 R V$
- Complete heart block

Chest X-ray/CMR/CT
- Clear lungs
- CMR allows evaluation of right ventricular global/segmental function

Cardiac Catheterization
- Coronary arteriography
- Elevated right atrial (12 to 20mmHg) and right ventricular diastolic pressures

Medical/Surgical Treatment
- Plasma expanders to maintain right ventricular preload/cardiac output
- Avoid diuretics/nitrates/morphine
- Positive inotropes (e.g., Dobutamine, dopamine)
- AV sequential pacing
- Thrombolytic therapy
- Intra-aortic balloon pump/pulmonary artery balloon counterpulsation
- PTCA/stenting
- Right ventricular assist device
- Coronary artery bypass graft (tricuspid valve annuloplasty/repair may be indicated)

2D
- Use multiple on-axis and modified off axis views to evaluate the right ventricle (the right ventricle may be visualized in almost every standard 2D echocardiographic view)
- Segmental wall motion abnormality (look for associated wall motion abnormality of inferior wall and/or posterior septum) (W-shaped infarct)
- Right ventricular dilatation (normal Basal RV diameter 25 to 41mm)
- Right atrial dilatation (upper limits of normal RA values: major dimension <53mm, minor dimension <44mm, end-systolic area <18cm^2) [13]
- Hyperdynamic wall motion of unaffected right ventricular wall segments
- Inferior vena cava dilatation with lack of inspiratory collapse
- Paradoxical septal motion (may indicate significant tricuspid regurgitation)
- Bowing of the interatrial septum towards the left atrium

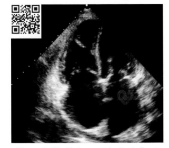

Figure 8.16: **Right ventricular infarct**

- Papillary muscle dysfunction (e.g., "tenting" of the tricuspid valve, papillary muscle rupture)
- Determine:
  - Right ventricular wall thickness, dimension(s), systolic function (RV strain has been shown to provide prognostic value)
  - Presence of complications of myocardial infarction (e.g., true aneurysm, pseudoaneurysm, ventricular septal rupture, thrombus)

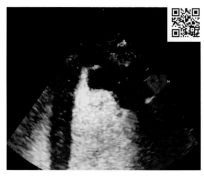

Figure 8.17: Apical 4-chamber view with ultrasound enhancing agent demonstrating thrombus in the left ventricular apex following acute myocardial infarction. As the left ventricle fills with the enhancing agent, the thrombus will appear as an echolucent area. A thrombus is not vascular and will not uptake the enhancing agent. Notice there is also a smaller thrombus located slightly further into the ventricle along the lateral wall, enhancing agent can be visualized filling the space in between.

Doppler

- Tricuspid regurgitation (if present, pulmonary artery pressures should be unexpectedly low)
- Right-to-left shunting through a patent foramen ovale (associated with hypoxemia and large right ventricular infarctions)
- Evaluate coexisting complications (e.g., ventricular septal rupture)
- Determine:
  - RV/LV stroke volume, cardiac output, cardiac index
  - Right ventricular grade of diastolic dysfunction

Important to Note

- Right ventricular infarction reduces venous return to the left ventricle due to right ventricular pump failure. This decrease in left ventricular preload is the principal mechanism for a decrease in cardiac output.
- Right ventricular infarction may result in cardiogenic shock.
- Right ventricular infarction should be suspected in a patient with neck vein distention with clear lung fields, systemic hypotension and low cardiac output.
- The clinical presentation may resemble cardiac tamponade.

Cardiogenic Shock

Definition

Shock resulting from failure to maintain blood supply to the circulatory system and tissues due to inadequate cardiac output.

Etiology

Post Myocardial Infarction

- Severe left ventricular failure (85%)
- Mechanical complications (8%)
- Right ventricular infarct (2%)
- Other comorbidities (5%)

History/Physical Examination

- Acute myocardial infarction (5 to 15%)
- Hypotension
- Heart failure (dyspnea, orthopnea, paroxysmal nocturnal dyspnea, fatigue, cough, weight gain)
- Elevated filling pressures
- Pulmonary edema
- Compensatory tachycardia
- Evidence of hypoperfusion of vital organs (e.g., cool extremities, oliguria, acidosis, cyanosis)

Medical/Surgical Treatment

- Oxygen
- Intubation
- Fluid bolus (250mL)
- Positive inotropes (e.g., Dobutamine, norepinepherine)
- Vasodilators (e.g., nitroglycerin)
- Morphine
- Lasix (cardiogenic shock with pulmonary edema)
- Hemodynamic monitoring
- Intra-aortic balloon pump
- Left ventricular assist device (percutaneous, surgical)
- Revascularization (e.g., CABG, angioplasty)

2D/Doppler

- Evaluate for cause of cardiogenic shock (e.g., acute myocardial infarction, markedly reduced left/right ventricular systolic function, ventricular septal rupture, right ventricular infarction, cardiac tamponade, ruptured papillary muscle with severe mitral regurgitation)
- 50% of patients with cardiogenic shock will have normal size left ventricle, and some may present with normal left ventricular ejection fraction (left ventricular ejection fraction has prognostic value)

Important to Note

- Cardiogenic shock is characterized by hypotension (longer than 30 minutes) with systolic blood pressure less than 80mmHg with a reduction in cardiac index (<1.8 L/min/m²), increased right, left or both right and left sided filling pressures, low urine output.
- If more than 40% of the left ventricle is infarcted, cardiogenic shock is likely to result.
- Most common cause of death following AMI
- In hospital mortality has reduced to 51% due to improvement in revascularization treatment (previously 81%).
- Presence of mitral regurgitation in the setting of cardiogenic shock following AMI has poor prognosis.

Dynamic Left Ventricular Outflow Tract Obstruction

Definition

Obstruction of blood flow in the area of the left ventricular outflow tract due to systolic anterior motion of the mitral valve, progressively worsening in late systole. Most commonly observed in the setting of hypertrophic obstructive cardiomyopathy, but may also be present in volume depleted ventricles with increased basal septal thickness, or in the setting of compensatory hyperdynamic function of unaffected segments following AMI.

History/Physical Examination

- New systolic murmur following AMI
- Risk factors include women of advanced age, system hypertension with basal septal hypertrophy, acute anterior myocardial infarction, and single vessel disease
- Cardiogenic shock
- Pulmonary edema
- Hypotension

Medical Treatment

- Fluids
- Beta blockers
- Alpha antagonist

2D

- Segmental wall motion abnormalities typically at the apex, with compensatory hyperdynamic function of non-infarcted basal segments
- Systolic anterior motion of the mitral valve

Doppler

- Turbulent color flow in the left ventricular outflow tract
- Posteriorly directed mitral regurgitation (usually mid to late systole)
- High late peaking systolic Doppler velocity in the left ventricular outflow tract

Important to Note

Early recognition of a left ventricular outflow tract obstruction following AMI is important so that vasodilators and inotropics are not used in the medical management of the patient.

References

1. Anderson B. (2014). A Sonographer's Guide to the Assessment of Heart Disease. Australia: MGA Graphics.

2. Arnett DK, Blumenthal RS, Albert MA, et.al. 2019 ACC/AHA Guideline on the Primary Prevention of Cardiovascular Disease: Executive Summary. Circulation 2019. Doi:10.1161/cir0000000000000677

3. Heart.org. (2019). Obesity Information. [online] Available at: http://www.heart.org/HEARTORG/HealthyLiving/WeightManagement/Obesity-Information_UCM_307908_Article.jsp#.XTHV1-hKhaQ [Accessed 19 Jul. 2019].

4. Oh J, Kane G, Seward J, Tajik AJ. (2018). The Echo Manual, 4TH ed. Lippincott Williams & Wilkins.

5. Lang R, Badano L, Mor-Avi V, et al. Recommendation for Chamber Quantification by Echocardiography in Adults: An Update from the American Society of Echocardiography and the European Association of Cardiovascular Imaging. J Am Soc Echocardiogr 2015;28:1-39

6. Yingchoncharoe T, Agarwal S, Popvic ZB, Marwick TH. Normal Ranges of Left Ventricular Strain: A Meta-Analysis. J Am Soc Echocardiogr 2013;26(2): 185-191.

7. O'Gara PT, Kushner FG, Ascheim DD, et al. 2013 ACCF/AHA Guidelines for the Management of ST-Elevation Myocardial Infarction: a report of the American College of Cardiology Foundation/American Heart Association Task Force on Practice Guidelines. J Am Coll Cardiol 2013;61(4):e78-e140. Doi:10.1016/j.jacc.2012.11.019

8. Delewi R, Zijlstra F, Piek J. Left ventricular thrombus formation after acute myocardial infarction. Heart Journal 2012. Doi:10.1136/heartjnl-2012-301962

9. Serrano CV, Ramires JAF, de Matos Soeiro A, et al. Efficacy of aneurysmectomy in patients with severe left ventricular dysfunction: favorable short- and long-term results in ischemic cardiomyopathy. Clinics 2010;65(10):947-952. Doi:10.1590/S1807-59322010001000004

10. Shapira OM, Gersh BJ, Saperia GM. (2017) Left ventricular aneurysm and pseudoaneurysm following acute myocardial infarction. Up to Date. Retrieved July 20, 2019 from https://www.uptodate.com/contents/left-ventricular-aneurysm-and-pseudoaneurysm-following-acute-myocardial-infarction

11. Bisoyi S, Dash AK, Nayak D, Sahoo S, Mohapatra R. Left ventricular pseudoaneurysm versus aneurysm a diagnosis dilemma. Ann Card Anaesth 2016;19(1):169-172. doi 10.4103/0971-9784.173042

12. Frances C, Romero A, Grady D. Left ventricular pseudoaneurysm. J Am Coll Cardiol 1998;32:557-561. Doi:10.1016/s0735-1097(98)00290-3

13. Rudski LG, Lai WW, Afilalo J, et al. Guidelines for the Echocardiographic Assessment of the Right Heart in Adults: A Report from the American Society of Echocardiography. J Am Soc Echocardiogr 2010;23:685-713.

14. Jones BM, Kapadia SR, Smedira NG, et al. Ventricular septal rupture complicating acute myocardial infarction: a contemporary review. Eur Heart J 2014;35(31):2060-2068. Doi:10.1093/eurheartj/ehu248

15. Khan S, Kundi A, Sharieff S. Prevalence of right ventricular myocardial infarction in patients with acute inferior wall myocardial infarction. Int J Clin Pract 2004;58(4):354-357.

16. Thiele H, Ohman EM, Desch S, Eitel I, de Waha S. Management of cardiogenic shock. Eur Heart J 2015;36(20):1223-1230. doi:10.1093/eurheartj/ehv051

17. Reynolds HR, Hochman JS. Cardiogenic Shock. Circulation 2008;117(5):686-697. doi:10.1161/CIRCULATIOAHA.106.613596

18. Califf RM, Bengtson JR. Cardiogenic Shock. N Engl J Med. 1994;330(24):1724-1730, doi:10.1056/NEJM199406163302406

19. Lang RM, Goldstein SA, Kronzon I, Khanderia BK, Mor-Avi V. (2015). ASE's Comprehensive Echocardiography. Elsevier.

20. Diepen S, Katz JN, Albert NM, et al. Contemporary Management of Cardiogenic Shock: A Scientific Statement From the American Heart Association. Circulation. 2017;136:e232-e268. doi:10.1161/CIR.0000000000000525

Cardiomyopathies
Merri L. Bremer, Ed.D., RN, ACS, RDCS, FASE

Dilated Cardiomyopathy (DCM)

Definition

Disease of the myocardium characterized by dilatation and decreased systolic function of the left ventricle or both the left and right ventricles

Table 9.1: Most Common Etiologies for Dilated Cardiomyopathy
Idiopathic – specific cause cannot be delineated
Familial/genetic transmission (20 to 50% of cases) [1,2]
Ischemic heart disease
Hypertensive heart disease
Infectious (myocarditis) – viral, bacterial, fungal, parasites
Inflammatory disease (e.g., systemic lupus erythematosus, rheumatoid arthritis)
Peripartum cardiomyopathy
Left ventricular noncompaction
Cardiomyopathy due to valvular heart disease

Cardiac rhythm-related cardiomyopathy
  • Toxins
  • Alcohol
  • Chemotherapeutic agents
  • Cocaine

Endocrine abnormalities (e.g., thyroid dysfunction, acromegaly, pheochromocytoma)

Clinical Presentation

- Fatigue
- Decreased exercise tolerance
- Dyspnea
- Orthopnea
- Paroxysmal nocturnal dyspnea
- Chest discomfort

Physical Examination

- Evidence of left heart failure
  - Normal to low blood pressure
  - Diffuse, apical impulse displaced laterally and diminished in force
  - Pulsus alternans (severe left ventricular failure)
  - Tachycardia
  - Lung crackles (pulmonary edema)
- Evidence of right heart failure
  - Hepatomegaly
  - Elevated JVP
  - Peripheral edema
  - Ascites

Cardiac Auscultation

- Paradoxical splitting of the second heart sound with left bundle branch block
- Accentuated pulmonary component of the second heart sound if pulmonary hypertension is present
- S^3 with ventricular decompensation
- S^4
- Systolic murmurs of mitral and tricuspid regurgitation

Ancillary Diagnostic Testing

- Electrocardiogram
  - Sinus tachycardia
  - Nonspecific ST-T wave abnormalities
  - Atrial arrhythmias or atrial fibrillation
  - Ventricular arrhythmias
  - Left bundle branch block or other conduction abnormalities
  - Left atrial enlargement
- Chest X-ray
  - Cardiomegaly
  - Evidence of pulmonary congestion
- Cardiac Magnetic Resonance Imaging (MRI)
  - May be used to assess myocardial injury or inflammation
- Cardiac Catheterization
  - Coronary arteriography to evaluate for the presence of coronary artery disease
  - Endomyocardial biopsy may be considered
- Exercise Testing
  - May help determine cause of exercise limitation

Medical Treatment

- Pharmacologic therapy for heart failure
  - Angiotensin-converting enzyme (ACE) inhibitors
  - Angiotensin receptor blockers (ARBs)
  - Beta blockers
  - Aldosterone antagonists
  - Diuretics

Interventional/Surgical Treatment

- Implantable cardiac defibrillator (ICD) therapy (for ventricular arrhythmias)
- Biventricular pacing (CRT)

- Mitral valve and tricuspid valve surgery
- Ventricular reduction surgery
- Ventricular assist devices
- Cardiac transplantation

M-mode/2D

- Left ventricular enlargement
  - 2D or 3D quantitative end-diastolic and end-systolic dimensions or volumes
- Spherical configuration of the left ventricle
- Decreased global LV systolic function indices
  - Ejection fraction (preferred method is 2D or 3D volumetric technique)
  - Global or regional longitudinal strain
  - Fractional shortening
  - Systolic longitudinal motion of the mitral annulus
- Superimposed regional wall motion abnormalities may be present
- Increased left ventricular mass (often eccentric hypertrophy)
- Secondary features
  - Enlarged atria
  - Right ventricular enlargement
  - May exhibit decreased RV systolic function indices
    - Fractional area change (FAC)
    - Pulsed Doppler S wave (cm/sec)
    - Tricuspid annular plane systolic excursion (TAPSE)
    - RV longitudinal strain
    - RV 3D EF
  - Abnormal ventricular septal motion due to interventricular conduction delay (left or right bundle branch block)
  - Possible mural thrombus, especially at LV apex
  - Dilated mitral annulus and incomplete coaptation of the mitral valve leaflets
  - Tethering or tenting of the mitral valve leaflets due to LV remodeling
  - Dilated IVC with reduced inspiratory collapse
  - Evidence of ventricular dyssynchrony

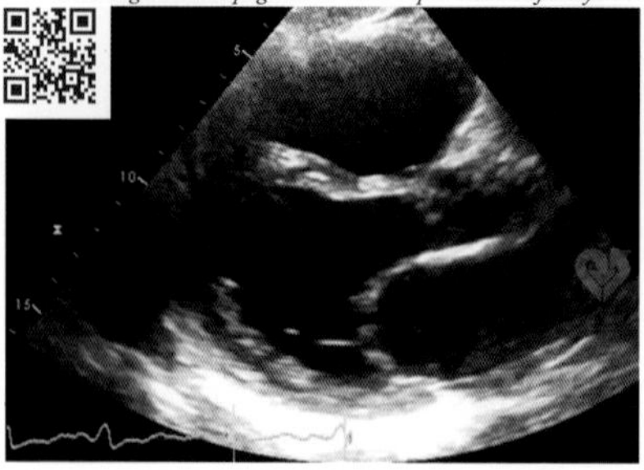

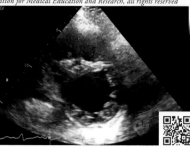

Figure 9.1: **Parasternal long-axis view typical of DCM**

Figure 9.2: **Parasternal short-axis view typical of DCM**

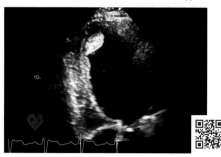

Figure 9.3: **Off-axis apical 2-chamber view of LV apical thrombus in the setting of DCM**

Table 9.2: Normal Values for 2D Echocardiographic Parameters of LV Size and Function According to Gender[3]				
Parameter	**Male**		**Female**	
	Mean ± SD	Range Additional Findings	Mean ± SD	Range Additional Findings
LV Internal Dimension				
Diastolic dimension (mm)	50.2 ± 4.1	42.0 to 58.4	45.0 ± 3.6	37.8 to 52.2
Systolic dimension (mm)	32.4 ± 3.7	25.0 to 39.8	28.2 ± 3.3	21.6 to 34.8
LV Volumes (biplane)				
LV EDV (mL)	106 ± 22	62 to 150	76 ± 15	46 to 106
LV ESV (mL)	41 ± 10	21 to 61	28 ± 7	14 to 42
LV Volumes Normalized by BSA				
LV EDV (mL/m²)	51 ± 10	34 to 74	45 ± 8	29 to 61
LV ESV (mL/m²)	21 ± 5	11 to 31	16 ± 4	8 to 24
LV EF (biplane)	62 ± 5	52 to 72	64 ± 5	54 to 74

BSA: body surface area; **EDV:** end-diastolic volume; **EF:** ejection fraction
ESV: end-systolic volume; **LV:** left ventricular; **SD:** standard deviation.

Table 9.3: Normal Values for LV Mass Indicies [3]		
Linear Method	**Male**	**Female**
LV mass (g)	88 to 224	67 to 162
LV mass/BSA (g/m²)	49 to 115	43 to 95
Relative wall thickness (cm)	0.24 to 0.42	0.22 to 0.42
Septal thickness (cm)	**0.6 to 1.0**	**0.6 to 0.9**
Posterior wall thickness (cm)	**0.6 to 1.0**	**0.6 to 0.9**
2D Method		
LV mass (g)	96 to 200	66 to 150
LV mass/BSA (g/m²)	50 to 102	44 to 88

Bold values: recommended and best validated.

Table 9.4: Values for Parameters of RV Function [3]		
Parameter	**Mean ± SD**	**Abnormality Threshold**
TAPSE (mm)	24 ± 3.5	<17
Pulsed Doppler S wave (cm/sec)	14.1 ± 2.3	<9.5
Color Doppler S wave (cm/sec)	9.7 ± 1.85	<6.0
RV fractional area change (%)	49 ± 7	<35
RV free wall 20 strain (%)	-29 ± 4.5	<-20 (<20 in magnitude with the negative sign)
RV 30 EF(%)	58 ± 6.5	<45
Pulsed Doppler MPI	0.26 ± 0.085	>0.43
Tissue Doppler MPI	0.38 ± 0.08	>0.54
E wave deceleration time (msec)	180 ± 31	<119 or >242
E/A	1.4 ± 0.3	<0.8 or >2.0
e'/a'	1.18 ± 0.33	<0.52
e'	14.0 ± 3.1	<7.8
E/e'	4.0 ± 1.0	<6.0

MPI: Mycocardial performance index.
*Limited data; values may vary depending on vendor and software version.

Doppler Echocardiography and Color Flow Imaging Findings

• Decreased global LV systolic function indices
  - Stroke volume
  - Cardiac output and index
  - Reduced rate of rise in ventricular pressure (dP/dt)
• Evidence of ventricular dyssynchrony

9

Cardiomyopathies / Dilated Cardiomyopathy (DCM)

• Left ventricular diastolic dysfunction
  - May range from abnormal relaxation to restrictive filling
• Associated functional mitral and/or tricuspid regurgitation
• Decreased RV systolic function indices
  - Tricuspid annulus tissue Doppler imaging (TDI)
• Elevated RVSP

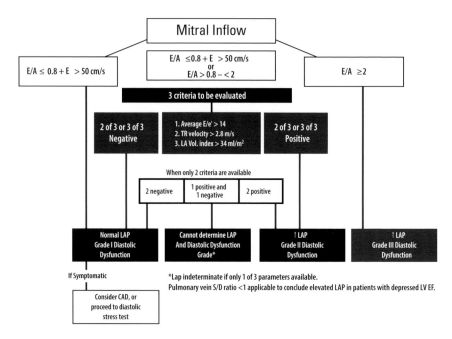

Figure 9.4: **Algorithm for estimation of LV filling pressures and grading LV diastolic function in patients with depressed LVEFs and patients with myocardial disease and normal LVEF** [4]

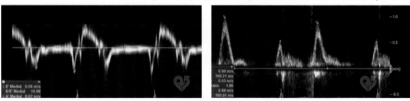

Figure 9.5: **Medial tissue Doppler and mitral inflow consistent with Grade 2/2 diastolic dysfunction**
(E/e' = 16)

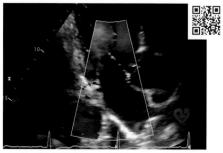

Figure 9.6: **Functional mitral regurgitation in a patient with DCM**

Left Ventricular Non-Compaction (LVNC)

Definition
- Genetic cardiomyopathy
- Frequently isolated to the left ventricle
- Characterized by prominent trabeculations and deep recesses that communicate with the ventricular cavity

Pathophysiology
- Occurs during fetal development when the normal compaction process of the endocardium and myocardium is halted
- Results in a two-layered LV myocardium
    - Compacted epicardial layer
    - Non-compacted endocardial layer with deep trabeculations and recesses
- May range from isolated LV non-compaction to coexistence with other congenital cardiac anomalies
- Manifests clinically as a dilated cardiomyopathy, with heart failure, embolic events and arrhythmias

Ancillary Diagnostic Testing
- Electrocardiogram
    - May be normal
    - Nonspecific repolarization abnormalities
    - Left bundle branch block
- Cardiac Magnetic Resonance Imaging (MRI)
    - May visualize the extent of the disease better than echocardiography, particularly at the apex
    - Confirms the presence of the anatomic features of LVNC
    - Provides accurate and reproducible measurement of the non-compacted and compacted myocardial layers
    - Evaluates the degree of myocardial fibrosis

Medical Treatment

Prevention and treatment of complications (heart failure, embolic events and arrhythmias)

Surgical Treatment

Cardiac transplantation

Table 9.5: Proposed Diagnostic Echocardiographic Criteria for Non-Compaction Cardiomyopathy
Chin et al [5]
• End-diastolic ratio of compacted to total myocardium <0.5
Jenni et al [6]
• Absence of coexisting cardiac abnormalities
• Two-layered LV myocardium; ratio of non-compacted to compacted layer >2.0
• Deep intertrabecular recesses filled by blood flow from the LV cavity
• Characteristic features are found predominantly in the apical and mid ventricular LV wall segments
Stöllberger et al [7]
• More than three trabeculations protruding from the LV wall, apically to the papillary muscles, visible in one image plane
• Evidence of perfusion of the intertrabecular spaces from the ventricular cavity by color flow imaging

M-mode/2D

• Features of dilated cardiomyopathy
  - Enlarged LV cavity
  - Reduced LV systolic function
• Bi-layered myocardium with deep trabeculations and recesses
• Predominantly apical involvement
• Use of echo enhancement agents may be useful for evaluation of LV systolic function, the ratio of non-compacted to compacted layers, and the presence or absence of thrombus

Doppler Echocardiography and Color Flow Imaging Findings

• LV diastolic dysfunction
  - Restrictive filling with advanced disease
• Varying degrees of mitral and tricuspid regurgitation
• Pulmonary hypertension

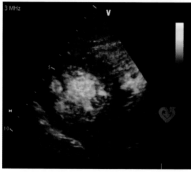

Figure 9.7: **Contrast echocardiography of the apical short-axis view in non-compaction cardiomyopathy**

Arrhythmogenic Right Ventricular Dysplasia or Cardiomyopathy (ARVD/C)

Definition
- Rare
- Progressive replacement of the RV myocardium by fibrous and fatty tissue
- Predominantly genetic; autosomal dominant inheritance
- Diagnosis includes major and minor criteria noted by imaging, tissue characterization, electrocardiographic, arrhythmic, and genetic features of the disease
- May be asymptomatic
- May present with ventricular arrhythmias, congestive heart failure, heart murmur, or sudden death

Pathophysiology
- Fibrofatty replacement of RV tissue results in wall thinning and aneurysm formation
- RV cavity gradually enlarges and systolic function decreases

Ancillary Diagnostic Testing
- Electrocardiogram
  - Arrhythmias
  - ST-T wave changes
- Cardiac Magnetic Resonance Imaging (MRI)
  - May identify fat in the RV myocardium
  - Evaluates RV size and function, presence of focal wall thinning or aneurysm

Medical Treatment

• Prevention and treatment of complications (heart failure, embolic events and arrhythmias)

Interventional/Surgical Treatment

• Implantable defibrillator (ICD) therapy
• Catheter ablation for arrhythmias
• Cardiac transplantation

M-mode/2D

• Findings are quite variable
• RV dilatation
• RV systolic dysfunction
• RV RWMA (typically anterior and apical)
• RV saccular aneurysms
• Abnormal RV trabeculation pattern
• Hyper-reflective moderator band
• LV is relatively normal, but may become involved in advanced disease
• Use of echo enhancement agents may be useful for evaluation of RV systolic function

Table 9.6: ARVD Echocardiographic Criteria[8]	
Major Criteria	**Minor Criteria**
Regional RV akinesia, dyskinesia, or aneurysm	Regional RV akinesia or dyskinesia
AND one of the following (in end diastole):	**AND** one of the following (in end diastole):
• Parasternal long-axis RV outflow tract dimension ≥32mm (corrected for body surface area ≥19mm/m^2)	• Parasternal long-axis RV outflow tract dimension ≥29 to <32mm (corrected for body surface area ≥16 to <19mm/m^2)
• Parasternal short-axis RV outflow tract dimension ≥36mm (corrected for body surface area ≥21mm/m^2)	• Parasternal short-axis RV outflow tract dimension ≥32 to <36mm (corrected for body surface area ≥18 to <21mm/m^2)
• Fractional area change ≤33%	• Fractional area change >33% to ≤40%

Doppler Echocardiography and Color Flow Imaging Findings

• Functional tricuspid regurgitation may be severe
  - Large color flow jet size
  - Increased tricuspid valve forward flow velocity
  - Systolic flow reversal in hepatic veins
  - Dense CW Doppler signal
  - TR velocity typically low due to large regurgitant orifice
• RV systolic pressure usually low due to RV failure

Echocardiographic views for diagnosis of arrhythmogenic right ventricular (RV) dysplasia. [9]

AoV, aortic valve; LA, left atrium; LV, left ventricle; RA, right atrium.

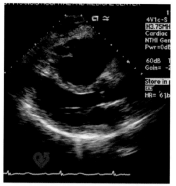

Figure 9.8: **Right ventricular outflow tract (RVOT) enlargement from the parasternal long-axis view**

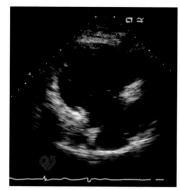

Figure 9.9: **RV inflow view showing right ventricular enlargement** [9]

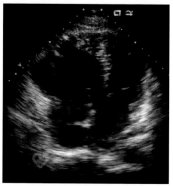

Figure 9.10: **Apical 4-chamber view showing a focal RV apical aneurysm**

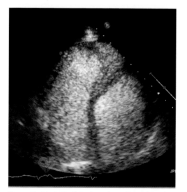

Figure 9.11: **Apical 4-chamber view showing right ventricular contrast**

Hypertrophic Cardiomyopathy (HCM)

Definition

Disease of the myocardium characterized by the presence of left ventricular hypertrophy (LVH) in the absence of another cause

Etiology

- Genetic disorder, typically an autosomal dominant trait
- Most common genetic cardiomyopathy (0.2%) [10]
- Many different mutations have been identified
- Variable expression of disease severity
- Echocardiographic screening of all first degree relatives is indicated

Pathophysiology

- Myocardial hypertrophy
- Myocardial disarray and fibrosis
- Small-vessel disease

Anatomic Features

- Asymmetric hypertrophy of the left ventricle (LV)
- Impaired diastolic LV function
- Dynamic LV outflow obstruction
  - May be labile at rest
  - May develop with provocation
- Associated mitral regurgitation

Mechanism of Dynamic Obstruction

- Narrowed LVOT due to hypertrophy
- Structural abnormalities of the mitral valve
  - Hypertrophy and anterior displacement of the papillary muscles
  - Intrinsic increase in mitral leaflet area and elongation
- Systolic anterior motion (SAM) of the mitral valve or chordae
  - Leaflets are predisposed to move into the LVOT by drag forces related to the hyperdynamic LV
  - Mitral leaflet coaptation is disrupted, resulting in mitral regurgitation of varying degree

Physiologic Variants

- "Classic" hypertrophic obstructive cardiomyopathy (HOCM)
- Non-obstructive HCM
- Mid-ventricular obstruction in hypertrophic cardiomyopathy
  - Intracavitary gradient often present
  - May also have LVOT obstruction
- Apical HCM
  - Less common
  - Predominantly involves the LV apex
  - May demonstrate an apical "pouch"
  - Ultrasound enhancement agents may be useful in delineating the anatomy
- Hypertensive cardiomyopathy in the elderly
  - Not a true HCM
  - May be due to systemic hypertension
  - Characterized by a basal septal bulge with associated increased outflow tract velocity

Clinical Presentation

- Wide variation in presentation
- May be asymptomatic (without obstruction)
- Dyspnea
- Chest pain
- Cardiac murmur
- Syncope/presyncope
- Sudden cardiac death
- Symptoms of heart failure

Physical Examination

- Unremarkable in many patients if no obstruction is present
- Rapid upstroke to the arterial pulse
- Sustained left ventricular impulse
- Prominent jugular venous *a* wave (decreased right ventricular compliance)

Cardiac Auscultation

- Left sided S^4
- Late-onset systolic murmur due to left ventricular outflow tract (LVOT) obstruction
- LVOT obstruction murmur is typically dependent on ventricular volume
  - May be enhanced with maneuvers that increase contractility or decrease cardiac chamber size (e.g., Valsalva maneuver (strain phase), amyl nitrite, standing, post-extrasystolic potentiation)
  - May be reduced with maneuvers that decrease contractility or increase cardiac chamber size (e.g., squatting, leg elevation)
- Many patients with LVOT obstruction also exhibit a murmur of mitral regurgitation
- Reversed splitting of S^2 may be noted with severe LVOT obstruction

Ancillary Diagnostic Testing

- Electrocardiogram
  - Majority of patient have abnormalities, but no patterns are specific to the disease
  - Voltage criteria for LVH
  - Repolarization abnormalities
  - Pathologic Q waves
  - Atrial enlargement
  - Giant negative T-waves in the mid-precordial leads is associated with apical HCM

- Chest X-ray
  - Cardiomegaly due to left ventricular and left atrial enlargement
  - Pulmonary congestion (late in course)
- Cardiac Magnetic Resonance Imaging (MRI)
  - Provides information about localization of hypertrophy (especially the apex)
  - Identifies thrombus, left ventricular non-compaction
  - May identify focal areas of fibrosis
  - Defines anatomic variations
    - Right ventricular structures
    - False tendons or trabeculae
    - Membranes
    - Complex multilevel obstruction
- Computed Tomography
  - Provides information concerning cardiac structure, ventricular volumes, LV wall thickness and mass, coronary artery anatomy
- Cardiac Catheterization
  - Largely superseded by echocardiography
  - Major use is exclusion of coronary atherosclerosis in older patients who have chest pain
  - May measure outflow tract gradients
  - May be utilized for septal ablation therapy
- Radionuclide Studies
  - May identify perfusion abnormalities
- Exercise Testing
  - Provides objective measure of functional capacity

Medical Treatment

Pharmacologic therapy

- Beta blockers
- Calcium channel blockers
- Diuretics
- Nitrates
- Antiarrhythmic agents
- Anticoagulants

Interventional/Surgical Treatment

- Implantable cardioverter defibrillator (ICD) for ventricular arrhythmias
- Electrical cardioversion of atrial fibrillation
- AV sequential pacemaker/Dual chamber permanent pacing to provide asynchronous activation of interventricular septum (which may reduce the LVOT gradient)
- Alcohol septal myocardial ablation
- Septal myotomy/myectomy
- Mitral valve replacement or repair during myotomy/myectomy

Table 9.7: Hypertrophic Cardiomopathy (HCM) [11]
1. Presence of hypertrophy and its distribution report should include measurements of LV dimensions and wall thickness (septal, posterior, and maximum)
2. LV EF
3. RV hypertrophy and whether RV dynamic obstruction is present
4. LA volume indexed to body surface area
5. LV diastolic function (comments on LV relaxation and filling pressures)
6. Pulmonary artery systolic pressure
7. Dynamic obstruction at rest and with Valsalva maneuver; report should identify the site of obstruction and the gradient
8. Mitral valve and papillary muscle evaluation, including the direction, mechanism, and severity of mitral regurgitation; if needed, TEE should be performed to satisfactorily answer these questions
9. TEE is recommended to guide surgical myectomy, and TTE or TEE for alcohol septal ablation
10. Screening

M-mode/2D

** Caveat: 2D features of HCM may be mimicked by chronic hypertension, cardiac amyloidosis, and Friedreich's ataxia, among other entities. Clinical context must be taken into account.

"Classic" HOCM

- Normal or slightly reduced ventricular cavity size by 2D or 3D volumes
- Normal to hyperdynamic ejection fraction with possible LV cavity obliteration in systole
- End-stage hypertrophic cardiomyopathy ("burnt-out" HCM) characterized by reduced ejection fraction
- Asymmetric septal hypertrophy
    - Consider use of ultrasound enhancement agents to delineate anatomy
    - Measure wall thickness in multiple views
    - Note location of the thickest walls and include measurements in the report
    - Septal thickness of >30mm holds a 40% cumulative risk for sudden death [12]
    - Characterize the variant of septal hypertrophy
- Right ventricular hypertrophy may also be present
- Speckle-tracking echocardiography
    - Characteristic patterns
    - Typically most abnormal in the thickest myocardial segments
- Enlarged left atrium due to elevated LV filling pressure and/or significant mitral regurgitation

- Mitral valve abnormalities
  - Systolic anterior motion of the mitral valve (SAM)
  - Thickened, elongated mitral valve leaflets
  - Coaptation point of the mitral valve leaflets in the body of the leaflets instead of at the leaflet tips
  - Anterior displacement of papillary muscles or anomalous papillary muscle with direct insertion of papillary muscle into mitral valve leaflet
- Endocardial plaque ("contact lesion") of the upper portion of interventricular septum due to SAM
- M-mode findings
  - Mid-systolic notching of the aortic valve – normal aortic flow is interrupted due to obstruction
  - B "bump" or "notch" of the mitral valve consistent with increased left ventricular end-diastolic pressure (LVEDP)

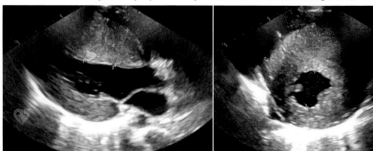

Figure 9.12: **Massive septal hypertrophy as measured in parasternal long-and short-axis views.**

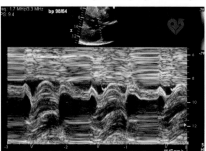

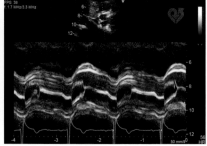

Figure 9.13: **M-mode example of systolic anterior motion**

Figure 9.14: **Mid-systolic notching of the aortic valve**

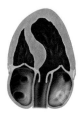
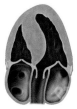
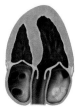
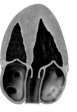

Figure 9.15:
Sigmoid

Figure 9.16:
Reverse curve

Figure 9.17:
Neutral

Figure 9.18:
Apical

Figure 9.19: **Depiction of ventricular septal morphologies in HCM.** [13]

- Septal geometry is defined in the apical long-axis view and categorized into sigmoid, reverse curve, neutral, and apical morphologies. [12]

Mid-ventricular Obstruction in Hypertrophic Cardiomyopathy

- Typically mid-ventricular hypertrophy is present at the papillary muscle level
- Typically SAM is not present

Apical HCM

- Localized apical hypertrophy with spade-like configuration of the left ventricle at end-diastole
- Best viewed from apical window, often from off-axis and short-axis views
- Apical aneurysm (pouch) present in 15% of patients [14]
- Consider use of ultrasound enhancement agents to evaluate for apical thrombus

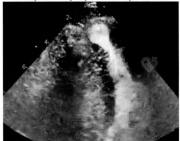

Figure 9.20: **Apical pouch visualized with use of UEA from off-axis apical 2-chamber view**

Doppler Echocardiography and Color Flow Imaging Findings
Systolic Function

Doppler stroke volume may be reduced due to the small LV cavity despite a normal EF

LVOT Obstruction

- Location of obstruction may be defined with color flow Doppler
  - Turbulent flow with aliasing
- Degree of obstruction may be assessed with CW Doppler
  - Characteristic late-peaking, dagger-shaped appearance
- Obstruction is dynamic in nature
  - No obstruction may be present at rest
  - Acquire peak gradient at rest and with provocation
    - Valsalva maneuver
    - Amyl nitrite
    - Squat-to-stand maneuver
  - Increased gradient may also be noted with a post-ectopic beat

Mitral Regurgitation (MR)

- Jet is typically directed posterolaterally if caused by SAM
- Presence of a central jet should prompt evaluation for intrinsic valve abnormalities (e.g., mitral valve prolapse, leaflet thickening, chordal rupture, endocarditis)
- Typically occurs after the onset of LVOT obstruction ("eject-obstruct-leak")
- High-velocity jet away from the apex is noted
  - May be confused with the LVOT velocity
  - Flow duration and Doppler spectral configuration may help to differentiate from LVOT obstruction
    - MR peak velocity is generally higher than the LVOT obstruction peak velocity due to the pressure gradient between the left atrium and the left ventricle
    - The LVOT velocity spectral display typically peaks in late systole
    - Duration of MR is longer
- Color M-mode may be utilized to determine the presence, duration and severity of mitral regurgitation
- MR should be evaluated with color flow to determine severity during provocative maneuvers that worsen LVOT obstruction

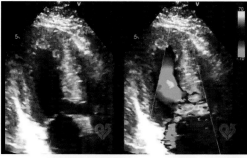

Figure 9.21: **Apical long-axis view of obstructive HCM with septal hypertrophy. Note the systolic anterior motion of the mitral apparatus, turbulent color flow in the LVOT due to obstruction, and the posteriorly directed mitral regurgitation.**

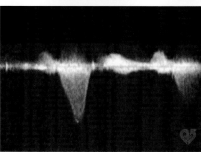
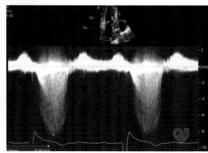

Figure 9.22: **Characteristic Doppler signal of LVOT obstruction compared with that of mitral regurgitation in the same patient with obstructive HCM.**

Diastolic Function

- Comprehensive assessment indicated
- Predominant abnormality is markedly impaired relaxation
- Relatively weak correlation between mitral inflow and pulmonary venous flow velocities and invasive parameters of LV diastolic function
- Variables to be evaluated in patients with HCM [4]
  - Average E/e' ratio (>14)
  - LA volume index (>34mL/m^2)
  - Pulmonary vein atrial reversal velocity (Ar-A duration >30 msec)
  - Peak velocity of TR jet by CW Doppler (>2.8 m/sec).
- Interpretation
  - If more than half of the variables meet cutoff values, then left atrial pressure (LAP) is elevated and grade II diastolic dysfunction is present
  - If <50% of the variables meet cutoff values, then LAP is normal and grade I diastolic dysfunction is present.
  - If 50% of the variables meet cutoff values, findings are inconclusive to estimate LAP
- In the presence of more than moderate MR, only Ar-A duration and peak velocity of TR jet are still valid

Echocardiography During and After Septal Reduction Procedures

Surgical Myectomy

- Pre-operative TEE determination of
  - Maximum septal wall thickness
  - Distance of maximum thickness from the aortic annulus
  - Presence/location of a contact lesion
  - Apical extent of the septal bulge
  - Further delineation of mitral valve and papillary muscle abnormalities for surgical decision-making
- Post-bypass TEE determination of residual
  - SAM/LVOT obstruction
  - Mitral regurgitation
- Post-operative TTE or TEE identification of
  - Complications/sequelae
    - Iatrogenic VSD
    - Unroofed septal perforator
    - Aortic regurgitation

Alcohol Septal Ablation

- Injection of alcohol into a proximal septal perforator branch of the left anterior descending coronary artery
- Produces a localized myocardial infarction of the thickened proximal ventricular septum
- Should result in reduced obstruction
- TTE is typically utilized during the procedure
- An ultrasound enhancement agent is used to visualize septal perforator distribution and guide administration of alcohol to the appropriate vessel
- Post-procedure evaluation
  - Presence of septal regional wall motion abnormalities (expected)
  - Residual severity of obstruction
  - Residual mitral regurgitation

Idiopathic Restrictive Cardiomyopathy (RCM)

Definition

- Idiopathic disorder
- May rarely be familial
- Diagnosis of exclusion
- Characterized by increased resistance to ventricular filling due to increased myocardial stiffness, decreased ventricular compliance, or both

Pathophysiology

- Non-dilated ventricle with normal wall thicknesses
- Stiff (non-compliant) ventricular walls result in severe diastolic dysfunction and restrictive filling with elevated filling pressures and dilated atria
- Typically normal ejection fraction

Clinical Presentation

- Symptoms of right and left heart failure
- Dyspnea
- Palpitations
- Fatigue
- Weakness
- Exercise intolerance

Physical Examination

- May be similar to that of constrictive pericarditis
- Jugular venous pressure is generally elevated with prominent y descent
- Peripheral edema
- LV apical impulse is typically normal

Cardiac Auscultation

- First and second heart sounds are typically normal
- S3 is frequently present due to abrupt cessation of the rapid ventricular filling phase
- Soft systolic murmurs of mitral and tricuspid regurgitation may be present

Ancillary Diagnostic Testing

- Electrocardiogram
  - Often nonspecific abnormalities
  - Atrial fibrillation
  - Conduction abnormalities
  - Ectopic atrial and ventricular beats
- Chest X-ray
  - Cardiomegaly secondary to atrial enlargement
  - Pulmonary venous congestion and pleural effusions
- Cardiac Magnetic Resonance Imaging (MRI)
  - May be used to assess myocardial fibrosis
  - May be used to determine other causes of restrictive physiology (e.g., sarcoidosis, amyloidosis, iron overload)
- Cardiac Catheterization
  - Right ventricular early diastolic dip and plateau (square root sign)

- Elevation with equalization of the following diastolic pressures: right atrial, right ventricular, pulmonary arterial, pulmonary capillary wedge and left ventricle
- Differentiate from constrictive physiology by lack of respiratory variation

• Endomyocardial biopsy may be considered

Medical Treatment

• Pharmacologic treatment of heart failure symptoms
- Beta blockers
- Calcium channel blockers
- Diuretics
- ACE inhibitors

Interventional/Surgical Treatment

• Pacemaker for advanced atrioventricular block
• Cardiac transplantation

M-mode/2D

• Normal left and right ventricular cavity size
• Preserved global systolic function (usually)
• Biatrial enlargement
• Dilated IVC
• Speckle-tracking echocardiography
- Reduced LV global longitudinal strain with better strain values in the basal segments

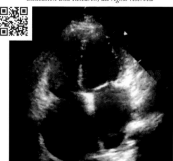

Figure 9.23: **RCM 4-chamber view**

Doppler Echocardiography and Color Flow Imaging Findings

• Diastolic dysfunction may vary
- Early in the disease – Grade I diastolic dysfunction with normal filling pressure or Grade II (pseudonormal)
- Later in the disease – Grade III (restrictive filling)

Hypereosinophilic Syndrome
Definition
- A hematologic disorder characterized by persistently elevated blood eosinophil counts (>6 months with >1500 eosinophils/mm^3) without an identifiable underlying etiology
- Both right and left heart cardiac involvement is common

Pathophysiology
- Necrotic Stage: Acute inflammatory stage with eosinophilic infiltration into the endomyocardium
- Thrombotic Stage: Thrombi may form on the affected portions of the endomyocardium and atrioventricular valves
- Fibrotic Stage: Endomyocardial fibrosis and scarring progresses; LV filling becomes restrictive

Ancillary Diagnostic Testing
- Electrocardiogram
    - Often nonspecific abnormalities
    - Atrial fibrillation
    - Conduction abnormalities
- Chest X-ray
    - Usually normal early in the disease
    - Cardiomegaly secondary to atrial enlargement (late)
    - Pulmonary venous congestion and pleural effusions (late)
- Cardiac Magnetic Resonance Imaging (MRI)
    - May be used to detect the presence of myocardial edema and/or fibrosis
    - May be used to detect thrombus
- Cardiac CT
    - Linear calcification (calcification of endocardial thrombus)
- Endomyocardial biopsy may be considered

Medical Treatment
- Corticosteroids
- Anticoagulation therapy

Surgical Treatment
- Valvular surgery
- Resection of the fibrous endocardium

M-mode/2D

- Global left ventricular systolic function is usually well preserved
- Apical obliteration by thrombus of the left ventricle, the right ventricle, or both
- Involvement of the posterior mitral and tricuspid valve leaflets, resulting in limited motion
- Biatrial dilatation
- Pericardial effusion

Doppler Echocardiography and Color Flow Imaging Findings

- Atrioventricular regurgitation due to valvular involvement and/or annular dilatation
- Restrictive physiology due to decreased compliance of affected myocardium
- Pulmonary hypertension due to elevated left-sided filling pressures

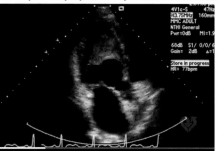

Figure 9.24: **Apical long-axis view showing apical obliteration of the left ventricle with thrombus and eosinophils**

Amyloidosis

Definition

- A multisystem disease with extracellular deposition of the amyloid protein in various tissues, which results in organ malfunction
- With cardiac disease progression, restrictive filling develops

Classification

Primary
- AL amyloidosis (light-chain)
- Most common type of cardiac amyloid
- Commonly involves extracardiac sites
    - Kidneys
    - Bone marrow
    - Tongue (macroglossia)
    - Gastric mucosa

Familial
- ATTR (amyloid transthyretin)
- Less common than AL amyloid
- Autosomal dominant disorder
- May be familial or wild-type mutation
- Common clinical features
    - Peripheral neuropathy
    - Carpal tunnel syndrome
    - Renal impairment
    - Autonomic dysfunction
    - Cardiomyopathy

Secondary (AA)
Associated with other inflammatory disorders (e.g., rheumatoid arthritis, tuberculosis, inflammatory bowel disease)

Senile
- Up to 25% of patients older than 80 years [15]
- Frequently confined to the heart

Pathophysiology
- Extracellular deposition of proteins
- Abnormal protein deposition leads to organ dysfunction
- Amyloid can also be found within the walls of intramural coronary arteries within the conduction system

Ancillary Diagnostic Testing
- Electrocardiogram
    - Atrial fibrillation
    - Conduction abnormalities
    - AL amyloid
        - Low QRS voltage
        - Pseudoinfarction pattern
- Chest X-ray
    - Pleural effusions and interstitial edema are common
- Cardiac Magnetic Resonance Imaging (MRI)
    - May be useful for tissue characterization
- Endomyocardial biopsy often required for diagnosis

Medical Treatment

- Aimed at reducing protein deposition
    - Prednisone
    - Melphalan
- Stem cell transplantation

Surgical Treatment

- Liver transplant with TTR amyloid
- Cardiac transplantation

M-mode/2D

- Increased LV and RV wall thickness
    - Increased wall thickness due to amyloid deposition, not hypertrophy
    - Typically concentric, although amyloid may mimic HCM with SAM and intracavitary obstruction
- Granular appearance of myocardium, although this may also be seen in patients without cardiac amyloid (e.g., chronic renal failure, HCM, hypertensive heart disease)
- Speckle-tracking echocardiography
    - Characteristic pattern with apical sparing
    - More sensitive than wall thickness
    - Apical longitudinal strain less than 14.5 % is associated with poor prognosis [16]
- Diffuse thickening of the cardiac valves and interatrial septum
- Normal to small LV cavity size
- With disease progression, ventricular systolic function worsens
- Biatrial enlargement due to elevated filling pressures
- Pericardial effusion (common)
- Intracardiac thrombi

Doppler Echocardiography and Color Flow Imaging Findings

- Multivalvular regurgitation with valvular involvement
- Diastolic function of varying degree
- With disease progression, ventricular diastolic function becomes restrictive
    - Deceleration time less than 150 msec associated with a poorer prognosis [17]

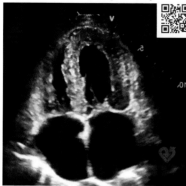

Figure 9.25: **Typical 2D appearance of cardiac amyloid**

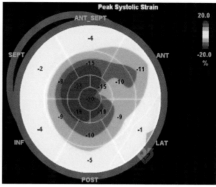

Figure 9.26: **Typical cardiac amyloid strain pattern with apical "sparing"**

Sarcoidosis

Definition

• Multisystem granulomatous disease of unknown cause
• More common in patient of Japanese or African-American descent
• Development of noncaseating granulomas in various tissues, including the lungs, lymph nodes, liver, spleen, skin, parotid glands and heart
• Most common involvement is pulmonary, which results in pulmonary hypertension and right-sided heart failure
• Pathologic cardiac involvement in 20 to 25% of patients, but only 5% of patients have symptomatic cardiac disease [18]
• May present clinically in young or middle-aged adults as high-grade AV block
• Ventricular arrhythmias are common and may result in sudden cardiac death

Pathophysiology

• Tissue fibrosis
• Can range from active granuloma to scar formation
• Conduction tissue may also be involved

Ancillary Diagnostic Testing

• Electrocardiogram
   - Complete heart block
   - Ventricular dysrhythmias
   - Pseudo-infarction pattern
• Chest X-ray
   - Typically normal

- Radionuclide Imaging
  - May reveal defects related to presence of scar or granulomas
- Cardiac Magnetic Resonance Imaging (MRI) and Positron Emission Tomography (PET)
  - May be useful for identification of edema (MRI) or disease activity (PET)
- Endomyocardial biopsy
  - May not be helpful due to patchy granulomatous involvement

Medical Treatment

- Corticosteroids
- Methotrexate

Interventional/Surgical Treatment:

- Permanent pacemaker
- Cardiac transplantation

M-mode/2D

- LV cavity normal or dilated
- LV systolic function may be preserved or reduced
- Regional wall motion abnormalities may not follow normal coronary distributions or may be present in the absence of coronary disease
- Ventricular septal thickness may be increased early in the disease
- Patchy LV wall thinning may be present later in the disease due to fibrosis
- Ventricular aneurysms, typically in the basal inferior and lateral walls

Doppler Echocardiography and Color Flow Imaging Findings

- LV diastolic dysfunction
  - Restrictive filling with advanced diseases
- Functional mitral regurgitation due to RWMA
- Pulmonary hypertension
  - Occurs frequently with pulmonary sarcoid, but may also be noted in the presence of restrictive LV filling

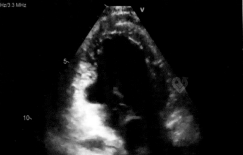

Figure 9.27: **Apical 2-chamber view of a patient with cardiac sarcoid. Note the small LV aneurysm in the mid-inferior wall.**

Hemochromatosis

Definition

- Iron storage disease that affects multiple organ and tissue systems
  - Most commonly the heart, liver, pancreas and pituitary gland
- May result in tissue damage and organ malfunction
- Typical onset is in the fifth or sixth decade of life
- Cardiac involvement typically noted in advanced disease

Types

- Primary (hereditary)
  - Autosomal recessive disorder
  - Abnormal increase in iron absorption
  - Men more commonly affected than women
- Secondary
  - Iron overload due to another disease or condition
    - Excess dietary iron
    - Multiple blood transfusions
    - Chronic liver disease

Pathophysiology

- Excessive intracellular deposition of iron
- Cardiac deposition most common in the subepicardial myocardium
- Results in a dilated cardiomyopathy with restrictive filling
- Severity of left ventricular dysfunction correlates with extent of myocardial iron deposition
- Most common cardiac presentation is heart failure

Ancillary Diagnostic Testing

- Serologic Testing
  - Elevated fasting transferrin saturation
  - Serum ferritin levels sensitive but non-specific for iron overload
- Electrocardiogram
  - Nonspecific repolarization abnormalities
  - Conduction abnormalities
  - Atrial fibrillation
  - First-degree atrioventricular block
- Chest X-ray
  - Cardiomegaly
  - Pleural effusions
- Cardiac Magnetic Resonance Imaging (MRI)

- Iron deposition detected by a reduction of myocardial signal intensity
• Genetic testing to evaluated for hereditary hemochromatosis

Medical Treatment

• Phlebotomy
• Iron chelating therapy
• Cardiomyopathy may be reversed with treatment

Surgical Treatment:

• Cardiac transplantation with or without liver transplantation

M-mode/2D

• Features of dilated cardiomyopathy
• LV cavity typically enlarged
• LV systolic function typically reduced
• Increased wall thickness may be seen early in the disease

Doppler Echocardiography and Color Flow Imaging Findings

• LV diastolic dysfunction
  - Restrictive filling with advanced disease
• Varying degrees of mitral and tricuspid regurgitation
• Pulmonary hypertension

References

1. Burkett EL, Hershberger RE. Clinical and genetic issues in familial dilated cardiomyopathy. Journal of the American College of Cardiology 45:969-981, 2005.

2. Hershberger RE, Cowan J, Morales A, Siegfried JD. Progress with genetic cardiomyopathies: screening, counseling, and testing in dilated, hypertrophic, and arrhythmogenic right ventricular dysplasia/cardiomyopathy. Circulation Heart Failure 2:253-261, 2009.

3. Lang et al, Recommendations for cardiac chamber quantification by echocardiography in adults: An Update from the American Society of Echocardiography and the European Association of Cardiovascular Imaging. J Am Soc Echocardiogr 28:1-39, 2015.

4. Nagueh SF et al. Recommendations for the Evaluation of Left Ventricular Diastolic Function by Echocardiography: An Update from the American Society of Echocardiography and the European Association of Cardiovascular Imaging. J Am Soc Echocardiogr 29:277-314, 2016.

5. Chin TK, Perloff JK, Williams RG, et al. Isolated noncompaction of left ventricular myocardium. A study of eight cases. Circulation 82:507–13, 1990.

6. Jenni R, Oechslin E, Schneider J, et al. Echocardiographic and pathoanatomical characteristics of isolated left ventricular non-compaction: a step towards classification as a distinct cardiomyopathy. Heart 86:666–71, 2001.

7. Stollberger C, Finsterer J, Blazek G. Left ventricular hypertrabeculation, noncompaction and association with additional cardiac abnormalities and neuromuscular disorders. Am J Cardiol 90:899–902, 2002.

8. Marcus FI, McKenna WJ, Sherrill D, et al. Diagnosis of arrhythmogenic right ventricular cardiomyopathy/dysplasia: proposed modification of the Task Force Criteria. European Heart Journal 31:806-814, 2010.

9. Yoerger DM, Marcus F, Sherrill D, et al. Echocardiographic findings in patients meeting task force criteria for arrhythmogenic right ventricular dysplasia: new insights from the multidisciplinary study of right ventricular dysplasia. J Am Coll Cardiol, 2005;45(6): 860-865.

10. Maron BJ, McKenna WJ, Danielson GK, Kappenberger LJ, Kuhn HJ, Seidman CE, et al. ACC/ESC clinical expert consensus panel on hypertrophic cardiomyopathy: a report of the American College of Cardiology Task Force on Clinical Expert Consensus Documents and the European Society of Cardiology Committee for Practice Guidelines (Committee to Develop an Expert Consensus Panel on Hypertrophic Cardiomyopathy). J Am Coll Cardiol 42:1687-713, 2003.

11. Nagueh SF, Bierig SM, Budoff MJ, et al. American Society of Echocardiography Clinical Recommendations for Multimodality Cardiovascular Imaging of Patients with Hypertrophic Cardiomyopathy. J Am Soc Echocardiogr 24:473-98, 2011.

12. Spirito P, Bellone P, Harris KM, Bernabo P, Bruzzi P, Maron BJ. Magnitude of left ventricular hypertrophy and risk of sudden death in hypertrophic cardiomyopathy. New England Journal of Medicine 342:1778-1785, 2000.

13. Geske JB, Bos JM, Gersh BJ, et al. Deformation patterns in genotyped patients with hypertrophic cardiomyopathy. Eur Heart J Cardiovasc Imaging 15(4):456-465, 2014.

14. Klarich KW, Attenhofer Jost CH, Binder J, et al. Risk of death in long-term follow-up of patients with apical hypertrophic cardiomyopathy. American Journal of Cardiology 111:1784-1791, 2013.

15. Pereira NL, Dec GW: Restrictive and Infiltrative Cardiomyopathies. In Cardiology. Philadelphia, Elsevier, 2010, pp. 1113-1124.

16. Ternacle J, et al. Causes and consequences of longitudinal LV dysfunction assessed by 2D strain echocardiography in cardiac amyloidosis. JACC: Cardiovascular Imaging 9: 126-138, 2016.

17. Klein AL, Hatle LK, Taliercio CP, Oh JK, Kyle RA, Gertz MA, Bailey KR, Seward JB, Tajik AJ. Prognostic significance of Doppler measures of diastolic function in cardiac amyloidosis. A Doppler echocardiography study. Circulation 83(3):808-16, 1991.

18. Pereira NL, Dec GW: Restrictive and Infiltrative Cardiomyopathies. In Cardiology. Philadelphia, Elsevier, 2010, pp. 1113-1124.

9

Cardiomyopathies / Select Systemic Diseases Resulting in Restrictive Physiology / Hemochromatosis

Cardiac Auscultation

- Harsh, systolic ejection murmur, crescendo-decrescendo in shape, best heard at the right upper sternal border, which may radiate into the carotid arteries
- Gallivardin's phenomenon (radiation of mitral regurgitation murmur to aortic area) may be present
- High-pitched, early diastolic decrescendo murmur heard best along the left sternal border (indicates aortic regurgitation)
- Early systolic ejection click (most commonly detected in bicuspid aortic valve)
- Soft, absent aortic component of S2
- Prominent S4 (indicates decreased left ventricular compliance) (common)
- S3 (left heart failure)

Electrocardiogram

- Left ventricular hypertrophy with ST segment depression and T wave inversion (strain pattern or systolic overload pattern)
- Left atrial enlargement
- Atrial fibrillation (uncommon: suggests coexisting mitral valve disease or seen late in course)
- Conduction defects (e.g., first degree AV block, left bundle branch block)

Chest X-ray/CMR/CT

- Left ventricular hypertrophy (rounding of left ventricular border)
- Left atrial enlargement (may indicate co-exsiting mitral valve disease)
- Post-stenotic dilatation of the ascending aorta (common feature) (CT may be useful)

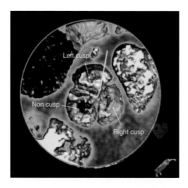 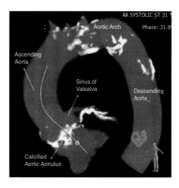

Figure 10.1: **Aortic valve calcification and root best seen with fluoroscopy/CT**

- CMR allows evaluation of peak velocity, pressure gradients, valve area, ventricular volumes, function and mass

10

Valvular Heart Disease / **Aortic Stenosis**

Cardiac Catheterization

- Determines the presence and severity of coronary artery disease (50% of adults will have concomitant coronary artery disease) (principal role)
- Determines peak-to-peak pressure gradient
- Determines mean transvalvular pressure gradient
- Determines aortic valve area by the Gorlin formula
- Transcatheter aortic valve replacement (TAVR) (percutaneous or transapical)
- Aortic valve balloon valvotomy (uncommon in adults)

Medical Treatment

- Rheumatic fever prophylaxis (when indicated)
- Digitalis/Diuretics (heart failure)
- ACE inhibitors/Nitrates/Beta blockers should be used with caution
- Cholesterol lowering drugs
- Cardioversion (atrial fibrillation)
- Activity should be limited in patients with significant stenosis
- Screening of first degree relatives (congenital aortic stenosis)

Surgical Treatment

- Surgical Aortic valve replacement (SAVR)
- TAVR
- Aortic balloon valvuloplasty (disappointing results in adults) (provides temporary relief ≤6 months)
- Ross procedure (pulmonic valve transplantation to aortic valve position, reimplantation of the coronary arteries and placement of a homograft in the pulmonary position)
- Aortic debridement (mechanical, ultrasonic) (rare due to development of significant aortic regurgitation post procedure)

Bicuspid Aortic Valve

M-mode

- Eccentric diastolic closure line of aortic valve leaflets
- Normal systolic valve opening may be present (especially in younger patients)

2D

- Thickened aortic valve leaflets (thickness increases with age)

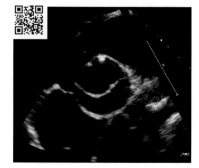

Figure 10.2: **Bicuspid Aortic Valve**

- Elliptical "football"-shaped opening (versus normal triangular-shaped systolic opening) of the aortic valve best seen in the parasternal/subcostal short-axis view of the aortic valve
- Systolic "doming" (best seen in parasternal long-axis view)
- Diastolic "doming" (aortic valve prolapse) (best seen in parasternal long-axis view)
- Eccentric diastolic closure line (best seen in parasternal long-axis view)
- Post-stenotic dilatation of the aorta (bicuspid aortic valve syndrome)
- Concentric left ventricular hypertrophy (may indicate significant aortic stenosis, coarctation and/or systemic hypertension) (normal IVSd and LVPWd: men 0.6 to 1.0cm; women 0.6cm to 0.9cm)
- Left ventricular dilatation (may indicate significant aortic regurgitation and/or left ventricular failure)
- Left atrial dilatation (may indicate decreased left ventricular compliance)
- Evaluate:
  - Aortic valve commissural attachment to the aorta in parasternal short-axis view of the aortic valve (two commissures attach to the aorta in bicuspid aortic valve instead of three) number of sinuses of Valsalva present (there may be only two sinuses instead of three in bicuspid aortic valve)
- Determine:
  - Anatomic aortic valve area by planimetry of the aortic valve orifice in the parasternal short-axis view of the aortic valve using 2D and 3D methods *(ASE Level 2 Recommendation)*
  - Left ventricular global and segmental systolic function presence and severity of possible coexisting lesions such as aortic regurgitation, coarctation of the aorta, ventricular septal defect, patent ductus arteriosus, aortic aneurysm, aortic dissection, infective endocarditis, and Shone's syndrome

Degenerative/Rheumatic (Inflammatory)
M-mode/2D
- Increased thickness with reduced systolic excursion of aortic valve leaflets
- Decreased systolic maximal aortic cusp separation
- Leaflet edge thickening, commissural fusion, systolic doming and coexisting mitral valve disease suggest rheumatic etiology
- Post-stenotic dilatation of the ascending aorta
- Left ventricular hypertrophy (suggests significant aortic stenosis, coarctation and/or systemic hypertension) (normal IVSd and LVPWd: men 0.6 to 1.0cm; women 0.6cm to 0.9cm)
- Increased left ventricular mass index (normal LV Mass Index: men 49 to 115g/m^2; women 43 to 95g/m^2)

- Decreased left ventricular global systolic function (suggests significant aortic regurgitation and/or left ventricular failure)
- Left atrial dilatation (may indicate decreased left ventricular compliance and/or coexisting mitral regurgitation)
- Mitral annular calcification
- Determine:
  - Anatomic aortic valve area by planimetry of the aortic valve orifice in the transthoracic short-axis view of the aortic valve *(ASE Level 2 Recommendation)*
  - Left ventricular global and segmental systolic function.

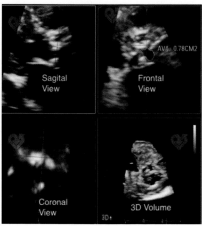

Figure 10.3: **3D TTE**

Doppler

- Determine:
  - Peak aortic valve velocity [1]
  - Peak instantaneous pressure gradient
  - Mean transvalvular pressure gradient *(ASE Level 1 Recommendation)* [1]
  - Aortic valve area (continuity equation) *(ASE Level 1 Recommendation)* [1]
  - Aortic valve area index or velocity ratio (LVOT$_{VTI}$ ÷ Aortic Valve$_{VTI}$) *(ASE Level 2 Recommendation)* [1]
  - Presence and severity of coexisting valvular regurgitation left ventricular stroke volume/stroke volume index, cardiac output, cardiac index
  - Grade of diastolic dysfunction
  - Left ventricular systolic pressure

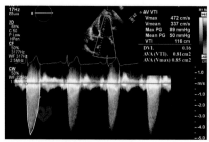

Figure 10.4: **Apical 5-chamber aortic valve CW Doppler**

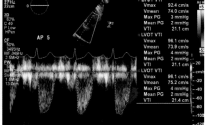

Figure 10.5: **Apical 5-chamber LVOT PW Doppler**

Table 10.1: **Evaluation of Aortic Stenosis** (ASE Recommendations) [1]

Level 1

- Aortic stenosis jet peak velocity
- Mean transaortic gradient
- Valve area by the continuity equation using VTI's

Table 10.2: **Aortic Stenosis Severity Scales** (ASE Recommendations) [1]

	Aortic sclerosis	Mild	Moderate	Severe
Peak velocity (m/s)	≤2.5m/s	2.6 to 2.9	3.0 to 4.0	≥4.0
Mean gradient (mmHg)	-	<20	20 to 40	≥40
AVA (cm^2)	-	>1.5	1.0 to 1.5	<1.0
Indexed AVA (cm^2/m^2)	-	>0.85	0.60 to 0.85	<0.6
Velocity ratio	-	>0.50	0.25 to 0.50	<0.25

Stress Echocardiography

With caution, low dose Dobutamine infusion may be used in patients where there is a thickened aortic valve, poor systolic function (EF <50%), low pressure gradients (mean pressure gradient <30 to 40mmHg), reduced aortic valve area (<1.0cm^2) and the question is if the valve excursion is decreased due to aortic stenosis valve excursion decreased due to aortic stenosis (low-flow, low-gradient aortic stenosis) or is there limited motion due to a low transaortic volume (e.g., "paradoxical" low flow, low gradient aortic stenosis – a "small" left ventricle which has a normal ejection fraction but a decreased volume due to hypertrophy) [1]

Table 10.3: **Dobutamine Stress Echo in Aortic Stenosis** (ASE Recommendations) [1]

Starting dobutamine dose of 2.5 to 5mcg/kg/min

Increase dose 2.5 to 5 mcg/kg/min every 3-5 minutes

Maximum dobutamine dose of 20mcg/kg/min

Infusion stopped when:

1) Maximum dobutamine dose reached (20 mcg/kg/min)

2) Positive result obtained

3) Heart rate rises 10 to 20 bpm over baseline or exceeds 100 bpm

4) Symptoms, blood pressure fall, or significant arrhythmias

Positive Result:

- An increase in effective AVA to a final valve area >1.0cm^2 suggests that stenosis is not severe.

- Severe stenosis is suggested by an AS jet velocity ≥4.0m/s or a mean gradient >30-40mmHg provided that valve area does not exceed 1.0cm^2 at any flow rate.

- Absence of contractile reserve (failure to increase stroke volume by >20%) is a predictor of a high surgical mortality and poor long-term outcome although valve replacement may improve LV function and outcome even in this subgroup.

Transesophageal Echocardiography

- Provides structural information in the patients in which transthoracic echocardiography cannot reliably quantify. The distal transgastric views are very useful in acquiring the continuous wave Doppler assessment of the aortic valve.

- TEE may provide adjunct information in patients with suspected aortic dissection, coarctation, discrete subaortic stenosis, left ventricular outflow tract tunnel, suspected infective endocarditis, or coexisting mitral valve disease.

- Planimeter the aortic valve in the aortic valve short-axis view (multiplane or 3D acquisition at aortic valve level 30 to 60° with slight retroflexion of the probe). Trace should occur at the aortic valve leaflet tips including the orifice within the commissures. *(ASE Recommendation)* [1]

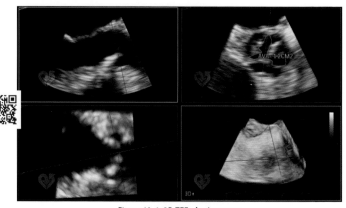

Figure 10.6: **3D TEE planimmetry**

- Useful during aortic valve balloon valvuloplasty in determining aortic valve annulus diameter, integrity of the aortic root, directing balloon placement, degree of disruption of the aortic valve leaflets, residual aortic regurgitation and ventricular systolic/diastolic function.

- Determine the end-diastolic diameter of the aortic annulus, sinuses of Valsalva and sinotubular junction for sizing of TAVR, aortic homograft, or stentless valve.

Important to Note

- Valvular aortic stenosis is initially a left ventricular pressure overload.

- Predominantly affects males (2:1).

- It has been suggested that valvular aortic stenosis may be due to age related degenerative changes as well as an active disease process. [4]

- LVOT is measured in a zoomed parasternal long axis view in mid systole using the inner edge to inner edge method parallel to the aortic valve plane. Some experts prefer to measure within 0.3 to 1.0cm of the valve orifice whereas others prefer the measurement at the aortic valve annulus (hinge points) level

- It is most important that the LVOT PW Doppler sample volume is placed at the same location as the measurement of the LVOT diameter

- Left ventricular systolic function is preserved by the development of concentric left ventricular hypertrophy

- Dilatation of the left ventricle does not occur until the contractile state of the myocardium is significantly depressed. [1]

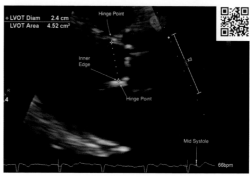

Figure 10.7: **LVOT measurement**

- Other causes of valvular aortic stenosis include severe familial hypercholesterolemia, diabetes, systemic lupus erythematosus, Pagets disease and ochronosis.

- Aortic sclerosis is present when there is aortic valve fibrosis/calcification without obstruction.

- If one aortic valve cusp is seen to move to the periphery (up against the aortic root wall) in either a long-axis or short-axis view, severe aortic stenosis is unlikely. Conversely, if aortic valve motion appears significantly reduced, severe aortic stenosis is most likely present (assuming preserved left ventricular global systolic function).

- Left ventricular intracavitary systolic gradients may be present in post-op aortic valve replacement for aortic stenosis patients. Patients with small, hypertrophied, hyperdynamic ventricles are most likely to have intracavitary gradients. Patients with intracavitary gradients post-op have a higher post-operative mortality and may be treated with volume loading or afterload reduction.

- The aortic valve should be examined from several windows (e.g., apical, right parasternal, suprasternal, supraclavicular, subcostal, left parasternal) with CW Doppler to confirm that the ultrasound beam is parallel to flow; this ensures that the highest velocity across the aortic valve is obtained. A minimum of three windows using a Pulsed Echo Doppler Flow (PEDOF) (dedicated CW Doppler) probe are required for laboratory accreditation.

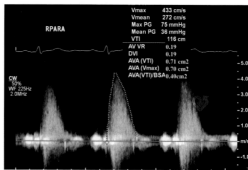

Figure 10.8: **Right parasternal CW Doppler (PEDOF)**

- it has been demonstrated that asymptomatic patients are unlikely to develop symptoms due to aortic stenosis over the next five years with an aortic jet velocity of <3.0 m/s, while those with a jet velocity of >4.0m/s have a 50% likelihood of symptom onset or death within two years. Those with a jet velocity between 3 and 4m/s have an intermediate likelihood of symptom onset. [4]

- Cardiac catheterization measures the peak-to-peak gradient, while Doppler determines the peak maximum instantaneous pressure gradient. To confirm the Doppler results, compare the mean gradient and aortic valve area with the catheterization findings. They should be nearly equal.

- The phenomena of pressure recovery may result in a discrepancy between the cardiac Doppler determined transvalvular pressure gradient and the pressure gradient determined by cardiac catheterization. Cardiac Doppler determines the pressure gradient at the vena contracta (location of the smallest flow area and the highest velocity). Beyond the vena contracta flow becomes turbulent and the pressure increases distal to the vena contracta. Cardiac catheterization may inadvertently place the catheter distal to the vena contracta therefore measuring a lower pressure gradient. This discrepancy is important especially in patients with small aortic roots (<2.9cm at the sinuses of Valsalva and <2.30cm at the sinotubular junction) and moderate pressure gradients.

- Evaluate left ventricular global systolic function. It has a direct effect on the peak velocity and pressure gradients of the aortic valve.

- Significant mitral regurgitation and/or significant mitral stenosis may affect the peak aortic valve velocity by reducing forward flow across the aortic valve.

- When aortic regurgitation is severe, determine the aortic valve area. Significant aortic regurgitation increases velocity across the aortic valve, causing stenosis to be overestimated.

- Be careful not to confuse mitral regurgitation with the aortic stenosis jet. Mitral regurgitation is longer in duration because there is no flow during the isovolumic contraction or isovolumic relaxation period through the aortic valve. In addition, mitral regurgitation usually has a greater velocity than aortic stenosis because the pressure gradient between the left ventricle and aorta is less than that between the left ventricle and left atrium.

- When utilizing a suprasternal or right supraclavicular continuous wave Doppler recording position, be careful not to confuse the returning high velocity signal with peripheral vascular disease such as subclavian artery stenosis.

- An asymmetric triangular contour with an early peaking of the jet usually indicates mild aortic stenosis.

- Symmetric and rounded velocity contour with a late peaking jet velocity (peak >50% of total ejection time) is usually seen in severe aortic stenosis.

- To evaluate whether a bicuspid aortic valve is present, use the parasternal short-axis view of the aortic valve and evaluate the valve during systole. A "raphe" (an underdeveloped aortic cusp) may give the appearance of three leaflets during diastole.

- A bicuspid AOV most commonly arises from fusion of the right and left coronary cusps (>80%) [4]

- It may be difficult to differentiate a bicuspid aortic valve from acquired aortic stenosis. Aortic stenosis due to a bicuspid aortic valve usually becomes symptomatic at age 20 to 50, while calcific aortic stenosis occurs in the elderly.

- The average rate of increase in aortic stenosis peak velocity is 0.32 ± 0.34m/s per year, an increase in the mean pressure gradient of 7 ± 7mmHg per year and a decrease in aortic valve area of 0.12 ± 0.19cm^2 per year. [4]

Table 10.4: **Criteria That Increase the Likelihood of Severe AS in Patients with AVA <1.0cm^2 and Mean Gradient <40mmHg in the Presence of Preserved EF** *(ASE Recommendations)* [1]		
1. Critical criteria		
• Physical examination consistent with severe aortic stenosis		
• Typical symptoms without other explanation		
• Elderly patient (>70 years)		
2. Qualitative imaging data		
• LVH (additional history of hypertension to be considered)		
• Reduced LV longitudinal function without other explanation		
3. Quantitative imaging data		
• Mean gradient 30 to 40mmHg*		
• AVA ≤0.8cm^2		
• Doppler technique (LVOT measurement by 3D TEE, MSCT, CMR, or Invasive data)		
• Calcium score by MSCT [a]		
• Severe AS likely:	Men ≥2000	Women ≥1200
• Severe AS very likely:	Men ≥3000	Women ≥1600
• Severe AS unlikely:	Men <1600	Women <800

AS = aortic stenosis; AVA = aortic valve area; CMR = cardiac magnetic resonance imaging; EF = ejection fraction; LVOT = left ventricular outflow tract; MSCT = multislice computed tomography; SVI = stroke volume index; TEE = transesophageal echocardiography.

* Hemodynamics measured when the patient is normotensive

a) Values are given in arbitrary units using Agatston method for quantification of valve calcification

10

Valvular Heart Disease / **Aortic Stenosis** / Degenerative/Rheumatic (Inflammatory)

Table 10.5: Data Recording and Measurements for Aortic Stenosis Quantitation
(ASE Recommendations) [1]

Recording	Measurement
LVOT Diameter	
• 2D parasternal long-axis view • Zoom mode • Adjust gain to optimize the blood tissue interface	• Inner edge to inner edge • Mid-systole • Parallel and adjacent to the aortic valve or at the site of velocity measurement • Diameter is used to calculate a circular CSA
LVOT Velocity	
• Pulsed-wave Doppler • Apical 5-chamber or long-axis view • Sample volume positioned just on LV side of valve and moved carefully into the LVOT if required to obtain laminar flow curve • Velocity baseline and scale adjusted to maximize size of velocity curve • Time axis (sweep speed) increase to 50 to 100mm/sec • Low wall filter setting • Smooth velocity curve with a well-defined peak and a narrow velocity range at peak velocity	• Maximum velocity from peak of dense velocity curve • VTI traced from modal velocity
AS Jet Velocity	
• CW Doppler (dedicated transducer) • Multiple acoustic windows (e.g., apical, suprasternal, right parasternal) • Decrease gains, increase wall filter, adjust baseline, and scale to optimize signal • Time axis (sweep speed) 100mm/sec • Gray scale spectral display with expanded time scale • Velocity range and baseline adjusted so velocity signal fits but fills the vertical scale	• Maximum velocity at peak of dense velocity curve • Avoid noise and fine linear signals • VTI traced from outer edge of dense signal curve • Mean gradient calculated from traced velocity curve • Report window where maximum velocity obtained
Valve Anatomy	
• Parasternal long- and short-axis views • Zoom mode	• Identify number of cusps in systole, raphe if present • Assess cusp mobility and commissural fusion • Assess valve calcification

Table 10.6: Resolution of Discrepancies in the Evaluation of Aortic Stenosis *(ASE Recommendations)* [1]

AS Velocity >4m/s and AVA >1.0cm^2

1. Check LVOT diameter measurement and compare with previous studies
2. Check LVOT velocity signal for flow acceleration
3. Calculate indexed AVA when
   a. Height is <135cm (5'5")
   b. BSA <1.5 m^2
   c. BMI <22 (equivalent to 55 kg or 120 lb at this height)
4. Evaluate AR severity
5. Evaluate for high cardiac output
   a. LVOT stroke volume
   b. LV EF and stroke volume

Likely causes: high output state, moderate-severe AR, large body size

AS Velocity ≤4m/s and AVA ≤1.0cm^2

1. Check LVOT diameter measurement and compare with previous studies
2. Check LVOT velocity signal for distance from valve
3. Calculate indexed AVA when
   a. Height is <135cm (5'5")
   b. BSA <1.5 m^2
   c. BMI <22 (equivalent to 55 kg or 120 lb at this height)
4. Evaluate for low transaortic flow volume
   a. LVOT stroke volume (e.g., reduced ejection fraction, "paradoxical"– normal ejection fraction with "small" hypertrophied left ventricle)
   b. LV EF and stroke volume (e.g., reduced ejection fraction, "paradoxical"– normal ejection fraction with "small" hypertrophied left ventricle)
   c. MR severity
   d. Mitral stenosis
5. When EF <55%
   a. Assess degree of valve calcification
   b. Consider Dobutamine stress echocardiography

Likely causes: low cardiac output, small body size, severe MR

Table 10.7: **Aortic Stenosis Classifications (Tracks)**

High Gradient ("Easy") Track

- Peak aortic valve velocity $\geq$4m/s and a mean pressure gradient $\geq$40mmHg:

  - Indicates severe high gradient aortic stenosis in the presence of normal flow (Stroke volume index $\geq$35mL/m^2) or low flow (Stroke volume index <35mL/m^2), normal ejection fraction or abnormal ejection fraction

  - Exclude high flow states (Stroke volume index $\geq$58mL/m^2) (e.g., significant aortic regurgitation, anemia, hyperthyroidism, arteriovenous shunts) If high flow state is present determine reason and if reversible

  - If not reversible (e.g., significant aortic regurgitation, hemodialysis) – Severe aortic stenosis

  - If reversible (e.g., anemia, hyperthyroidism, arteriovenous shunts) – Re-assess at restored normal flow

Low Gradient ("Difficult") Track

- Peak aortic valve velocity <4m/s and a mean pressure gradient <40mmHg and an AVA >1.0cm^2: Moderate AS (assumes accurate measurements)

- Peak aortic valve velocity <4m/s and a mean pressure gradient <40mmHg: AVA $\leq$1.0cm^2

  - Exclude measurement errors

  - Determine stroke volume index (SVI)

    - If SVI $\geq$35mL/m^2 – Severe AS is unlikely

    - If SVI <35mL/m^2 – Determine ejection fraction (EF)

      - Reduced EF (<50%) – Dobutamine stress test indicated

      - Normal EF ($\geq$50%) – Most challenging group – Use integrated approach (e.g., review measurements, evaluate extent of calcification

References

1. Baumgartner H, Hung J, Bermejo J, Chambers J, Edvardsen T, Goldstein S, Lancellotti P, LeFevre M, Miller F: Recommendations on the Echocardiographic Assessment of Aortic Valve Stenosis: A Focused Update from the European Association of Cardiovascular Imaging and the American Society of Echocardiography. Journal of the American Society of Echocardiography 30: 372-92, 2017

2. Lancellotti P, Pellikka PA, Budts, W, Chaudhry FA, Donal E, Dulgheru R, Edvardsen T, Garbi M, Won Ha J, Kane GC, Kreeger J, Mertens L, Pibarot P, Picano E, Ryan T, Tsutsui J, Varga A: The Clinical Use of Stress Echocardiography in Non-Ischaemic Heart Disease: Recommendations from the European Association of Cardiovascular Imaging and the American Society of Echocardiography. Journal of the American Society of Echocardiography 30: 101-38, 2017

3. Feigenbaum H, Armstrong WF, Ryan T: Aortic Valve Disease. Feigenbaum's Echocardiography. Philidelphia, LW&W, 2005, 271-288

4. Otto, K. Valvular Stenosis. Textbook of Clinical Echocardiography. Philidelphia, Saunders, 2013, 271-289

Valvular Heart Disease
Aortic Regurgitation
Alicia Armour, MA, BS, ACS, RDCS, FASE

Definition

The backflow of blood through the aortic valve during diastole; may be acute or chronic.

Etiology

American Society of Echocardiography Recommendations[1]

- Congenital/leaflet abnormalities
  - Bicuspid
  - Unicuspid
  - Quadricuspid aortic valve
  - Ventricular septal defect
- Acquired leaflet abnormalities
  - Senile calcification
  - Infective endocarditis
  - Rheumatic disease
  - Radiation-induced valvulopathy
  - Toxin-induced valvulopathy: anorectic drugs, 5-hydroxytryptamine (carcinoid)

- Congenital/genetic aortic root abnormalities
  - Annuloaortic ectasia
  - Connective tissue disease: Loeys Deitz, Ehlers-Danlos, Marfan syndrome, osteogenesis imperfecta
- Acquired aortic root abnormalities
  - Idiopathic aortic root dilatation
  - Systemic hypertension
  - Autoimmune disease: systemic lupus erythematosis, ankylosing spondylitis, Reiter's syndrome
  - Aortitis: syphilitic, Takayasu's arteritis
  - Aortic dissection
  - Trauma

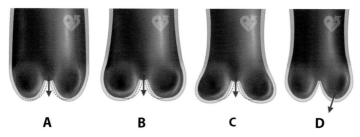

A   **B**   **C**   **D**

Figure 10.9: **Type I. Normal cusp motion with aortic dilation or cusp perforation**

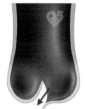

Figure 10.10: **Type II. Cusp prolapse**

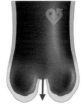

Figure 10.11: **Type III. Cusp restriction**

Suggested classification of aortic regurgitation morphology, depicting the various mechanisms of aortic regurgitation.

- **Type Ia** – Sinotubular junction enlargement and dilatation of the ascending aorta
- **Type Ib** – Dilatation of the sinuses of Valsalva and sinotubular junction
- **Type Ic** – Dilatation of the ventriculoarterial junction (annulus). Type Id denotes aortic cusp perforation.

History

- Heart failure (dyspnea, orthopnea, paroxysmal nocturnal dyspnea, fatigue, cough, weight gain)
- Chest pain (angina pectoris) prominent late in course
- Syncope (uncommon)
- Right heart failure (e.g., jugular venous distention, hepatomegaly, peripheral edema, ascites, anasarca)
- Pulmonary edema (suggests acute aortic regurgitation)

Physical Examination

- Wide pulse pressure (>50% of peak systolic pressure or diastolic blood pressure <50mmHg may indicate significant regurgitation)
- Bounding peripheral pulses (e.g., Corrigan's pulse, Quincke's pulse, de Musset's sign, Müller sign, Traube's sign, Duroziez's sign, pistol-shot pulse, Rosenbach's sign, Gerhardt's sign, Landolfi's sign) (peripheral signs not present in acute aortic regurgitation)
- Displaced, hyperdynamic left ventricular impulse

Cardiac Auscultation

- A high-pitched, blowing, diastolic decrescendo murmur heard best with the diaphragm of the stethoscope along the left sternal border (suggests aortic valve disease) and/or right sternal border (suggests aortic root dilatation) with the patient sitting upright, leaning forward with held in deep exhalation
- An Austin Flint murmur, associated with severe aortic regurgitation and described as a low-pitched mid to late diastolic rumble at the cardiac apex
- Musical, "cooing dove" diastolic murmur (associated with aortic valve perforation/prolapse due to infective endocarditis)
- Systolic ejection murmur secondary to increased flow volume across the aortic valve
- Systolic ejection click (dilated aorta or bicuspid aortic valve)
- Soft S1 (premature mitral valve closure)
- S3
- S4 (suggests left ventricular hypertrophy in chronic/absent in acute)

Electrocardiogram

- Left ventricular hypertrophy (80 to 85%) with ST segment elevation and peaked T waves (diastolic overload pattern) or ST segment depression with T wave inversion (strain pattern or systolic overload pattern)
- Left atrial enlargement/atrial fibrillation (uncommon until late in course/if early may indicate coexisting mitral valve disease)
- Arrhythmias (ventricular ectopy, ventricular tachycardia)
- PR interval prolongation (late stages; inflammatory process)
- Sinus tachycardia (acute aortic regurgitation)
- Atrioventricular block (suggests acute aortic regurgitation due to infective endocarditis)

Chest X-ray/CMR/CT

- Cardiomegaly due to left ventricular dilatation (cor bovinum)
- Dilatation of the ascending aorta (suggests Marfan's, Ehlers-Danlos, aortic valve stenosis, aortic dissection)
- Widened mediastinum suggests aortic dissection
- Aortic valve calcification (suggests valvular aortic stenosis)
- Egg shell calcification confined to the ascending aorta (syphilitic aortitis)
- Pulmonary edema (acute aortic regurgitation)
- CMR allows determination of regurgitant volume, effective regurgitant orifice, ventricular volumes, ventricular function and ventricular mass, indicated if TTE is suboptimal. Discordance between echo and Doppler findings, discordance between clinical findings and severity of aortic regurgitation by echocardiography, bicuspid aortic valve and the morphology of the aortic sinuses, sinotubular junction or ascending aorta (at least 4cm above the aortic plane) cannot be assessed or in setting of multivalvular regurgitation when echocardiographic assessment may be challenging.

Cardiac Catheterization

- Coronary arteriography (primary role)
- Supravalvular aortography allows assessment of presence, etiology and severity (improved with Valsalva maneuver)

Medical/Surgical Treatment

- Beta blockers (e.g., Marfan syndrome, Ehlers-Danlos)
- Vasodilator therapy (e.g., hydralazine, nifedipine, ACE inhibitors)
- Antiarrhythmic (atrial fibrillation, bradyarrhythmias)
- Digitalis and/or diuretics for heart failure
- Sodium nitroprusside/Dobutamine (acute aortic regurgitation)
- Avoidance of isometric exercise, competitive sports, heavy physical exertion (moderate or greater aortic regurgitation)

• Aortic valve repair or replacement (with aortic root replacement when indicated) for significant chronic aortic regurgitation:

  - Acute aortic regurgitation (hemodynamic instability)
  - Symptomatic with normal EF (>50%)
  - Asymptomatic with EF <50%
  - Asymptomatic with normal EF (≥50%), but with severe LV dilatation (>50mm LVESD)
  - Asymptomatic with EF ≥50% but with progressive LVEDD >65mm if low surgical risk

M-mode

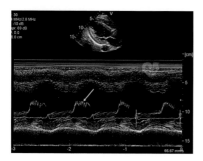 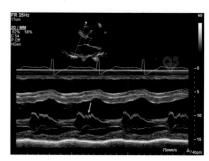

Figure 10.12: **Fine Diastolic Flutter of the Mitral Valve**

• Fine diastolic flutter of the anterior mitral valve leaflet (90%), posterior mitral valve leaflet, chordae tendineae, papillary muscle and/or the interventricular septum (50%)

• Premature closure of the mitral valve (defined as the C point of the mitral valve occurring on or before the onset of the QRS complex)* (indicates increased left ventricular end-diastolic pressure (LVEDP))

• Premature opening of the aortic valve is defined as occurring when the aortic valve opens on or before the onset of the QRS complex. Associated with severe acute aortic regurgitation and indicates increased LVEDP

• Color M-mode demonstrates the timing and thickness of the aortic regurgitation jet

• Color M-mode may be helpful in detecting the presence, timing and duration of diastolic flow reversal in the descending thoracic aorta/abdominal aorta (holodiastolic flow reversal may indicate significant aortic regurgitation)

2D

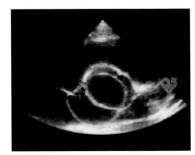

Figure 10.13: **Bicuspid Aortic Valve**

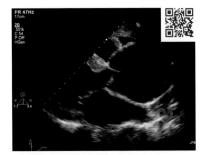

Figure 10.14: **Ascending Aortic Aneurysm**

- Anatomic basis for the presence of aortic regurgitation (e.g., ascending aortic aneurysm, bicuspid aortic valve, aortic valve vegetation)
- Incomplete closure of the aortic valve cusps (≥2mm) as seen on the parasternal short-axis view of the aortic valve
- Reverse "doming" of the anterior mitral valve leaflet is associated with severe aortic regurgitation
- Left ventricular volume overload pattern (left ventricular dilatation with hyperkinesis)
- Globular, spherical-shaped left ventricle suggests eccentric hypertrophy
- Left ventricular dilatation with decreased systolic function late in course. Normal: men LVIDd 4.2 to 5.8cm; women 3.8 to 5.2cm
- Left atrial dilatation late in course or due to coexisting mitral valve disease. Normal LA volume: ≤34mL/m^2
- 3D validates ventricular volumes, ventricular function, measurement of vena contracta, PISA
- Determine:
  - Left ventricular mass index
    Normal LV Mass Index: men 49 to 115g/m^2; female 43 to 95g/m^2
  - Left ventricular dimensions, fractional shortening, end-diastolic and end-systolic volumes, ejection fraction and presence of segmental wall motion abnormalities, global longitudinal strain (GLS)

PW Doppler

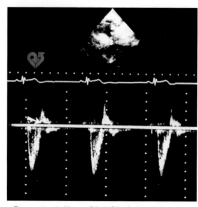

Figure 10.15: **Normal Brief Early Diastolic Flow Reversal in the Descending Thoracic Aorta**

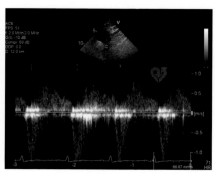

Figure 10.16: **Abnormal Holodiastolic Flow Reversal in the Descending Thoracic Aorta**

- Holodiastolic flow reversal in the descending thoracic aorta (velocity ≥20cm/s may indicate significant aortic regurgitation)
- Holodiastolic flow reversal detected in the abdominal aorta may indicate severe aortic regurgitation
- Increased left ventricular outflow tract velocity and velocity time integral due to increased flow volume
- Determine regurgitant volume and regurgitant fraction

CW Doppler

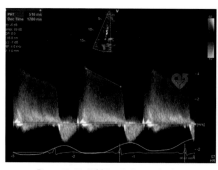

Figure 10.17: **Mild Aortic Regurgitation**

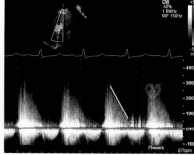

Figure 10.18: **Severe Aortic Regurgitation**

- Jet density (spectral strength) indicates severity
- Determine:
    - Pressure half-time of the aortic regurgitation spectral display (mild >500 msec; severe <200 msec)
    - Slope of the aortic regurgitation spectral display. In general, the steeper the slope, the more severe the aortic regurgitation; a slope of 3m/s^2 may indicate significant aortic regurgitation

- Effective regurgitant orifice area
- Left ventricular end-diastolic pressure (LVEDP)

Color Flow Doppler

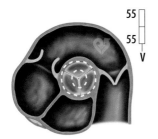

Figure 10.19: **AR Jet Area/LVOT Area Ratio**

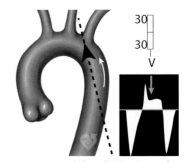

Figure 10.20: **Holodiastolic Flow Reversal in Descending Thoracic Aorta**

- Determine:
  - Blood pressure, appropriate color gain settings, velocity scale settings (50 to 70cm/s)
  - Jet width/LVOT width ratio in the parasternal long-axis view (mild <25%; severe ≥65%)
  - Vena contracta width (mild <0.3cm; severe >0.6cm)
  - Holodiastolic flow reversal in the descending thoracic aorta and/ or abdominal aorta indicates aortic regurgitation is significant. May also be detected by PW/CW Doppler and color M-mode

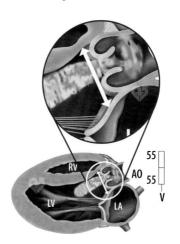

  - Regurgitant volume and effective regurgitant orifice area by the PISA method

Figure 10.21: **AR Jet Width /LVOT Width Ratio**

  - Jet CSA/LVOT CSA in the parasternal short-axis view of the aortic valve (mild <5%; moderate 5 to 20%; moderately severe 21 to 59%; severe ≥60%)
  - Jet direction, eccentric or central, in the parasternal long-axis view (eccentric jet implies aortic valve prolapse, central jet implies aortic root dilatation or restricted valve motion such as in aortic valve stenosis or valve perforation)

Transesophageal Echocardiography

- Test of choice in aortic dissection
- Primary use is to determine the etiology of aortic regurgitation (e.g., infective endocarditis)
- Severe mitral annular calcification or mitral prosthetic valve may make it difficult to evaluate aortic regurgitation due to the artifact of flow masking

Important to Note

- Significant chronic aortic regurgitation is a left ventricular volume overload
- Significant acute aortic regurgitation is a left ventricular pressure overload
- Systolic aortic regurgitation may occur in patients with continuous flow LVAD, cardiac arrhythmias (e.g., atrial fibrillation), Damus-Kaye-Stansel surgery, and heart failure
- In patients with significant chronic aortic regurgitation, carefully evaluate left ventricular dimensions, volumes, and global systolic function
- In patients with severe acute aortic regurgitation, note the presence or absence of premature closure of the mitral valve (M-mode), premature opening of the aortic valve (M-mode) and/or a mitral valve deceleration time <140 msec with increased E/A ratio (PW Doppler) (suggests increased left ventricular end-diastolic pressure (LVEDP))
- Causes for holodiastolic flow reversal in the descending thoracic aorta include severe aortic regurgitation, patent ductus arteriosus, aortopulmonary window, ruptured sinus of Valsalva aneurysm, aorta-LV tunnel, cerebral arteriovenous fistula, and upper extremity dialysis shunt
- It is important to always identify the reason for the presence of aortic regurgitation (e.g., aortic valve pathology, ascending aorta disease, infective endocarditis, discrete subaortic stenosis (DSS), outlet VSD, perimembranous VSD, supravalvular aortic stenosis)
- Aortic regurgitation is rare (<1%) in young individuals (<40 years of age) and presence increases with age (10 to 20%) in older individuals (>60 years of age)

Table 10.8: Classification of Aortic Regurgitation Severity (ASE Recommendations) [1]	
Specific Criteria for Mild AR	**Specific Criteria for Severe AR**
• Abnormal or normal leaflets	• Abnormal/flail leaflets, or wide coaptation defect
• Vena contracta width <0.3cm	• Vena contracta width >0.6cm
• Central Jet, width <25% of LVOT	• Central Jet, width ≥65% of LVOT
• Small or no flow convergence	• Large flow convergence
• Soft or incomplete jet by CW	• Dense jet by CW
• PHT Slow, >500 msec	• PHT Steep, <200 msec
• Brief, early diastolic flow reversal in the descending aorta	• Prominent holodiastolic flow reversal in the descending aorta
• Normal LV size	• Usually dilated LV size
≥4 criteria definitely mild (quantification not needed)	≥4 criteria definitely severe (may still quantitate)

Table 10.9: Classification of Aortic Regurgitation Severity (*ASE Recommendations*) [1]

	AR severity		
	Mild	**Moderate**	**Severe**
Structural parameters			
Aortic leaflets		Normal or abnormal	Abnormal/flail, or wide coaptation defect**
LV size	**Normal***	Normal or dilated	Usually dilated [a]
Qualitative Doppler			
Jet width in LVOT, color flow	Small in central jets**	Intermediate	Large in central jets**; variable in eccentric jets
Flow convergence, color flow	None or very small**	Intermediate	Large
Jet density, CW	Incomplete or faint**	Dense	Dense
Jet deceleration rate, CW (PHT, msec) [b]	Incomplete or faint Slow, >500	Medium, 500 to 200	Steep, <200**
Diastolic flow reversal in descending aorta, PW	Brief, early diastolic reversal**	Intermediate	Prominent holodiastolic reversal**
Semiquantitative parameters			
VCW (cm)	<0.3	0.3-0.6	>0.6
Jet width/LVOT width, central jets (%)	<25	25 to 45 / 46 to 64	≥65
Jet CSA/LVOT CSA, central jets (%)	<5	5 to 20 / 21 to 59	≥60
Quantitative parameters			
RVol (mL/beat)	<30	30 to 44 / 45 to 59	≥60
RF (%)	<30	30 to 39 / 40 to 49	≥50
EROA (cm^2)	<0.10	0.10 to 0.19 / 0.20 to 0.29	≥0.30

PHT, Pressure half-time; PW, pulsed wave Doppler.

** Qualitative and semiquantitative signs are considered specific for their AR grade. Color Doppler usually performed at a Nyquist limit of 50 to 70cm/s.

*Unless there are other reasons for LV dilation.

a) Specific in normal LV function, in absence of causes of volume overload. Exception: acute AR, in which chambers have not had time to dilate.

b) PHT is shortened with increasing LV diastolic pressure and may be lengthened in chronic adaptation to severe AR

c) Quantitative parameters can subclassify the moderate regurgitation group.

10

Valvular Heart Disease / **Aortic Regurgitation**

Referernces

1. Zoghbi WA, Adams DB, Bonow RO, Enriquez-Sarano M, Foster E, Grayburn PA, Hahn RT, Han Y, Hung J, Lang RM, Little SH, Shah DJ, Shernan S, Thavendiranathan P, Thomas JD: Recommendations for Noninvasive Evaluation of Native Valvular Regurgitation A Report from the American Society of Echocardiography Developed in Collaboration with the Society for Cardiovascular Magnetic Resonance. J Am Soc Echocardiogr 30:305-371, 2017.

2. Nishimura RA, Otto CM, Bonow RO, Carabello BA, Erwin JP 3rd, Guyton RA, et al.: 2014 AHA/ACC Guideline for the Management of Patients with Valvular Heart Disease: A Report of the American College of Cardiology/American Heart Association Task Force on Practice Guidelines. J Am Coll Cardiol 63:2438-88, 2014.

3. Lancellotti P, Tribouilloy C, Hagendorff A, Moura L, Popescu BA, Agricola E, Monin J-L, Pierard LA, Badano L, Zamorano JL: European Association of Echocardiography Recommendations for the Assessment of Valvular Regurgitation. Part 1: Aortic and Pulmonary Regurgitation (Native Valve Disease). Eur J Echocardiogr 11:223-244, 2010.

4. Lang RM, Badano LP, Mor-Avi V, Afilalo J, Armstrong A, Ernande L, Flachskampf FA, Foster E, Goldstein SA, Kuznetsova T, Lancellotti P, Muraru D, Picard MH, Rietzschel ER, Rudski L, Spencer KT, Tsang W, Voigt J-U: Recommendations for Cardiac Chamber Quantification by Echocardiography in Adults:

5. Recommendations for Cardiac Chamber Quantification by Echocardiography in Adults: An Update from the American Society of Echocardiography and the European Association of Cardiovascular Imaging. J Am Soc Echocardiogr 28:1-39, 2015.

Valvular Heart Disease
Mitral Regurgitation (MR)
Brad Roberts, BS, ACS, RCS, RDCS, FASE

Definition

The backward flow of blood from the left ventricle (LV) through the mitral valve (MV) and into the left atrium (LA) during ventricular systole; may be acute, chronic, or intermittent and vary in duration and timing in the systolic cardiac cycle (early, late, or holosystolic); etiology may be categorized as Primary (degenerative), Secondary (functional) or Mixed.

Etiology

American College of Cardiology Recommendations

• When MR is detected, the first task at hand is to meticulously evaluate the entire MV complex — including left ventricular (LV) size and function, papillary muscles, chordae tendineae, all segments of both leaflets, and MV annulus – to determine the underlying cause, or etiology, of the regurgitation.

• The etiology, along with the Carpentier classification, should be defined and clearly stated in the echocardiography report.

• In addition to etiology, other important goals of echocardiography include assessment of LA size (volume), estimation of right ventricular systolic pressure (RVSP) and confirming MR severity through a composite of echo Doppler parameters.

Table 10.10: **Mitral Regurgitation Etiology**	
Primary MR	(Degenerative, etiology isolated to part(s) of valvular complex only)
MV myxomatous changes	Prolapse (most common), flail, ruptured or elongated chordae
Papillary muscle rupture	Secondary to coronary ischemia or physical trauma
Degenerative changes	Calcification, thickening of valve components
Infectious	Endocarditis resulting in destructive vegetations, leaflet perforation or aneurysm
Inflammatory	Rheumatic, collagen vascular disease, radiation, adverse medical side effects
Congenital	Cleft leaflet, parachute MV (both very rare)
Secondary MR	(Functional, etiology due to ventricular dilation or segmental wall motion abnormality)
Ischemic	Secondary to coronary artery disease, especially posteroinferior LV territories
Nonischemic	Dilated, viral or idiopathic cardiomyopathy
Annular dilatation	Atrial fibrillation, restrictive cardiomyopathy
Mixed	Primary and secondary etiologies may coexist (e.g. ischemic cardiomyopathy and new ruptured chordae)

Carpentier Classification of Mitral Regurgitation

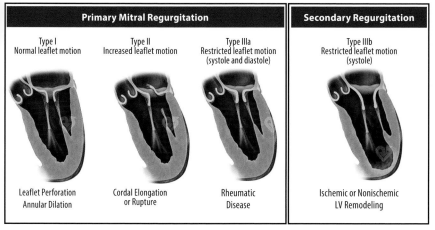

Figure 10.22: **The motion observed by the MV leaflets should be defined per the Carpentier classification system and stated on the echo report**

History/Physical Examination

- Fatigue (earliest symptom)
- Dyspnea upon exertion (most common)
- Angina pectoris (may indicate coronary artery disease)
- Palpitations (suggests atrial fibrillation)
- Severe, sudden orthopnea and frank pulmonary edema suggests severe acute MR
- Heart failure symptoms (dyspnea, orthopnea, paroxysmal nocturnal dyspnea, fatigue, cough, weight gain)
- Right heart failure in advanced stages (jugular venous distention, hepatomegaly, peripheral edema, ascites)

Cardiac Auscultation

- Blowing, high-pitched holosystolic murmur, heard best at the cardiac apex radiating to the axilla (best heard with patient in left decubitus position)
- S3 (common)
- Accentuated P2 (pulmonary hypertension)
- Decrescendo systolic murmur (suggests acute MR)
- S4 (may indicate acute MR or appears late in course)

Electrocardiogram

- May be normal in mild cases or in acute MR
- LA enlargement, atrial fibrillation
- LV hypertrophy with ST segment elevation and peaked T waves (diastolic volume overload pattern)
- Right ventricular (RV) hypertrophy (15%) (suggests pulmonary hypertension)
- Ischemia or infarction patterns (suggests MR due to coronary artery disease)

Chest X-ray/CMR/CT

- Heart size may be normal in mild cases or in acute regurgitation
- Cardiomegaly (due to LA and LV enlargement) in significant chronic MR
- Pulmonary congestion (vascular redistribution, interstitial edema, pleural effusion)
- Acute pulmonary edema (acute or intermittent regurgitation)
- CMR assesses chamber dimensions, mass, jet length, jet area, volumetric flow, may be indicated when TTE is suboptimal, mechanism of significant MR is not clear, echo and/or Doppler parameters are discordant or inconclusive, or there is a discrepancy between the TTE findings and patient symptoms.

Cardiac Catheterization

- Coronary angiography demonstrates coronary flow traits and anatomy
- Degree of regurgitation is determined during ventriculography (injection of contrast into the LV) by observing reflux of contrast into the LA
- Elevated v-wave in the pulmonary capillary wedge pressure tracing with significant MR

Medical/Surgical Treatment

- Vasodilators for afterload reduction (e.g., sodium nitroprusside, hydralazine, nitrates, ACE inhibitors)
- ACE inhibitors (e.g., enalapril) (severe chronic MR with LV dysfunction)
- Anti-arrhythmic agents (e.g., beta blocker, calcium channel blocker)
- Direct current cardioversion (DCCV) (new-onset atrial fibrillation)
- Digitalis (atrial fibrillation, LV failure)
- Diuretics (heart failure)
- Anticoagulation (warfarin) (atrial fibrillation)
- Resynchronization (dual ventricular chamber pacing)
- Intra-aortic balloon pump (severe acute MR)
- Treatment of underlying condition (e.g., revascularization for CAD)
- Valvular repair should always be the first consideration, then valvular replacement.

Surgical Indications

Class I

- Symptomatic acute MR
- Symptomatic chronic MR
- Asymptomatic chronic MR with EF <60% and/or LVESD ≥40mm
- Asymptomatic: EF ≥60%, LVESD ≥40mm

Class IIa

- Asymptomatic chronic MR with EF >60% and/or LVESD <40mm (valvular center of excellence)

- Asymptomatic chronic MR with EF >60% and LVESD <40mm with new atrial fibrillation or pulmonary hypertension >50mmHg at rest or >60mmHg when active
- Chronic MR with EF <30% or LVESD >55mm where repair is feasible

Class IIb

- Chronic secondary MR (ischemic) with EF <30% and functional class (NYHA) III-IV in spite of medical treatment including resynchronization and only if valve can be repaired

M-mode/2D

- It's important to understand that all cardiac valves leak due to malcoaptation of opposing leaflet tissues and the etiology must be clearly understood in order for the safest and most effective treatment strategy to be implemented, be it surgical treatment, medical therapy or both.
- Determine LA volume index (LAVi)
- Normal LAVi: ≤34 mL/m²; normal LA dimension: men ≤4.0cm; women ≤3.8cm)

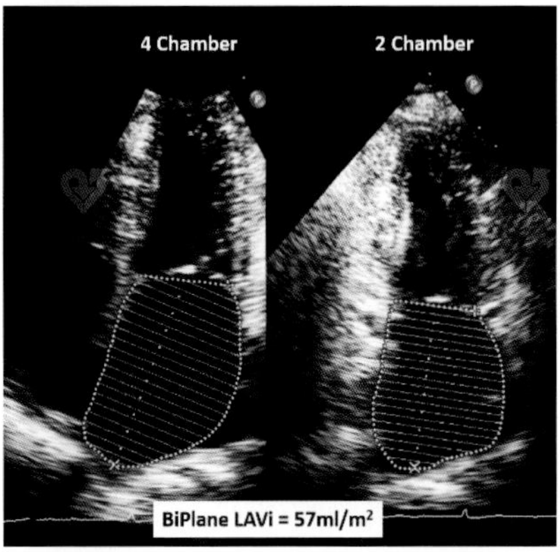

Figure 10.23: Biplane LA volume index (LAVi) is an important goal of echocardiography in the assessment of MR. (Normal ≤34mL/m²)

- Assess LV size (normal LV end-diastolic volume: men ≤74 mL/m², women ≤61mL/m²; normal LV end-diastolic dimension: men ≤5.8cm; women ≤5.2cm)

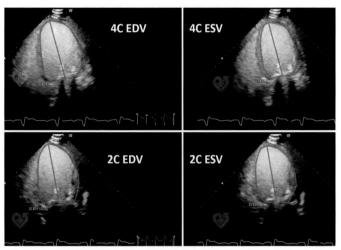

Figure 10.24: **LV biplane Simpson's method-of-disks volume tracings utilizing ultrasound enhancement agent (UEA) in a patient with ischemic cardiomyopathy and MR. Calculated LVOT stroke volume can be subtracted from LV stroke volume to determine MR regurgitant volume. (LV$_{sv}$ = 82, LVOT$_{sv}$=31, MR RegV=51mL, which is within the moderate, Grade III MR range)**

10

Valvular Heart Disease / **Mitral Regurgitation (MR)**

- Identify LV volume overload pattern (LV enlargement with hyperkinetic wall motion)
- Consistent billowing of the atrial septum into right atrium in systole
- Dilation of the mitral annulus
- Assess PASP
- Color M-mode may be useful in determining the presence, duration and timing of MR in the systolic cycle (early, late, or holosystolic)

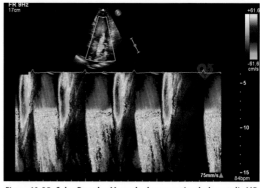

Figure 10.25: **Color Doppler M-mode documenting holosystolic MR**

PW Doppler

- Increased MV E velocity >1.2 m/s (in the absence of stenosis) suggests significant MR. *(ASE Recommendation)* [4]
- Decreased MV deceleration time (<140 msec) may indicate significant regurgitation (assumes normal LV systolic function and diastolic function)
- A-wave dominant LV inflow pattern virtually excludes severe MR
- Systolic flow reversal in more than one pulmonary vein is specific for severe MR *(ASE Recommendation)* [4]
- Normal pulmonary vein pattern suggests low LA pressure and, therefore, non-severe MR
- Increased MV E/A ratio >2.0 suggests significant MR (assumes ejection fraction >40%)
- Determine:
  - MR regurgitant volume and regurgitant fraction *(ASE Recommendation)* [4]

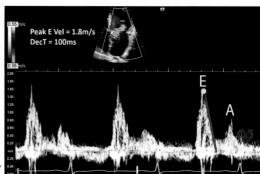

Figure 10.26: **Increased MV E-wave velocity and short deceleration time suggest significant MR**

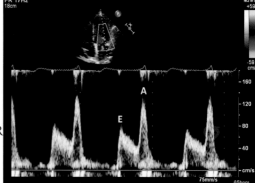

Figure 10.27: **A-wave dominant LV filling pattern in a patient with moderate MR**

- MV forward flow velocity time integral (VTI) is increased with significant MR
- LVOT VTI (<15cm may indicate significant regurgitation due to decreased forward stroke volume)
- MV VTI/LVOT VTI ratio >1.0 may indicate significant regurgitation
- E/e' (average) >14 suggests LV increased filling pressures

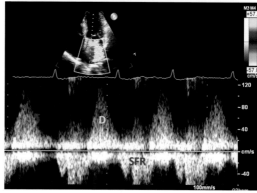

Figure 10.28: **Pulmonary vein systolic flow reversal (SFR).** (D-Diastolic wave)

- Presence of diastolic MR (common in atrial fibrillation, post-premature ventricular contractions, first- and second-degree atrioventricular block, complete heart block, increased LV end-diastolic pressure)

CW Doppler

• Jet density (spectral brightness) is directly proportional to the number of red blood cells reflecting the signal and therefore is a surrogate for MR severity *(ASE Recommendation)* [4]

• Dense, triangular shaped (V-wave cutoff sign) MR Doppler envelope denotes a large regurgitant pressure wave into the left atrium and hemodynamic significance

• Low velocity of the MR jet (≤4 m/s) may indicate elevated LA pressure due to significant regurgitation in the setting of normal LV function

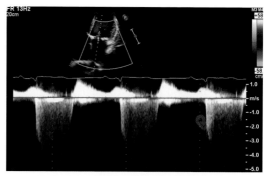

Figure 10.29: **Mild MR with sparse Doppler profile and parabolic shape**

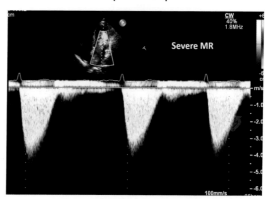

Figure 10.30: **Severe MR with bright, dense Doppler profile and triangular shape**

Color Flow Doppler

Color flow Doppler is invaluable in the assessment of blood flow in the heart and great vessels. With it we are able to visualize hemodynamic flow patterns which offer insight to the morphology, location(s) and number of regurgitant lesions. In addition to assisting with alignment of the Doppler cursor with both regurgitant jets and LV inflow, it also enables the sonographer to quantitate the degree of severity using vena contracta width measurement and proximal isovelocity surface area (PISA) techniques. This modality is very sensitive to technical settings, however, and care should be taken to ensure proper settings are used, including color Doppler gain, Nyquist limit and color box size.

An important concept to understand is that color Doppler does not represent the actual volume of blood produced by a regurgitant lesion, but rather displays the spatial distribution of velocities on the ultrasound screen. This is particularly important for very directional, laminated MR jets that spread most of their blood volume across a large area of the LA wall, thus making them appear "thin" and less severe in standard imaging planes. Conversely, the size of a strong, central MR jet may be overestimated due to entrainment of the surrounding blood pool which produces velocities yet does not make up a portion of the regurgitant volume. This entrainment moves blood already within the LA and causes a "blooming" effect on the color Doppler image.

Understanding the "anatomy" of a regurgitant lesion, as it is displayed with color flow Doppler, requires a knowledge of the conservation of mass (or continuity) principle and the resulting hemodynamic phenomena which occur as a result of blood passing through the regurgitant orifice. The fluid dynamics are much the same for both stenotic and regurgitant lesions. As blood flow nears the orifice, it begins to continuously accelerate until the maximum velocity is reached at the level of the vena contracta, which is just downstream from the anatomic orifice and corresponds to the instantaneous pressure difference across the valve. Once past the vena contracta, the jet quickly loses velocity and definition as it is absorbed into the LA blood pool, forming the "jet" of regurgitation as seen with color flow Doppler.

Image courtesy of Brad Roberts

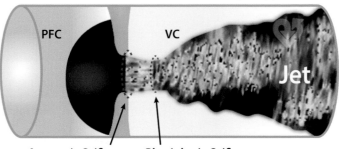

Figure 10.31: **Components of a regurgitation jet with anatomic (actual) and physiologic (calculated) orifices detailed. (PFC — Proximal flow convergence, VC — Vena contracta, Jet — Body of regurgitant jet)**[1]

MR Quantitation

- Blood pressure should always be recorded at the time of the echocardiographic examination, regardless of whether or not regurgitation exists. Elevated blood pressure may exacerbate (worsen) MR due to increased afterload on the LV, while hypotensive patients, common with anesthesia, often diminishes MR.

- Nyquist limit (aliasing velocity) should be set between 50 to 70cm/s for general color Doppler imaging.

- Optimize color Doppler gain settings by first increasing the gain until color speckling appears, then decrease until the speckling is just eliminated. This maximizes sensitivity for displaying flow within the color Doppler box while eliminating gain artifact.

- Duration of the color flow Doppler jet should be noted (Color M-mode, PW Doppler, CW Doppler)

- Considerations in eccentric, wall impinging jet(s):

  - Presence of an eccentric jet strongly suggest a structural abnormality of the MV (e.g., prolapse, flail, vegetation, perforation)

  - May result in underestimation of MR severity due to the Coanda effect (lamination of jet body against LA wall, diminishing visible jet area)

  - Constraining LV wall effects often enlarge the PFC, confounding PISA quantitation.

Jet Area

Color Doppler jet area is an excellent method for excluding MR, but is not reliable for grading MR severity, even when indexed to body surface area. It can be useful, however, for qualitative grading in obvious cases of mild or severe MR. (Mild: small, central, and narrow; Severe: large central jet >50% of LA area or eccentric wall-impinging jet of variable size.

Vena Contracta

- Vena contracta width (VCW) is a semi-quantitative technique which measures the diameter of the high-velocity vena contracta, which is just downstream from the PFC. Measurement should be performed only in a long axis plane, with the parasternal plane preferred over the apical plane due to better axial resolution and closer proximity to the imaging probe.

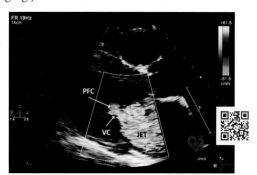

Figure 10.32: MR jet components as viewed in the parasternal long-axis plane. (PFC — Proximal flow convergence, VC-Vena contracta, Jet-Tail of regurgitant jet)

- It is important to note that VCW measurement represents a single point in time in the systolic cycle and may be overestimate MR if the regurgitation is not holosystolic.

PISA

- PISA quantitation of MR calculates the effective regurgitant orifice area (MREROA) by using color flow Doppler to exploit the phenomena produced as flow passes through a regurgitant orifice and measuring the maximum velocity of the regurgitant jet.

- This technique poses a number of technical demands on the sonographer, but there are only two measurements that the sonographer actually needs to make:

    - measurement of the radius of the baseline-shifted PFC and,

    - measure MR peak velocity.

    - Once the EROA is known, MR regurgitant volume (MR RegV) can then be calculated by multiplying the EROA by MR VTI.

- It is important to understand that, just like VCW measurement, PISA quantitation represents a single snapshot of systole and the timing and duration of MR should be taken into account.

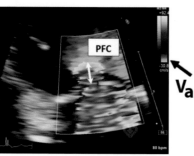
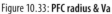
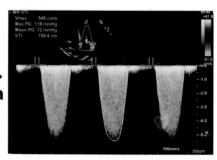

Figure 10.33: **PFC radius & Va**   Figure 10.34: **MR Peak Velocity & VTI**

- PISA formula for EROA and graphics of color Doppler proximal flow convergence (PFC) and CW Doppler. Color Doppler baseline should be shifted in the direction of MR to a velocity to create a hemispheric PFC, usually between 20-40cm/s. The only two measurements required from the sonographer are highlighted in red in the formula – PISA radius and MR peak velocity.

$$\text{Pisa MR}_{EROA} = \frac{2\pi r^2 \times Va}{MRPKV}$$

PISA Important Tips

Color Doppler Map

It is imperative that the sonographer select a velocity color Doppler map when utilizing the PISA method to quantify regurgitation from any valve. *(Figure 10.27)*

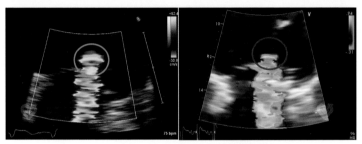

Figure 10.35: **Examples of two different color Doppler maps using identical baseline shift to quantitate MR with PISA in the same patient**

A velocity color Doppler map (left image) *must* be used to create a measurable flow convergence zone (green circle). A variance color Doppler map (right image) cannot create a flow convergence at all (red circle), as it is designed to display turbulent flow and will not work in this application of color Doppler.

Considerations in Functional MR

Functional MR will often have a wide regurgitant orifice along the coaptation line of the mitral valve and this should be understood when quantifying MR in this patient population. *(Figure 10.4)*

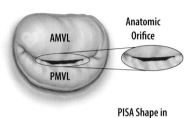

• The PISA formula assumes that the regurgitant orifice is perfectly round and, consequently, consistently underestimates MR EROA with functional MR. In light of these facts, ASE guidelines specify the cutoff for severe MR at ≥ 0.20cm^2 in patients with functional MR.[1]

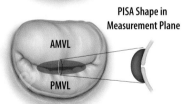

• 3-D TEE and color Doppler can avoid the geometric assumptions of the PISA formula by orienting imaging planes across the regurgitant orifice, then directly measuring the area of the vena contracta.

Figure 10.36: **A wide regurgitant orifice is common with functional MR and creates a wide proximal flow convergence (PFC) across the orifice (bottom image, blue zone).**

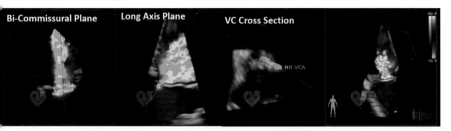

Figure 10.37: **3-D TEE color Doppler imaging in a patient with functional MR and a wide regurgitant orifice (lower left panel). Vena contracta area (VCA) measures 0.52cm^2 (upper right)**

10

Valvular Heart Disease / **Mitral Regurgitation (MR)**

Impact of PISA Radius on EROA Calculation

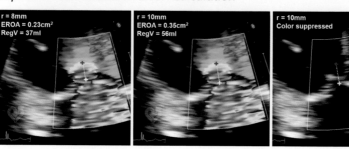

Figure 10.38: Small changes in PISA radius have a profound effect on the resulting calculated area. Color Doppler image suppression is instrumental in avoiding measurement error at the proximal end of the radius

- A difference of only 2mm in the PISA radius has a profound impact on the calculated effective regurgitant orifice area (EROA). Figure 10.28 demonstrates the impact of this error on EROA and underscores the usefulness of color Doppler suppression in defining the distal end of the radius.

- PISA radii measured incorrectly at 8mm **(left image)** and correctly at 10mm **(center image)** yield large differences in EROA and regurgitant volume due to squaring error.

- The distal caliper point of the proximal flow convergence (PFC) radius is easily defined by the blue to yellow interface (red calipers), but the proximal caliper point is obscured by the color Doppler signal (white calipers) and placement is an estimation, at best.

- Once the distal caliper has been placed, however, color Doppler is no longer needed and the color overlay may be suppressed **(right image)**, revealing the underlying regurgitant orifice and enabling accurate placement of the proximal measurement caliper.

MR Severity Values

- Vena contracta width (VCW) in the parasternal (preferred) or apical long-axis plane (Mild ≤0.3cm; Severe ≥0.7cm (>0.8cm for biplane))

- PISA radius: (Mild: absent or ≤0.3cm at Nyquist at 30 to 40cm/s) (Severe: ≥1.0cm at Nyquist 30 to 40cm/s)

- PISA EROA (mild: <0.20cm^2) (Severe: ≥0.40cm^2) or ≥0.20cm^2 in functional MR)

- MR regurgitant volume: (Mild: <30mL) (Severe: ≥60mL)

- 3-D may improve evaluation of jet size, number, direction, flow convergence (PISA) region and VCA and VCW

Stress Echocardiography

May be used to evaluate:

- Severity of regurgitation with exercise

- Presence of co-existing coronary artery disease (CAD)

- Functional capacity and unmask symptoms

- Pulmonary artery systolic pressures and RV systolic function
- LV systolic contractile reserve (LVEF should increase with exercise; predicts postoperative outcomes)

Transesophageal Echocardiography

- Indicated when TTE is inconclusive in identifying underlying mechanism and/or MR severity; strategical planning for MV surgery.
- Higher resolution, multiplane and 3-D imaging capabilities, and physical proximity to MV makes VC imaging, PISA quantification and color Doppler mapping of the MR jet easier and more accurate than TTE

- Superior to TTE for determining the presence of chordal rupture and ruptured papillary muscle

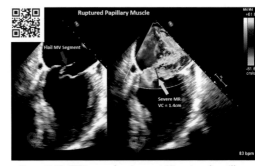

Figure 10.39: **TEE image showing post-MI ruptured papillary muscle and severe MR**

- Quantitation of the severity of MR by TEE is accomplished by assessing:
  - VC width
  - Size of the PFC zone for PISA
  - Jet geometry
  - Pulmonary venous flow evaluation by PW Doppler for all pulmonary veins (usually only one assessed by TTE)
  - Jet density by CW Doppler
  - Regurgitant volume, regurgitant fraction and effective regurgitant orifice area (EROA)
- Due to shadow artifacts common with prosthetic heart valves and severe mitral annular calcification (MAC), TEE is often more accurate than TTE in determining the severity of MR in those patients
- "Off axis" views are often needed in assess
- An eccentric jet that sweeps around the left atrium may indicate significant regurgitation (Coanda effect)

Important to Note

- Chronic MR subjects the LV and LA to long-standing volume overload conditions, leading to chamber dilatation with significant regurgitation. Longstanding MR can arise from many causes, including LV dysfunction (regional or global) and any disease process of the MV complex.
- Acute MR imposes an abrupt pressure overload in the LA and pulmonary venous system secondary to an acute failure of one or more components of the mitral valve complex, which often leads to flash pulmonary edema. The most common causes of acute MR include chordal rupture secondary to myxomatous degeneration, acute LV ischemia (especially posteroinferior), papillary muscle rupture and infective endocarditis.

Table 10.11: Specific Criteria for Mild vs Severe Chronic MR *(ASE Recommendations)* [4]

Mild MR	Severe MR
• Small, central, narrow, often brief color flow jet	• Flail leaflet
• Vena contracta width ≤0.3cm	• Vena contracta width ≥0.7cm (biplane >0.8cm)
• PISA radius absent or ≤0.3cm at Nyquist 30 to 40cm/s	• PISA radius ≥1.0cm at Nyquist 30 to 40cm/s
• Mitral A wave dominant inflow	• Central large jet >50% of LA area
• Soft or incomplete jet by CW Doppler	• Pulmonary vein systolic flow reversal
• Normal LV and LA size	• Enlarged LV with normal function
≥4 criteria definitely mild	**≥4 criteria definitely severe**

Table 10.12: Grading the Severity of Chronic MR by Echocardiography *(ASE Recommendations)* [4]

	Mild	Moderate	Severe
MV morphology	**None or mild leaflet abnormality** (e.g., mild thickening, calcifications or prolapse, mild tenting)	Moderate leaflet abnormality or moderate tenting	**Severe valve lesions** (primary: flail leaflet, ruptured papillary muscle, severe retraction, large perforation; secondary: severe tenting, poor leaflet coaptation)
LV and LA size [a]	Usually normal	Normal or mild dilated	Dilated [b]
Qualitative Doppler			
Color flow jet area [c]	**Small, central, narrow, often brief**	Variable	Large central jet (>50% of LA) or eccentric wall-impinging jet of variable size
Flow convergence [d]	**Not visible, transient or small**	Intermediate in size and duration	**Large throughout systole**
CWD jet	Faint/partial/parabolic	Dense but partial or parabolic	Holosystolic/dense/**triangular**
Semiquantitative			
Vena contracta width (cm)	≤0.3	<0.7	≥0.7 (biplane >0.8cm) [i]
Pulmonary vein flow [e]	**Systolic dominance** (may be blunted in LV dysfunction or A-fib)	Normal or systolic blunting [e]	Minimal to no systolic flow, **systolic flow reversal**
Mitral inflow [f]	**A-wave dominant**	Variable	E-wave dominant (>1.2 m/s)
Quantitative			
EROA; 2D PISA (cm²)	<0.20	0.20 to 0.29; 0.30 to 0.39	≥0.40 (≥0.20 functional MR with elliptical ROA)
RegVol (mL)	<30	30 to 44; 45 to 59 [g]	≥60 (may be lower in low flow conditions)
RegF (%)	<30	30 to 39; 40 to 49	≥50

EROA, Effective regurgitant orifice area.
ROA, Regurgitant orifice area.
Bolded qualitative and semiquantitative signs are considered specific for their MR grade.
*   All parameters have limitations, and an integrated approach must be used that weighs the strength of each echocardiographic measurement. All signs and measures should be interpreted in an individualized manner that accounts for body size, sex, and all other patient characteristics.

a) This pertains mostly to patients with primary MR.
b) LV and LA can be within the "normal" range for patients with acute severe MR or with chronic severe MR who have small body size, particularly women, or with small LV size preceding the occurrence of MR.
c) With Nyquist limit 50 to 70cm/s.
d) Small flow convergence is usually ≤0.3cm, and large is ≥1cm at a Nyquist limit of 30 to 40cm/s.
e) Influenced by many other factors (LV diastolic function, atrial fibrillation, LA pressure).

f) Most valid in patients >50 years old and is influenced by other causes of elevated LA pressure.
g) Discrepancies among EROA, RF, and RVol may arise in the setting of low or high flow states.
h) Quantitative parameters can help subclassify the moderate regurgitation group.
i) For average between apical two- and four-chamber views.

Table 10.13: Key Points in Mitral Regurgitation Assessment *(ASE Recommendations)* [4]

When MR is detected, **the underlying mechanism must first be determined and classified** as Primary, Secondary or Mixed etiology, especially when the MR is more than mild. Both the etiology and Carpentier classification should be reported.

No single echocardiographic parameter should be used to determine MR severity. An **integrated approach of multiple parameters** provides more accurate assessment, especially for mild or severe MR.

LV and LA volumes, indexed to body surface area, are important measures to determine chamber enlargement (or lack thereof) and account for patient body size in patients with chronic severe MR.

With color Doppler and MR, it is important to assess the **three components of the regurgitant jet**: 1. Proximal flow convergence, 2. Vena contracta, and 3. Downstream jet. Beware of eccentric jets.

Determine the **systolic duration of MR** and take this into account when quantifying MR.

Quantify MR when qualitative and semiquantitative measures of MR are unclear or ambiguous.

Systemic blood pressure at the time of exam is a very important variable which can significantly impact the size of an MR jet in the LA, independent of EROA or RVol.

Acute severe MR can be more challenging to assess than chronic severe MR. TEE should be utilized if TTE 2D and Doppler measures suggest significant MR.

Consider additional testing, such as TEE or CMR, when MR mechanism and severity are not clearly defined with conventional TTE imaging and analysis.

Chronic Mitral Regurgitation by Doppler Echocardiography [3]

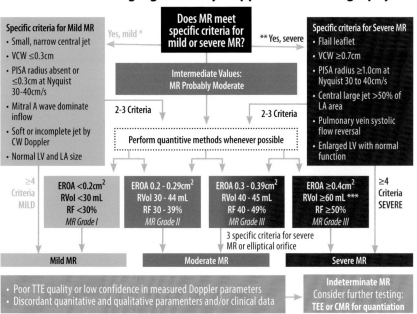

Specific criteria for Mild MR
- Small, narrow central jet
- VCW ≤0.3cm
- PISA radius absent or ≤0.3cm at Nyquist 30-40cm/s
- Mitral A wave dominate inflow
- Soft or incomplete jet by CW Doppler
- Normal LV and LA size

Does MR meet specific criteria for mild or severe MR?

Yes, mild * → ** Yes, severe

Specific criteria for Severe MR
- Flail leaflet
- VCW ≥0.7cm
- PISA radius ≥1.0cm at Nyquist 30 to 40cm/s
- Central large jet >50% of LA area
- Pulmonary vein systolic flow reversal
- Enlarged LV with normal function

Intermediate Values: MR Probably Moderate

2-3 Criteria   2-3 Criteria

Perform quantitive methods whenever possible

| ≥4 Criteria MILD | EROA <0.2cm² RVol <30 mL RF <30% *MR Grade I* | EROA 0.2 - 0.29cm² RVol 30 - 44 mL RF 30 - 39% *MR Grade II* | EROA 0.3 - 0.39cm² RVol 40 - 45 mL RF 40 - 49% *MR Grade III* | EROA ≥0.4cm² RVol ≥60 mL *** RF ≥50% *MR Grade III* | ≥4 Criteria SEVERE |

3 specific criteria for severe MR or elliptical orifice

Mild MR   **Moderate MR**   **Severe MR**

- Poor TTE quality or low confidence in measured Doppler parameters
- Discordant quanitative and qualitative paramenters and/or clinical data

→ **Indeterminate MR** Consider further testing: **TEE or CMR for quantiation**

* Beware of underestimation of MR severity in eccentric, wall impinging jets; quantification is advised.

** All values for EROA by PISA assume holosystolic MR; single frame EROA by Pisa and VCW overstimate non-holsystolic MR.

*** Regurgitant volume for severe MR may be lower in low flow conditions

Mitral Valve Prolapse

Definition

Abnormal systolic valve motion of one or both mitral valve (MV) leaflets ≥2mm beyond the long-axis plane of the MV annulus.

Etiology

Also known as *degenerative* or *myxomatous* MV disease, mitral valve prolapse (MVP) is the most common cause of primary mitral regurgitation (MR) in developed countries and is comprised of a spectrum of valvular lesions with the mildest form being fibroelastic deficiency (FED) and the most severe being Barlow's disease. Intermediate forms also exist which share similarities of both FED and Barlow's Disease and are termed FED+ and forme fruste.

MVP is also a common finding in patients with Marfan syndrome, the most common of the hereditary connective tissue disorders.

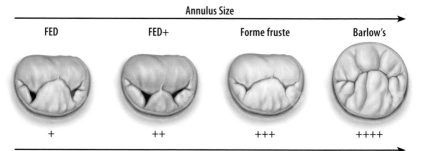

Figure 10.40: **Spectrum of degenerative mitral valve disease from fibroelastic deficiency (FED) to Barlow's disease.**

In isolated FED (far left figure), there is a deficiency of fibrillin which results in very thin, transparent leaflets and often includes one or more ruptured chordae. In long-standing MVP, secondary myxomatous pathologic changes may occur which result in leaflet thickening and expansion (FED+). Forme fruste designates myxomatous degenerative disease with excess MV tissues in usually more than one leaflet segment, but valve size is typically normal, distinguishing it from Barlow's disease. Barlow's disease (right figure) has a distinctive valvular appearance with diffuse myxomatous changes in one or both leaflets, excess leaflet tissue and dilated MV annulus, distinguishing it from the other three forms of degenerative MV disease. Note the size and shape of the annulus when compared to the other forms of disease. [1]

10

Valvular Heart Disease / **Mitral Regurgitation (MR)** / Mitral Valve Prolapse

Fibroelastic Deficiency (FED)

FED is characterized by a deficiency of fibrillin which results in elongation and thinning of the MV chordae, often leading to chordal rupture and frank appearance of significant MR. The middle scallop of the posterior leaflet (P2) is the segment most often affected, with the majority of the unaffected leaflet tissue appearing thin and of relatively normal size. Most patients present in their 6th decade of life with a short clinical history of MR due to the sudden onset of symptoms.

Barlow's Disease

In contrast, Barlow's disease is characterized by diffuse thickening of multiple scallops of one or both MV leaflets due to an abnormal accumulation of mucopolysaccharides. This myxomatous infiltration leads to thick, redundant leaflets and elongation of the chordae, causing MVP. Due to the chronic accumulation of myxomatous infiltrates, Barlow's disease is usually discovered in young adulthood with patients presenting with a MR murmur. Billowing, bileaflet MVP is a common finding and patients are usually followed for decades until indications for surgical repair manifest. Surgical repair with this disease is more sophisticated and technically challenging for the surgeon than repair for FED.

Table 10.14: Comparisons between fibroelastic deficiency (FED) and Barlow's Disease of the MV Apparatus		
	Fibroelastic Deficiency (FED)	**Barlow's Disease**
Pathology	Impaired production of connective tissue results in weakening of MV leaflets and chordae	Thickening of MV leaflets and chordae due to abnormal accumulation of mucopolysaccharides
Typical Age of Patient	Older (>60 years)	Younger (<40 years)
Manifestation of MR	Acute, days to months	Chronic, years to decades
Leaflet Segment(s) Involved	Usually single segment	Multiple segments of one or both leaflets
Leaflet Appearance	Diffusely thin segments with focal thickening of affected segment	Diffuse thickening with redundant (excess) leaflet tissue
Observed Dysfunction	Prolapse with or without flail leaflet	Bileaflet prolapse
Chordal Rupture	Common	Rare
Carpentier Classification	Class II (excessive leaflet motion)	Class II excessive leaflet motion)
Complexity of Surgical Repair	Average, typical techniques	High, skilled techniques

History/Physical Examination

- Most patients asymptomatic
- Blood pressure normal/low
- Orthostatic hypotension
- Family history of cardiac disease
- Palpitations (most common presenting symptom) (due to cardiac arrhythmias)
- Chest pain (usually atypical, non-exertional) ("stabbing pain at the apex")
- Dyspnea, fatigue, lassitude, exercise intolerance
- Neuropsychiatric symptoms (anxiety, panic attacks)
- Presyncope/syncope
- Amaurosis fugax, transient ischemic attack, cerebral vascular accident
- Heart failure due to significant mitral regurgitation

Complications

- Progressive mitral regurgitation (most common reason for MV repair/replacement in the United States)
- Infective endocarditis (MVP is the leading predisposing cardiovascular diagnosis for infective endocarditis)
- Embolic events (transient ischemic attack, cerebral vascular accident due to fibrin emboli)
- Ruptured chordae tendineae with acute mitral regurgitation (more common in males older than 50 years of age)
- Arrhythmias/conduction disturbances (paroxysmal supraventricular tachycardia most common, atrial fibrillation)
- Heart failure (due to significant mitral regurgitation)
- Pulmonary hypertension (due to significant mitral regurgitation)
- Acute pulmonary edema (due to ruptured chordae tendineae with significant mitral regurgitation)
- Sudden death (least common) (due to ventricular arrhythmias) (severe mitral regurgitation, myxomatous MV)

Physical Appearance

- Normal (asthenic)
- Loss of normal thoracic configuration (e.g., straight-back syndrome, scoliosis, pectus excavatum, pectus carinatum, kyphosis)

Cardiac Auscultation

- Mid-late systolic click(s) (due to sudden tensing of chordae tendineae) with or without a medium to high-pitched late systolic murmur due to mitral regurgitation
- S1 may be accentuated
- S3 (may suggest significant mitral regurgitation)
- Early diastolic rumble (may suggest significant mitral regurgitation)

Dynamic Cardiac Auscultation

- Maneuvers which reduce left ventricular volume (e.g., supine to standing, Valsalva, amyl nitrite inhalation) cause the click and murmur to occur earlier in ventricular systole
- Maneuvers which increase left ventricular volume (e.g., standing to supine, standing to squatting) cause the click and murmur to move toward the second heart sound

Electrocardiogram

- Normal (in asymptomatic patients)
- Flat, inverted or biphasic T waves in leads II, III, aVF (most common finding 20 to 60%)
- Nonspecific ST segment changes (leads II, III, aVF)
- Arrhythmias (e.g., paroxysmal supraventricular tachycardia (most common), premature atrial or ventricular contractions, bradyarrhythmias)
- Conduction disturbances (first degree AV block, WPW syndrome, prolonged QT interval, RBBB)
- Left atrial enlargement (significant mitral regurgitation)

Chest X-ray/CMR/CT

Normal

- Thoracic abnormalities (e.g., straight back, kyphosis, scoliosis, pectus excavatum, pectus carinatum)
- Cardiomegaly due to left atrial enlargement and left ventricular enlargement suggests significant mitral regurgitation
- Pulmonary venous congestion (suggests left heart failure due to significant mitral regurgitation)
- Acute pulmonary edema (suggests chordal rupture with significant acute mitral regurgitation)
- CMR provides information concerning the presence of MVP, the severity of the mitral regurgitation, chamber dimension and function (e.g., left atrial size, left ventricular size and function)

Cardiac Catheterization

• Coronary arteriography (to exclude coronary artery disease, congenital anomalies of the coronary vessels)

Medical/Surgical Treatment

• Holter monitor (syncope, palpitations, serious arrhythmia)

• Exercise stress test

• Beta blockers, antiarrhythmic, electrophysiologic testing

• Cessation of catecholamine stimulants (e.g., caffeine, alcohol)

• Radiofrequency ablation of atrioventricular bypass tracts

• Prophylaxis for volume depletion

• Anticoagulation therapy (daily aspirin therapy/warfarin for MVP patients with documented focal neurologic events or post-stroke patients with MVP)

• Transcatheter edge-to-edge MV repair (e.g.; MitraClip™, PASCAL)

M-mode

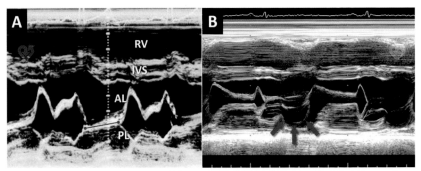

Figure 10.41: **Parasternal M-mode tracings of the MV. Panel A – Normal motion of the MV with coaptation of both leaflets throughout systole (red line). Panel B – M-mode demonstrating late-systolic posterior MVP (arrows) with normal coaptation in early systole (red line).**

2D

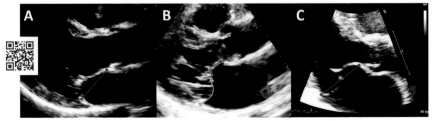

Figure 10.42: **2D parasternal long axis views of the MV in three patients. Panel A – Normal MV with coaptation point and both leaflets remaining on ventricular side of annular plane (red line) throughout systole. Panel B – Posterior MVP with thickened, redundant leaflets and chordal elongation in a patient with Barlow's disease of the MV. Note the excessive leaflet lengths, thickness, and enlarged size of the MV annulus (red dot, line — anterior MV annulus and leaflet; green dot, line — posterior MV annulus and leaflet). Panel C – Isolated P2 prolapse with very thin leaflet tissue and elongated chordae in a patient with FED of the MV. Note that only the posterior MV leaflet prolapses beyond the annular plane (red line).**

• MVP is considered present when any portion of the leaflet protrudes beyond the mitral annular plane ≥2mm in the long-axis plane. If poor parasternal windows exist, the apical long axis view can be used.

• It is important to understand that the *apical 4-chamber view should not be used* to determine the presence or absence of MVP. The MV annulus has a hyperbolic paraboloid ("saddle") shape and can often create the appearance of MVP though the leaflets and chordae are structurally normal.

• Degenerative MV disease:

- Barlow's disease – Diffuse thickening of multiple segments of one or both leaflets creates the appearance of "floppy leaflets" on 2D echo with redundant leaflet tissues and elongated chordae.

- FED – Patients often present with acute rupture of one or more chordae from a single segment of the mitral valve. Adjacent MV segments are usually normal in thickness or thinned with a normal size.

• Left atrial dilatation secondary to significant mitral regurgitation. (normal LA volume: ≤34mL/m² for both men and women; normal anteroposterior dimensions: men 3.0 to 4.0cm; women 2.7 to 3.8cm).

• Left ventricular volume overload pattern secondary to significant MR (left ventricular dilatation with hyperkinesis).

• Determine:

- Leaflet morphology of each segment of both MV leaflets, including thickness, length, and presence of prolapse beyond the plane of the MV annulus in long axis.

- Mitral annulus diameter in the parasternal long-axis view (normal end-diastolic 2.91cm ± 0.34; normal end-systolic 2.68cm ± 0.39) (increased in MVP)

- Left atrial volume, dimension and area

- Left ventricular volumes, diastolic and systolic dimensions, and ejection fraction

Doppler

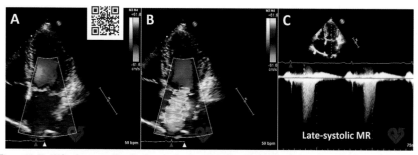

Figure 10.43: **Mid to late systolic mitral regurgitation. Panel A – No MR in mid-systole and antegrade right upper pulmonary venous flow. (Red triangle, ECG R-wave; White triangle, current color Doppler imaging frame) Panel B – Large MR jet begins at mid-systole and extends into right upper pulmonary vein. Panel C – Continuous wave Doppler demonstrating late onset and short duration of MR over systolic cycle.**

10

Valvular Heart Disease / **Mitral Regurgitation (MR)** / Mitral Valve Prolapse

- Mitral regurgitation (often late-systolic)
- Determine:
  - Which segment(s) of the MV are prolapsing or flail using 2D echo.
  - The direction of the MR jet with color Doppler:
    - Posterior MVP creates an anteriorly-directed MR jet.
    - Anterior MVP creates a posteriorly-directed MR jet.
    - Bileaflet MVP can create one or more MR jet(s) that are directional, but often creates a centrally-directed jet.

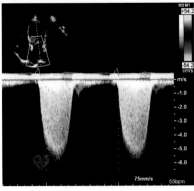

Figure 10.44: **Mitral regurgitation demonstrated**

- Presence and severity of associated MR, paying careful attention to MR duration (holosystolic or late-systolic)
- Other hemodynamics to consider (rest and exercise):
  - Systolic pulmonary artery pressure (SPAP)
  - Mean pulmonary artery pressure (MPAP)
  - Pulmonary artery end-diastolic pressure (PAEDP)
  - Pulmonary vascular resistance (PVR)

Transesophageal Echocardiography

- 3-Dimensional transesophageal echocardiography (3D TEE) has evolved into an incredibly powerful tool in the assessment of both degenerative and acquired MV disease. Leaflet morphology and motion can be determined by quickly and accurately reproducing both the "surgeon's view" of the MV from the atrial perspective, as well as a view from the ventricular aspect. Improvements in probe design and software can now provide highly detailed information about all segments of the valve, including any prolapsing segments and/or ruptured chordae.

- All patients with degenerative MV disease resulting in MVP and MR should be considered for surgical repair over prosthetic valve replacement. It is imperative to perform a complete TEE and describe the MV anatomy and pathophysiology completely, including:
  - Morphology and size of the MV annulus, leaflets, and chordae
  - Describe all three segments of the anterior (A1, A2, A3) and posterior (P1, P2, P3) MV leaflets, noting those that are normal and any affected by degenerative disease.
  - Determine where on the spectrum of degenerative MV disease each valve exists, from FED to Barlow's disease, and report the findings.
  - Perform quantitative measures to determine the severity of MR

- Not the presence and severity of mitral annular calcification. This can significantly impact both surgical repair and prosthetic valve replacement.
- Left and right ventricular systolic function
- Pulmonary artery systolic pressures

• Allows for assessment of possible complications postoperative valve repair/replacement:
  - Residual mitral regurgitation (> mild post-op is undesirable)
  - Systolic anterior motion with left ventricular outflow tract obstruction (6% to 9%)
  - Dehisced ring; Perivalvular leak (PVL)
  - Leaflet perforation
  - Residual mitral stenosis
  - Significant tricuspid regurgitation (> mild is unacceptable)
  - Global and segmental left and right ventricular systolic dysfunction

2-Dimensionally, the MV annulus has a "D" shape with the straight section positioned anteriorly. Long axis and midcommissural imaging planes intersect the MV annulus in minor and major axis planes, respectively, and the leaflet segments imaged in each plane are shown (green dotted lines). The anterior MV leaflet has a semicircular shape and is continuous with the fibrosa of the aortic valve along its base. For descriptive purposes, it is divided into three segments numbered from lateral to medial – A1, A2 and A3. Anterior leaflet occupies one-third of the circumference of the MV annulus anteriorly. Posterior leaflet has a quadrangular shape and occupies the remaining two-thirds of the MV annulus. It is also divided into segments numbered from lateral to medial (P1, P2 and P3) and form true scallops. Though posterior MV leaflet occupies more of the MV annulus it is considerably shorter than anterior leaflet and both leaflets end up having approximately the same surface areas. The coaptation line of each leaflet terminates at the anterolateral and posteromedial commissures (*).

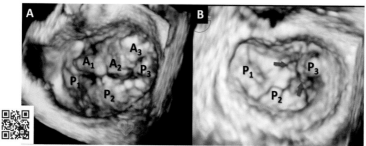

Figure 10.45: Examples of Barlow's disease and FED of the MV from the "surgeon's view" in the left atrium. Panel A – Bileaflet, billowing MVP in a patient with Barlow's disease which affected all segments of both leaflets. (A1-3 – anterior leaflet segments, P1-3 – posterior leaflet segments) Panel B – P3 isolated MVP with flail chordae (arrows) causing severe eccentric MR in a patient with FED. Single segment involvement with sudden structural failure is a common presentation in mitral valves with FED, though the P2 segment is most commonly involved.

10

Valvular Heart Disease / **Mitral Regurgitation (MR)** / Mitral Valve Prolapse

Important to Note

- Degenerative MV disease is a common disorder affecting around 2% of the population, with the most common finding in degenerative disease being MVP and MR.

- The posterior MV leaflet is made up of three scallops: the middle (P_2, largest), lateral (P_1) and medial (P_3, smallest). The middle scallop is best visualized in the parasternal and apical long-axis views, the lateral scallop is best seen in the apical four-chamber view, the medial scallop is visualized best in the apical two-chamber view. Multiple views are required to evaluate the posterior MV leaflet.

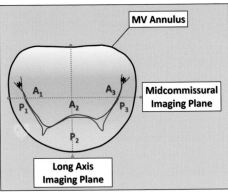

Figure 10.46: **Graphic of MV anatomy and intersecting tomographic echocardiography planes.**
A = Anterior MV leaflet,
P = Posterior MV leaflet,
* = MV commissures

- Rupture of the chordae to the P_2 scallop due to FED is the most common chordal rupture.

- The parasternal and apical long-axis views allow the evaluation of both the A_2 and P_2 scallops of the MV.

- The transducer should be tilted medially and laterally from the long axis plane to assess all portions of both MV leaflets.

References

1. Adapted from David H. Adams et al. Eur Heart J 2010;31:1958-1966 – Degenerative mitral valve regurgitation: best practice revolution (Publication permission process can be found here.)

2. Adapted from Roberts, BJ, Grayburn, PA. Color Flow Imaging of the Vena Contracta in Mitral Regurgitation: Technical Considerations, J Am Soc Echocardiogr 16:1002-106, 2003.

3. Adapted from Journal of the American Society of Echocardiography; Volume 30, Number 40

4. Zoghbi WA, Adams DB, Bonow RO, Enriquez-Sarano M, Foster E, Grayburn PA, Hahn RT, Han Y, Hung J, Lang RM, Little SH, Shah DJ, Shernan S, Thavendiranathan P, Thomas JD: Recommendations for Noninvasive Evaluation of Native Valvular Regurgitation A Report from the American Society of Echocardiography Developed in Collaboration with the Society for Cardiovascular Magnetic Resonance. J Am Soc Echocardiogr 30:305-371, 2017.

Valvular Heart Disease
Mitral Stenosis
Marsha L. Roberts, BS, ACS, RCS, RDCS (AE/PE), FASE

Definition

A narrowing of the mitral valve orifice impeding the diastolic flow of blood from the left atrium into the left ventricle.

Etiology

- Rheumatic fever (most common) (99%)
- Congenital (e.g., parachute mitral valve, cor triatriatum, Shone's syndrome, double orifice mitral valve)
- Non-rheumatic acquired mitral stenosis
- Severe mitral annular calcification
- Left atrial ball-valve thrombus (usually associated with mitral stenosis)
- Left atrial tumor (e.g., myxoma)
- Infective endocarditis with obstructive vegetation
- Systemic lupus erythematosus
- Ergotamine induced; methysergide induced
- Antiphospholipid antibody syndrome
- Whipple's disease
- Pseudoxanthoma elasticum
- Rheumatoid arthritis
- Infiltrative diseases
- Carcinoid heart disease
- Iatrogenic (e.g., prosthetic mitral valve, mitral valve clip (e.g.; MitraClip®), mitral valve annuloplasty, radiation valvular injury)

History

- Dyspnea at rest or upon exertion (principal symptom) (80%)
- Hemoptysis (second most common presenting symptom) (30%)
- Chest pain (15%)
- Palpitations (due to atrial fibrillation)
- Syncope
- Heart failure (dyspnea, orthopnea, paroxysmal nocturnal dyspnea, fatigue, cough, weight gain)
- Right heart failure (e.g., jugular venous distention, hepatomegaly, peripheral edema, ascites, anasarca)

Physical Examination

- Irregularly irregular pulse (atrial fibrillation)
- Malar flush (mitral facies)
- Small/absent left ventricular impulse
- Parasternal right ventricular heave (pulmonary hypertension)
- Blood pressure low normal
- Ortner's syndrome (hoarseness)
- Apical diastolic thrill

Complications

- Mitral regurgitation (coexistent)
- Passive/reactive pulmonary hypertension
- Left atrial thrombus (7 to 15%)
- Systemic embolization (20%) (80% of those in atrial fibrillation)
- Infective endocarditis (more common in mild mitral stenosis)
- Pulmonary edema, hemorrhage, embolism and/or infarction
- Decreased stroke volume, cardiac output, cardiac index
- Right heart failure (e.g., jugular venous distention, hepatomegaly, peripheral edema, ascites, anasarca)

Cardiac Auscultation

- Opening snap (important physical sign)
- Low pitched diastolic rumble best heard at the cardiac apex (pan-diastolic, mid-diastolic, pre-systolic)
- Crescendo pre-systolic accentuation of the diastolic rumble (due to atrial systole)
- Loud S1
- Accentuated P2 (pulmonary hypertension)
- Murmur of mitral, aortic, tricuspid and/or pulmonic regurgitation

Electrocardiogram

- Left atrial enlargement (P-mitral) (90%)
- Atrial fibrillation (50%)
- Evidence of pulmonary hypertension (e.g., right ventricular hypertrophy, P pulmonale)

Chest X-ray/CMR/CT

- Left atrial enlargement with normal left ventricular size (pure mitral stenosis) ("double density")
- Pulmonary venous hypertension with flow redistribution from the bases to the apices ("cephalization")
- Pulmonary edema (Kerley A lines, Kerley B lines)
- CMR determines valve morphology, chamber dimensions, peak velocity, pressure gradient(s) and mitral valve area with planimetry

Cardiac Catheterization

- Coronary arteriography to identify underlying coronary artery disease (25%) (primary role)
- Transvalvular diastolic pressure gradient across the mitral valve (hallmark finding)
- Determines mitral valve area by the Gorlin formula
- Exercise may be utilized to evaluate the change in the transmitral mean pressure gradient and pulmonary artery pressures
- Percutaneous mitral balloon valvuloplasty (PMBV) may be performed

Medical/Surgical Treatment

- Prophylactic antibiotic therapy to prevent recurrences of rheumatic fever
- Electrical cardioversion for atrial fibrillation (duration of arrhythmia <12 months and left atrial dimension <5cm)
- Atrial fibrillation ablation
- Digitalis (atrial fibrillation, heart failure)
- Beta-adrenergic blocking agent (e.g., atenolol)
- Calcium antagonist (e.g., diltiazem, verapamil)
- Antiarrhythmic (e.g., amiodarone)
- Anticoagulation (e.g., warfarin) (increased risk of embolic event if LA dimension >55mm; spontaneous echo contrast present)
- Diuretics (relieves pulmonary congestion)
- Restriction of activity corresponding to degree of severity of stenosis
- Sodium restriction (pulmonary congestion)
- Left atrial appendage occlusion- Watchman device
- Maze procedure (atrial compartment operation) (chronic atrial fibrillation)
- Percutaneous mitral balloon valvuloplasty (PMBV) (trans-septal; retrograde) (treatment of choice)
- Surgical commissurotomy (open or closed)
- Mitral valve replacement

10

Valvular Heart Disease / **Mitral Stenosis**

M-mode

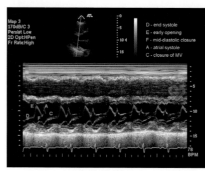

Figure 10.47: **Normal Mitral Valve M-mode**

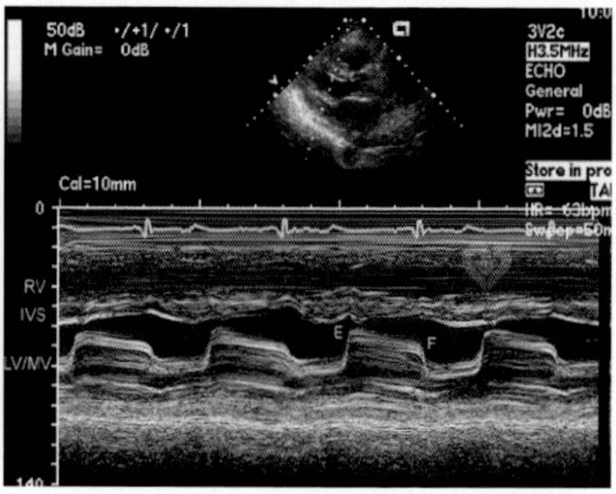

Figure 10.48: **Thickened mitral valve leaflets**

- Decreased E-F slope of the anterior mitral valve leaflet (0 to 30mm/s) indicates severe mitral stenosis)
- Anterior motion of the posterior mitral valve leaflet (83 to 90%)

2D

Planimetry for Mitral Valve Area in parasternal short axis view

- Diastolic "doming" of the anterior mitral valve leaflet ("hockey-stick" appearance) (best seen in parasternal long-axis view)
- Shortening and fibrosis of chordae tendineae

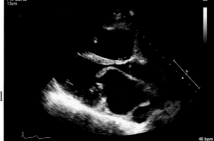

Figure 10.49: **Diastolic Doming of Anterior MV Leaflet**

- Commissural fusion (best seen in parasternal short-axis of mitral valve)
- Left atrial dilatation/ Left atrial spontaneous echo contrast ("smoke")/Left atrial thrombus (especially in atrial appendage)
- "Small"/"protected" left ventricle
- Pulmonary hypertension
- Right atrial dilatation (normal RA volume index: men 25 ± 7mL/m²; women 21 ± 6mL/m²)

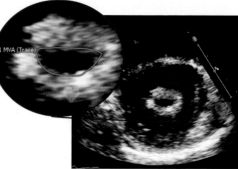

Figure 10.50: **Thickened mitral valve leaflets (>3mm), especially at the leaflet tips and chordae with restricted valve motion**

- 3D confirms 2D findings with improved evaluation of mitral valve commissures, chordal structures, extent of fibrosis/calcification, planimetry of the mitral valve orifice
- Determine:
  - Anatomic mitral valve area by planimetry of the mitral valve orifice in the parasternal short-axis view of the mitral valve in mid-diastole [1]
  - Whether aortic stenosis, tricuspid stenosis and/or pulmonic stenosis (rare) is present
  - Whether Lutembacher's syndrome (mitral stenosis with ostium secundum atrial septal defect) is present (may effect Doppler hemodynamics)
  - Echo score index

PW/CW Doppler

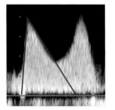

Figure 10.51: **Mild Mitral Stenosis**

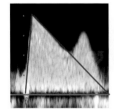

Figure 10.52: **Moderate Mitral Stenosis**

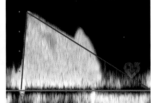

Figure 10.53: **Severe Mitral Stenosis**

- Increased mitral valve E velocity (CW Doppler from the apical window recommended) (>1.3 m/s)
- Decreased E-F slope of the mitral valve inflow Doppler tracing (indicates an increased deceleration time and increased pressure half-time)
- Evaluate the pulmonary venous flow pattern (decreased systolic flow with a prolonged duration and increased pressure half-time of diastolic flow)
- Determine:
  - Mitral valve mean transvalvular pressure gradient [1]
  - Mitral valve area by the pressure half-time method [1]
  - SPAP/MPAP/PAEDP/PVR at rest and exercise [1]
  - Mitral valve area utilizing the continuity equation (cannot be used in patients with atrial fibrillation, significant mitral regurgitation, significant aortic regurgitation [1]
  - Mitral valve resistance (ratio of mitral valve mean pressure gradient to transmitral diastolic flow rate) (CSA_{LVOT} x VTI_{LVOT} / DFT) [1]
  - Mitral valve end-diastolic pressure gradient
  - Mitral valve area index
  - Whether aortic stenosis, tricuspid stenosis and/or pulmonic stenosis (rare) is present

- Presence and severity of coexisting valvular regurgitation

Color Flow Doppler

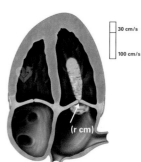
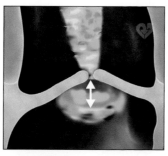

Figure 10.54: **Mitral Stenosis Flow with PISA**

- May be useful in guiding CW Doppler exam especially in patients with eccentric mitral valve diastolic jets

- Narrow, "flame-shaped" turbulent (mosaic) jet at mitral valve leaflet tips which extends into the left ventricle in diastole

- Determine:

  - Mitral valve area by the PISA method must be corrected for MV leaflet angle

Figure 10.55: **Mitral Valve PISA Radius**

$$MVA = \pi\,(r^2)(V_{aliasing})/Peak\;V_{mitral}\;\alpha\,/\,180°$$

  - Mitral valve area qualitatively by examining how narrow the color flow jet is at the mitral valve leaflet tips (vena contracta)

  - Presence and severity of valvular regurgitation (e.g., mitral, aortic)

Stress Echocardiography

- Recommended for patients with a mitral valve area <1.5cm^2 who claim to be asymptomatic or with doubtful symptoms [1]
- Semi-supine exercise echocardiography preferred to post-exercise echocardiography
- Simple supine leg lifts (30 to 60 seconds) may be useful to evaluate transmitral pressure gradients
- Dobutamine may be useful in patients who cannot exercise
- Increased cardiac Doppler peak E mitral valve velocity with exercise

- Increased cardiac Doppler mitral valve mean transvalvular gradient with exercise (an increase in mean transmitral pressure gradient >15mmHg is significant)
- Decreased mitral valve pressure half-time with exercise
- Increased mitral valve area by pressure half-time method with exercise
- Determine:
  - Mean pressure gradient (>15mmHg is significant)
  - SPAP/MPAP/PAEDP/PVR at rest and exercise (an increase in systolic pulmonary artery pressure >60mmHg is significant)
  - Severity of valvular regurgitation with exercise

Transesophageal Echocardiography

- Recommended only when transthoracic evaluation is suboptimal, to determine the presence of infective endocarditis, to detect left atrial thrombus before balloon valvuloplasty or following a thromboembolic event [1]
- Defines mitral valve anatomy: leaflet mobility, leaflet thickness, location and extent of calcification of the body of the leaflets or commissures, involvement of chordae tendineae and the subvalvular apparatus
- Superior to TTE in identifying LA spontaneous echo contrast and thrombus located in the appendage, atrial septum and the body of the left atrium
- Transgastric short-axis useful in approximately 50% of cases for planimetry of the mitral valve
- Affords the opportunity to determine mitral valve peak E velocity, peak pressure gradient, mean pressure gradient, end-diastolic pressure gradient, mitral valve area and mitral valve area index by cardiac Doppler
- Mitral balloon valvuloplasty is generally not recommended in patients with immobile mitral valve leaflets with significant valvular calcification, significant (moderate) mitral regurgitation or tricuspid regurgitation, left atrial thrombus and/or a dilated left atrium (>6cm)
- Provides information during percutaneous mitral balloon valvuloplasty concerning:
  - Guidance of trans-septal puncture site (contrast injection may be required to identify the location of the needle in the left atrium)
  - Proper placement of the balloon across the mitral valve
  - Planimetry of mitral valve area
  - Degree of commissural splitting
  - Extent of pre- and post-mitral valve regurgitation, (an increase in mitral regurgitation one grade is an indication to stop the procedure)
  - Detection of eccentric commissural mitral regurgitation
  - Detection of catheter complications (e.g., myocardial and atrial wall perforation, pericardial effusion, cardiac tamponade, mitral valve leaflet tear, papillary muscle rupture)

10

Valvular Heart Disease / **Mitral Stenosis**

- Measurement of the mitral valve annulus for proper balloon size
- Measurement of the interatrial septal thickness (normal 0.49cm ± 0.19)
- Evaluation of the degree of interatrial shunting post procedure
- Evaluation of the left and right ventricular global and segmental systolic function
- Evaluation of the associated valve disease (e.g., aortic stenosis, tricuspid regurgitation)
- Determination of the size of the atrial septal defect created by the trans-septal puncture (range 0.3 to 1.5cm, defects <0.7cm close within six months)
- Determination of the pulmonary artery pressure by cardiac Doppler (systolic pulmonary artery pressure may decrease by 10mmHg immediately post procedure)

Post Commissurotomy

- Allows evaluation of mitral valve area by two dimensional planimetry post balloon valvuloplasty. A valve area of 1.9cm^2 or greater predicts a long lasting benefit of percutaneous mitral balloon valvuloplasty.

- The pressure half-time method for calculation of the mitral valve area post percutaneous mitral balloon valvuloplasty tends to overestimate the valve area. The accuracy of the pressure half-time mitral valve area improves 72 hours post procedure.

- Allows for calculation of mitral valve area by the PISA method

Important to Note

- Mitral stenosis causes a pressure overload of the left atrium, pulmonary vascular tree and right ventricle.
- There are several pitfalls associated with the calculation of mitral valve area by the pressure half-time method.
- The following decrease pressure half-time, which increases mitral valve area:
  - Significant aortic regurgitation
  - Atrial septal defect
  - Decreased left ventricular compliance
  - Sudden change in left atrial compliance (e.g., fever, anemia, tachycardia, acute mitral regurgitation, exercise)
- The following increase pressure half-time, which decreases mitral valve area:
  - Decreased rate of left ventricular relaxation.
  - Immediate post mitral valve balloon valvuloplasty. The pressure half-time should not be employed immediately after percutaneous mitral balloon valvuloplasty (<72 hours).

Table 10.15: **Evaluation of Mitral Stenosis** *(ASE Recommendations)* [1]

	• CW Doppler tracings acquired from the apical window
	• In patients with atrial fibrillation, average five cycles with the least variation of R-R intervals and as close to possible normal heart rates
Level 1	• Determine mean pressure gradient
	• MVA planimetry using the parasternal short axis of the mitral level in mid-diastole
	• Determine MVA using the PHT method
Level 2	• Determine MVA by the continuity equation
	• Determine MVA by the PISA method
	• Determine MVA and SPAP with stress echocardiography
Level 3	• Determine mitral valve resistance
TEE	• Recommended when transthoracic approach is of poor quality, to detect left atrial thrombosis before mitral balloon commissurotomy or following a thromboembolic event

Table 10.16: **Mitral Stenosis Severity Scales** *(ASE Recommendations)* [1]

	Normal	Mild	Moderate	Severe
Specific Findings				
Valve Area (cm^2)	4 to 5	>1.5	1.0 to 1.5	<1.0
Supportive Findings				
Mean Pressure Gradient (mmHg)[a]		<5	5 to 10	>10
Systolic Pulmonary Artery Pressure		<30	30 to 50	>50

[a] At heart rates between 60 and 80 bpm and in normal sinus rhythm

Table 10.17: **Mitral Stenosis Severity Scales Additional Parameters**

Pressure Half-Time	Normal	30 to 60 msec
	Abnormal	90 to 400 msec
	Gray area	60 to 90 msec
	Mild	90 to 150 msec
	Moderate	150 to 219 msec
	Severe	≥220msec
Mitral Valve Area Index	Mild	1.5 to 2.3cm^2/m^2
	Moderate	1.0 to 1.5cm^2/m^2
	Moderately Severe	0.5 to 1.0cm^2/m^2
	Severe	<0.5cm^2/m^2
End-Diastolic Pressure Gradient	Normal	0 to 2mmHg
	Mild	2 to 6mmHg
	Moderate	7 to 10mmHg
	Severe	>10mmHg

Table 10.18: Echo Score Index for Mitral Stenosis

Mitral Valve Morphology

Leaflet Mobility

Grade 1	Highly mobile valve with leaflet tips only restricted
Grade 2	Leaflet mid and base portions have normal mobility
Grade 3	Valve continues to move forward in diastole, mainly from the base
Grade 4	No or minimal forward movement of the leaflets in diastole

Leaflet Thickening

Grade 1	Leaflets near normal in thickness (4 to 5mm)
Grade 2	Mid-leaflets normal, marked thickening of margins (5 to 8mm)
Grade 3	Thickening extending through the entire leaflet (5 to 8mm)
Grade 4	Marked thickening of all leaflet tissue (>8mm)

Subvalvular Thickening

Grade 1	Minimal thickening just below the mitral leaflets
Grade 2	Thickening of chordal structures extending up to one-third of the chordal length
Grade 3	Thickening extending to the distal third of the chords
Grade 4	Extensive thickening and shortening of all chordal structures extending down to the papillary muscles

Leaflet Calcification

Grade 1	A single area of increased echocardiographic brightness
Grade 2	Scattered areas of brightness confined to the leaflet margins
Grade 3	Brightness extending into the mid-portion of the leaflets
Grade 4	Extensive brightness throughout much of the leaflet tissue

To determine the echocardiographic score: Add the grades from the 4 categories; the minimum score is 4 and the maximum score is 16. Patients who score ≤8 are more favorable candidates for balloon valvuloplasty and patients with a score of ≥12 have a less favorable result.

Note: A successful balloon valvuloplasty includes an increase in mitral valve area >50%,
a mitral valve area >1.5cm^2 and <moderate mitral regurgitation.

Reference

1.   Baumgartner H, Hung J, Bermejo J, Chambers J, Edvardsen T, Goldstein S, Lancellotti P, LeFevre M, Miller F: Recommendations on the Echocardiographic Assessment of Aortic Valve Stenosis: A Focused Update from the European Association of Cardiovascular Imaging and the American Society of Echocardiography. Journal of the American Society of Echocardiography 30: 372-92, 2017

Valvular Heart Disease
Tricuspid Stenosis
Eric Kallstrom MBA, ACS, RDCS, FACVP, FASE

Definition

A narrowing of the tricuspid valve orifice, restricting blood flow from the right atrium to the right ventricle.

Etiology

- Rheumatic heart disease (most common, 90%)
- Carcinoid heart disease (always combined with tricuspid regurgitation)
    - Thickening of ventricular aspect of tricuspid valve leading to poor coaptation of leaflets [1]
    - Leaflets are fixed with unchanged position throughout cardiac cycle [2]
- Congenital Heart Disease [2]
- Pacemaker-induced adhesions
- Toxic (e.g., Phen-fen, methysergide)
- Infective endocarditis [3]
- Right atrial tumor/mass [3]
- Lupus valvulitis
- Coronary artery aneurysm (very rare instances) [4]
- Fabry's disease
- Whipple's disease
- Loeffler's syndrome
- Endocardial fibroelastosis
- Prosthetic valve dysfunction due to:
    - Leaflet degeneration [1]
    - Endocarditis [1]
    - Valve thrombosis/pannus formation [1]

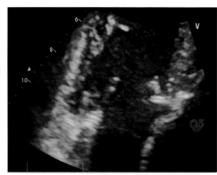

Figure 10.56: **TV Rheumatic heart disease demonstrating restricted TV leaflets in diastole**

History

- Rheumatic fever (two-thirds of patients)
- Female preponderance
- Right heart failure symptoms [1]
    - Fatigue, edema, palpitations

Physical Examination

- Signs and symptoms of associated mitral stenosis
- Peripheral cyanosis
- Elevated jugular venous pressure
- Neck vein distention with prominent a and v waves with slow y descent

Cardiac Auscultation

- Opening snap (may occur later than mitral valve opening snap)
- Diastolic rumble best heard along the lower left sternal border (higher frequency than mitral stenosis rumble) (may be accentuated with inspiration)
- Pre-systolic accentuation of the diastolic rumble (occurs earlier than mitral stenosis pre-systolic accentuation)
- Both the opening snap and the diastolic rumble may be accentuated with inspiration
- Possible tricuspid regurgitation murmur

Electrocardiogram

- Right atrial enlargement/biatrial enlargement
- Atrial fibrillation
- Right ventricular hypertrophy (suggests coexisting mitral stenosis with pulmonary hypertension)

Chest X-ray/CMR/CT

- Right atrial/left atrial enlargement
- Dilated superior vena cava, azygous vein without pulmonary artery dilatation

Cardiac Catheterization

- Increased mean diastolic pressure gradient between the right atrium and right ventricle (increases with inspiration)
- Persistence of end-diastolic gradient between right atrium and right ventricle (aids in differentiating tricuspid stenosis from tricuspid regurgitation)
- Determines tricuspid valve area by the Gorlin formula

Medical Treatment

- Treat possible underlying rheumatic fever prophylaxis
- Diuretic therapy due to volume overload
- Sodium restriction

Surgical Treatment [1]

- Surgical/Balloon commissurotomy
- Valve repair/valve replacement (mean pressure gradient >5mmHg and/or TVA ≤1.0cm^2) (large bioprosthetic is preferred choice)

M-mode[2]
- Thickened tricuspid valve leaflets
- Decreased E-F slope of the anterior tricuspid valve leaflet
- Anterior motion of the posterior tricuspid valve leaflet

2D
- Determines etiology (e.g., rheumatic)
- Thickened tricuspid valve leaflets, especially at leaflet tips and chordae tendineae with restricted motion[5]
- Diastolic "doming" of the tricuspid valve with commissural fusion of the tricuspid valve leaflets[2]
- Right atrial dilatation (normal RA volume: men 25 ± 7mL/m²; women 21 ± 6mL/m²)[1]
- Dilated inferior vena cava (normal ≤2.1cm), hepatic veins (normal 0.5 to 1.1cm)[1]
- Leftward protrusion of interatrial septum (indicates increased right atrial pressure)
- Increased right-sided pressures (due to coexisting mitral valve disease)

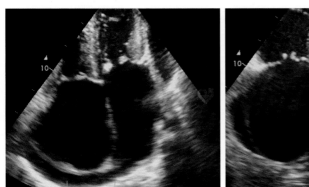
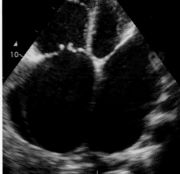

Figure 10.57: **TS in systole and diastole**

Doppler
- Assess structure and morphology of valve and surrounding anatomy[6]
- Increased tricuspid valve E velocity with PW Doppler recorded at the tricuspid valve leaflet tips (>1.0 m/s) (measure/average 5 cardiac cycles if atrial fibrillation is present)
  - Although measuring PW E velocity is not a routine measurement, labs should decide if this practice should be instituted in their organization's echo lab for all patients or just for patients with tricuspid stenosis[7]
- Helpful hint – Patient positioning and breath holding are techniques that can be used to better assess pathology
- Decreased E-F slope of the tricuspid inflow Doppler tracing (indicates increased deceleration time and an increased pressure half-time)[2]

- Increased or giant "a" wave of the hepatic vein by pulsed wave Doppler[8]
- Color flow Doppler will demonstrate a diastolic jet which is characterized as laminar aliased flow or candle flame-shaped with a mosaic center
- Because tricuspid stenosis is generally associated with tricuspid regurgitation, increased velocities and gradients contribute to higher right atrial pressure[9]
- Color flow Doppler will demonstrate flow convergence proximal to the tricuspid valve leaflets (seen on the right atrial side of the tricuspid valve)
- Determine:
  - Mean transvalvular pressure gradient using CW Doppler[9] (a mean gradient >2mmHg is diagnostic)

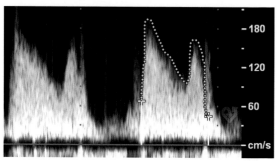

Figure 10.58: **Spectral Doppler with VTI measuring mean pressure gradient of TS**

  - Inflow velocity time integral (VTI)[9]
  - Helpful hint – Although not required from the IAC, practice using the Pedoff probe on all stenotic lesions, including tricuspid stenosis (looks similar to the mitral stenosis pattern)
  - Pressure half-time[9]
  - Tricuspid valve area utilizing the continuity equation[9]
  - Tricuspid valve area index
  - Presence and severity of tricuspid regurgitation
  - SPAP/MPAP/PAEDP/PVR at rest and exercise
  - Presence and severity of coexisting valve stenosis/regurgitation[9] (e.g., mitral)

Stress Echocardiography

- May be useful in enhancing transvalvular gradients (useful for mitral stenosis, too)
  - Record resting and post exercise mean gradients of tricuspid valve
    - Check with your lab's protocols regarding the sequence of regional wall motion analysis and valvular hemodynamic assessment

Transesophageal Echocardiography

- Generally not indicated solely for the evaluation of tricuspid stenosis. May be useful in difficult to image patients where there is a question of accuracy, or in evaluating the right atrium and appendage for thrombus formation.

3D Echocardiography

- 3D echocardiography allows sonographer/ cardiologist to obtain a direct view of the tricuspid valve orifice for calculation of TVA by way of planimetry [3]
  - The limits of 2D echocardiography prohibit visualization of tricuspid valve orifice

Important to Note

- Tricuspid stenosis is a pressure overload of the right atrium which will eventually produce peripheral edema and reduced cardiac output.

- Tricuspid stenosis almost never occurs as an isolated lesion; it generally accompanies mitral stenosis, so evaluate for mitral, aortic and pulmonic valve disease due to rheumatic fever [9]

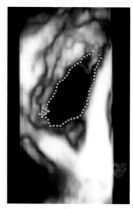

Figure 10.59:
3D TTE demonstrating planimetry of the TV to obtain a TVA

- Helpful hint – Refrain from focusing on just one lesion. Maintain the mindset of a complete echo on all valves and chambers.

- The incidence of rheumatic tricuspid valve stenosis is estimated to be <6% and has a striking female preponderance.

- The tricuspid valve in rheumatic heart disease is usually not as thickened or calcified as compared to mitral valve stenosis.

- In tricuspid valve stenosis the tricuspid valve peak E velocity is usually >1.0 m/s and this fact is helpful in separating patients who are normal or who have significant pure tricuspid regurgitation. [9]

- The tricuspid valve deceleration time is shorter in patients with tricuspid regurgitation as compared to the deceleration time of patients with tricuspid valve stenosis.

- Because respiration affects tricuspid stenosis waveforms, it is recommended to measure at end-expiration. [9]

- The constant 190 instead of 220 has been proposed for determining tricuspid valve area by the pressure half-time method: TVA (cm^2) = 190/PHT (msec)

Table 10.19: Significant Tricuspid Stenosis *(ASE Recommendations)* [9]

Specific Findings	
Mean pressure gradient	≥5mmHg
Inflow velocity time integral (VTI)	>60cm
Pressure half-time	≥190 msec
TVA (continuity equation)	≤1.0cm^2
Supportive Findings	
Dilated right atrium	≥ moderate
Inferior vena cava	dilated (>2.1cm)

References

1. Lang, R. M., Goldstein, S. A., Kronzon, I., Khandheria, B. K., Mor-Avi, V. (2016). ASE's Comprehensive Echocardiography. (2nd edition). Philadelphia, PA: Elsevier Saunders.

2. Dewitt, S. K. (2018). The Echo Notebook. (5th edition). St. Mary's, GA: Self Published.

3. Nanda, N. C., Karakus, G., Degirmencioglu, A. (2016). Manual of Echocardiography. Philadelphia, PA: Jaypee Brothers Medical Publishers (P) Ltd.

4. Wang, E., Fan, X., Qi, W., Song, Y., and Qi, Z. (2019). A giant right coronary artery aneurysm leading to tricuspid stenosis. Annals of Thoracic Surgery, , 108(3), 145-147

5. Feigenbaum, H., Armstrong, W. F., Ryan, T. (2005). Feigenbaum's Echocardiography. (6th ed.). Philadelphia, PA: Lippincott Williams & Wilkins.

6. Cuculich, P. S., Kates, A. M., Henderson, K. E., De Fer, T. M. (2009). The Washington Manual Cardiology Subspecialty Consult (2nd ed.). Philadelphia, PA: Lippincott Williams & Wilkins.

7. Mitchell, C., Rahko, P. S., Blauwet, L. A., Canaday, B., Finstuen, J. Foster, M. . .Velazquez, E. J. (2019). Guidelines for Performing a Comprehensive Transthoracic Echocardiographic Examination in Adults: Recommendation from the American Society of Echocardiography

8. Lilly, L. S. (2003). Pathophysiology of Heart Disease. (3rd. ed). Philadelphia, PA: Lipponcott Williams & Wilkins.

9. Baumgartner, H., Hung, J., Bermejo, J., Chambers, J., Evangelista, A., Griffin, B. . .Quinones, M. (2009). Echocardiographic Assessment of Valve Stenosis: EAE/ASE Recommendations for Clinical Practice. Journal of the American Society of Echocardiography, 22(1), 1-23.

Valvular Heart Disease
Tricuspid Regurgitation
Eric Kallstrom MBA, ACS, RDCS, FACVP, FASE

Definition

The reversal of blood flow from the right ventricle into the right atrium during ventricular systole; may be acute, chronic or intermittent, may be categorized as primary (degenerative) and secondary (ventricular remodeling, functional).

Etiology

Primary leaflet abnormality

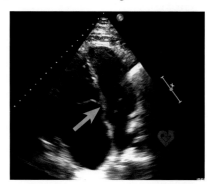

Figure 10.60: **TTE apical 4-chamber demonstrating Ebstein's anomaly and its characteristic downward displacement of the tricuspid valve**

• Acquired disease
   - Degenerative, myxomatous valve syndrome [1]
   - Rheumatic heart disease [2]
   - Infective endocarditis [2]
   - Carcinoid heart disease [2]
   - Endomyocardial fibrosis [2]
   - Toxins
   - Rheumatoid arthritis [3]
   - Trauma [3,4]
   - Iatrogenic (pacing leads, RV biopsy, cardiac transplantation) [2,4]
   - Radiation induced [4]
   - Congenital
   - Ebstein's anomaly (downward displacement of tricuspid valve "atrialized" ventricle)
• TV dysplasia [2]
• TV tethering associated with perimembranous ventricular septal defect and ventricular septal aneurysm
• Repaired tetralogy of Fallot
• Congenitally corrected transposition of the great arteries
• Marfan syndrome [3]
• Other (giant right atrium)

Secondary (ventricular remodeling, functional)

• Left heart disease
   - LV dysfunction or valve disease
• RV dysfunction [4]
   - RV myocardial infarction
   - RV volume overload

  - RV cardiomyopathy
- Pulmonary hypertension [4]
  - Chronic lung disease
  - Pulmonary thromboembolism
  - Left-to-right shunt
- Atrial fibrillation [5]
- Papillary/chordae rupture [1,4]

History

- Usually well tolerated in the absence of pulmonary hypertension
- Right heart failure (e.g., jugular venous distention, hepatomegaly, peripheral edema, ascites, anasarca)[2]

Physical Examination

- Jugular venous distention [2]
- Weight loss, cachexia, cyanosis, jaundice, edema [2]
- Thrill (lower left sternal border)
- Hyperdynamic right ventricular impulse along left sternal border

Complications [2]

- Severe right heart failure
- Renal failure when severe congestion is present

Cardiac Auscultation

- A holosystolic, high-pitched blowing murmur heard best in the xiphoid area along the left sternal border over the right ventricular apex
- Brief early systolic murmur (may suggest low pressure tricuspid regurgitation)
- The murmur of tricuspid regurgitation may be accentuated with inspiration; this is known as Rivero-Carvallo's sign
  - Venous return is increased due to the negative intrathoracic pressure from inspiration [6]
- Diastolic flow rumble (due to increased flow across the tricuspid valve)
- Right-sided S3 (accentuated with inspiration)

Electrocardiogram

- Right atrial enlargement [2]
- Atrial fibrillation (common finding)
- Right bundle branch block [3]

Chest X-ray/CMR/CT

- Right atrial enlargement [2,3]
- Right ventricular enlargement [2,3]

- Left heart enlargement (suggests functional tricuspid regurgitation)
- Pulmonary congestion (suggests functional tricuspid regurgitation)
- Pulmonary artery dilatation (suggests functional tricuspid regurgitation)
- CMR may be useful in determining the presence and severity of tricuspid regurgitation [7]

Cardiac Catheterization

- Right ventriculography to determine presence and severity
- Amplified right atrial v wave [3,6]
- Kussmaul's sign (increased right atrial pressure with inspiration)

Medical Treatment [3]

- None (tricuspid regurgitation may be well tolerated for years depending on severity)
- Treat underlying condition
- Digitalis/diuretics/sodium restriction
- Vasodilators (nifedipine, hydralazine, prazosin) in patients with pulmonary hypertension
- Anticoagulation (right heart failure)

Surgical Treatment [2,7]

- Tricuspid valve excision (drug addiction with infective endocarditis) (followed 6 to 9 months with bioprosthetic TVR)
- Annuloplasty (e.g., Carpentier ring, Kay ring, Duran ring, DeVega)
- Tricuspid valve replacement (usually with a bioprosthetic valve to reduce the risk of thrombus formation because of lower right sided pressures) transcatheter (e.g.; MitraClip™, TriCinch™, FORMA™, Cardioband™, Caval valve implantation)
- Bicuspidization

2D/M-mode [2,7]

- Assess the morphology of tricuspid valve/surrounding anatomy and identify the mechanism (primary vs. secondary)
- Physiologic to mild tricuspid regurgitation considered normal in healthy individuals
- Right atrial dilatation with systolic expansion
- Right ventricular diastolic expansion
- Right ventricular dilatation (normal basal RV diameter 25 to 41mm) with tenting of the tricuspid valve
- Right ventricular volume overload pattern (right ventricular dilatation with paradoxical septal motion)
- D-shaped left ventricle during ventricular diastole indicating a right ventricular diastolic volume overload

- Associated systolic D-shaped left ventricle during systole with right-sided pressure overload

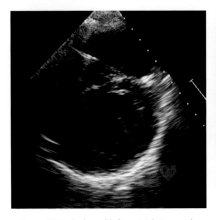

Figure 10.61: **D-shaped left ventricle in systole indicative of pressure overload**

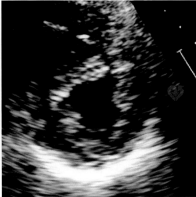

Figure 10.62: **D-shaped left ventricle in diastole indicative of volume overload**

• Globular (spherical-shaped) right ventricle which may form the cardiac apex
• Dilated:
   - Tricuspid valve annulus (significant annular dilatation defined as end-diastolic diameter ≥40mm or 21mm/m^2 acquired from the apical 4-chamber view) suggests severe tricuspid regurgitation
   - Inferior vena cava with lack of inspiratory collapse (normal ≤2.1cm)
   - Hepatic veins (normal: 0.5 to 1.1cm)
   - Coronary sinus
   - Superior vena cava/innominate vein
• Systolic bowing of the interatrial septum towards the left atrium
• Systolic reflux of saline contrast into the inferior vena cava and hepatic veins may indicate significant tricuspid regurgitation (may also be visualized by color flow Doppler)
• Persistent saline contrast echo may indicate significant tricuspid regurgitation
• Color M-mode may be useful in determining the presence, timing and duration of tricuspid regurgitation when combined with PISA
• Determine:
   - Tricuspid valve leaflet tethering distance (measured from plane of tricuspid annulus to coaptation point of the leaflets in apical 4-chamber view) (normal 1.6 ± 1.0mm)
   - Right atrial dimension(s) (normal: men 25 ± 7mL/m^2; women 21 ± 6mL/m^2)
   - Right ventricular wall thickness, dimension(s), systolic function

PW Doppler[7]

- Hepatic vein holosystolic flow reversal may indicate severe tricuspid regurgitation (peak systolic velocity usually ≥0.5 m/s)

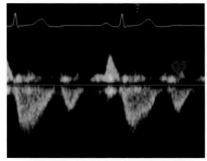
Figure 10.63: **Normal hepatic vein spectral Doppler**

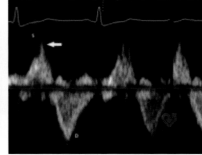
Figure 10.64: **Hepatic vein flow reversal (arrow)**

- Increased tricuspid E velocity (>1.0 m/s) with normal deceleration time may indicate significant tricuspid regurgitation
- Laminar tricuspid regurgitation flow may denote significant regurgitation (associated with lack of tricuspid leaflet coaptation)
- Determine:
  - Tricuspid valve velocity time integral (increased with significant tricuspid regurgitation)
  - Right ventricular outflow tract velocity time integral (decreased with significant tricuspid regurgitation)

CW Doppler[7]

- Jet density (spectral strength) indicates severity. Dense, triangular (asymmetrical) shape with early systolic peaking of the tricuspid regurgitation flow velocity envelope may indicate significant tricuspid regurgitation (due to large right atrial v wave)

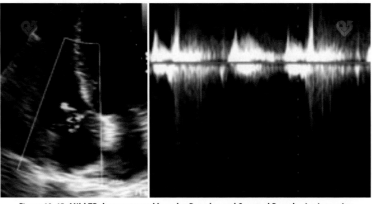
Figure 10.65: **Mild TR demonstrated by color Doppler and Spectral Doppler jet intensity**

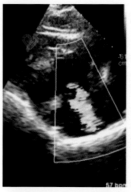
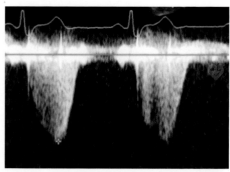

Figure 10.66: **Moderate TR demonstrated by color Doppler and Spectral Doppler jet intensity**

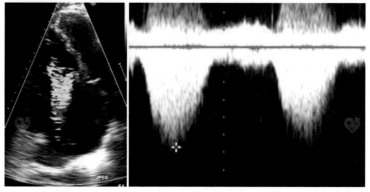

Figure 10.67: **Severe TR demonstrated by color Doppler and Spectral Doppler jet intensity**

• Determine the SPAP/MPAP/PAEDP/PVR at rest and exercise

Color Flow Doppler [7]

• Determine:

- Appropriate color gain setting, color velocity scale (50 to 70cm/s) are chosen

- Jet area- Mild <5cm²; Severe >10cm²

- Regurgitant jet area/right atrial area- mild <20%; severe >34%

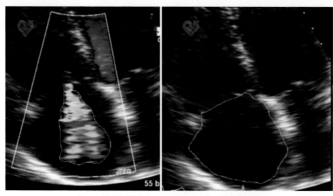

Figure 10.68: **TR jet area compared with RA area**

- Vena contracta width (Mild <0.3cm) (Severe ≥0.7cm)
- PISA radius (Mild: ≤0.5cm at velocity scale set at 30 to 40cm/s) (Severe: >0.9cm/s velocity scale set at 30 to 40cm/s)

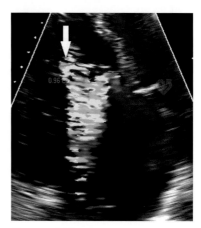

Figure 10.69: **TR vena contracta measuring .96 which is indicative of severe**

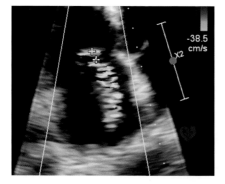

Figure 10.70: **Color Doppler demonstrating the diameter of the flow convergence to obtain PISA**

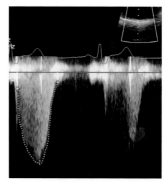

Figure 10.71: **Spectral Doppler VTI in calculating PISA of the TR jet**

- Presence of holosystolic flow reversal in the hepatic veins/inferior vena cava/ superior vena cava indicates severe tricuspid regurgitation (decrease color velocity scale, wall filter)
- Direction of jet (central jet: functional TR; eccentric jet: flail leaflet, leaflet impingement by an implanted device lead)
- Right to left shunt through patent foramen ovale (possible)

Transesophageal Echocardiography [2,7]

- May be indicated in patients with device leads, infective endocarditis, congenital abnormalities
    - Useful for challenging cases where valve coaptation is affected
- Useful post-operatively in mitral valve surgery to determine the severity of tricuspid regurgitation

3D Echocardiography

- Measurement of annulus size, right ventricular size, papillary muscle location and function, EROA, and vena contracta

Important to Note

- Chronic significant tricuspid regurgitation is a right heart volume overload [2]
- The most common etiology of tricuspid regurgitation is pulmonary hypertension due to left heart pathology (90% incidence when systolic pulmonary artery pressure is >40mmHg).
- The classic clinical triad of prominent jugular venous distention, holosystolic murmur at the lower left sternal border increasing with inspiration and a pulsatile liver is present in only 40% of patients with severe tricuspid regurgitation.
- The tricuspid regurgitant jet is frequently baffled towards the interatrial septum because the anterior leaflet is longest. The jet may be baffled towards the interatrial septum when there is significant left atrial dilatation as well. The baffling of the jet may make the subcostal 4-chamber useful in acquiring the CW Doppler tracing of tricuspid regurgitation.
- Tricuspid regurgitation is the most common physiologic regurgitation (57% in individuals <50 years of age; 74% >50 years of age). Normal tricuspid valve apparatus, normal chamber dimensions, peak tricuspid regurgitation velocity (2.0 m/s ± 0.2) with a short duration (<100 msec) and small regurgitant jet area are indicators of physiologic flow [7]
- Helpful hint--Look to the right atrium and right ventricle for clues on whether acute or chronic tricuspid regurgitation
    - Chronic, severe tricuspid regurgitation leads to enlargement of RA/RV
- Helpful hint—Avoid measuring opening clicks. Measure the modal velocity of tricuspid regurgitation spectral Doppler waveforms

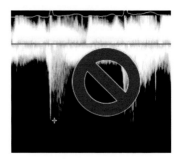

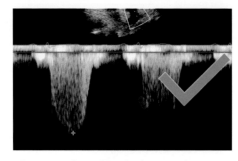

Figure 10.72: **Spectral Doppler demonstrating improper measurement of TR peak velocity**

Figure 10.73: **Spectral Doppler demonstrating proper measurement of TR peak velocity**

- Helpful hint—Always assess tricuspid regurgitation in multiple windows, regardless if one acquisition is technically excellent.
  - Can be obtained from PLAX, PSAX, A4C, or SC 4-chamber [8]

- Helpful hint--Severe tricuspid regurgitation will often give a low Spectral Doppler velocity
  - Don't always expect high velocity profiles with wide open tricuspid regurgitation

- Helpful hint--If tricuspid regurgitation jet is difficult to align with Doppler beam, utilize an RV Modified view to obtain best results. To do this, from the apical 4 position, move your transducer medially and up one or two rib spaces [8]

- Helpful hint: Not all patients with pulmonary hypertension have significant tricuspid regurgitation [2]

- Helpful hint—In challenging cases, ultrasonic enhancing agents can be used to augment Spectral Doppler profiles [8]

- Helpful hint—If multiple attempts are made from different angles for a patient in normal sinus rhythm, remember to keep the highest and best quality tricuspid regurgitation jet velocity for final calculations into the patient's right ventricular systolic pressure [8]

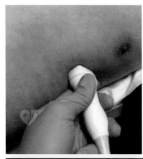

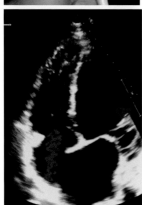

Figure 10.74: **Modified apical 4 window demonstrating proper alignment of TR jet with Doppler beam**

  - Lower, poorer quality signals should be deleted from the report page before transmission to PACS as to not give erroneous results

Table 10.20: Classification of Tricuspid Regurgitation Severity *(ASE Recommendations)* [7]

Specific Criteria for Mild TR	Specific Criteria for Severe TR
Thin, small, central color jet	Dilated annulus with no valve coaptation or flail leaflet
Vena contracta width <0.3cm	Large central jet >50% of RA
PISA radius ≤0.5cm at Nyquist 30 to 40cm/s	VC width ≥0.7cm
Incomplete or faint CW jet	PISA radius >0.9cm at Nyquist 30 to 40cm/s
Systolic dominant hepatic vein flow	Dense, triangular CW jet or sine wave pattern
Tricuspid A-wave dominant inflow	Systolic reversal of hepatic vein flow
Normal RV/RA	Dilated RV with preserved function
	Jet area >10cm^2

Table 10.21: Classification of Tricuspid Regurgitation Severity

Parameters	Mild	Moderate	Severe
Structural			
TV morphology	**Normal or mildly abnormal leaflets**	Moderately abnormal leaflets	**Severe valve lesions** (e.g., flail leaflet, severe retraction, large perforation)
RV and RA size	Usually normal	Normal or mild dilatation	Usually dilated*
Inferior vena cava diameter	Normal <2cm	Normal or mildly dilated 2.1 to 2.5cm	Dilated >2.5cm
Qualitative Doppler			
Color flow jet area [a]	**Small, narrow, central**	Moderate central	**Large central jet** or eccentric wall-impinging jet of variable size
Flow convergence zone	**Not visible, transient or small**	Intermediate in size and duration	**Large throughout systole**
CWD jet	Faint/partial/parabolic	Dense, parabolic or triangular	Dense, often triangular
Semiquantitative			
Color flow jet area (cm^2) [a]	Not defined	Not defined	**>10**
VCW (cm) [a]	<0.3	0.3 to 0.69	**≥0.7**
PISA radius (cm) [b]	≤0.5	0.6 to 0.9	**>0.9**
Hepatic vein flow [c]	Systolic dominance	Systolic blunting	**Systolic flow reversal**
Tricuspid inflow [c]	**A-wave dominant**	Variable	E-wave >1.0 m/s
Quantitative			
EROA (cm^2)	<0.20	0.20 to 0.39 [d]	**≥0.40**
RVol (2D PISA) (mL)	<30	30 to 44 [d]	**≥45**

RA, Right atrium.
Bolded signs are considered specific for their TR grade.

* RV and RA size can be within the "normal" range in patients with acute severe TR.

a) With Nyquist limit 50 to 70cm/s.
b) With baseline Nyquist limit shift of 28cm/s.
c) Signs are nonspecific and are influenced by many other factors (RV diastolic function, atrial fibrillation, RA pressure).
d) There are little data to support further separation of these values.

Tricuspid Valve Prolapse

Definition

• Referred to as a considerable amount of tricuspid valve billowing into the right atrium with redundant leaflets [9]

• Nominal tricuspid valve prolapse is considered normal

Echocardiographic Types [10]

• Mid to late systolic

• Holosystolic (pansystolic)

2D

• The best views are the apical 4-chamber view (anterior and septal leaflets) and the parasternal right ventricular inflow tract view (anterior and posterior leaflets)

• Prolapse of the anterior, septal and posterior leaflets, individually or together, superior to the tricuspid annulus >2mm (usually the anterior tricuspid valve leaflet)

• Myxomatous, redundant appearance of the involved tricuspid valve leaflet(s)

• Tricuspid annular dilatation (normal 2.2cm ± 0.3) (apical 4-chamber)

Doppler

• Tricuspid regurgitation (often predominantly late systolic and mild)

• Determine:
  - Severity of tricuspid regurgitation
  - SPAP/MPAP/PAEDP/PVR at rest and exercise

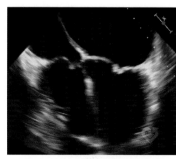

Figure 10.75: **TEE apical 4-chamber demonstrating TV prolapse**

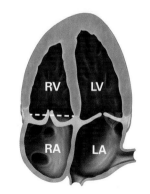

Figure 10.76: **Anterior and Septal Leaflet**

Important to Note

- Due to the inconstant anatomy and size of the tricuspid valve, its leaflet motion during systole and diastole is more difficult to expect, as opposed to other valves [11]

- Isolated tricuspid valve prolapse is rare. It is usually associated with mitral valve prolapse (19 to 50%).

- Tricuspid valve prolapse is a common finding in Marfan syndrome, ostium secundum atrial septal defect and Ebstein's anomaly.

- Anterior TV leaflet prolapse is the most common followed by septal and posterior leaflet prolapse.

Surgical Treatment [12]

- Edge-to-edge suture

References

1. Feigenbaum, H., Armstrong, W. F., Ryan, T. (2005). Feigenbaum's Echocardiography. (6th ed.). Philadelphia, PA: Lippincott Williams & Wilkins.

2. Lang, R. M., Goldstein, S. A., Kronzon, I., Khandheria, B. K., Mor-Avi, V. (2016). ASE's Comprehensive Echocardiography. (2nd edition). Philadelphia, PA: Elsevier Saunders.

3. Cuculich, P. S., Kates, A. M., Henderson, K. E., De Fer, T. M. (2009). The Washington Manual Cardiology Subspecialty Consult (2nd ed.). Philadelphia, PA: Lippincott Williams & Wilkins.

4. Nanda, N. C., Karakus, G., Degirmencioglu, A. (2016). Manual of Echocardiography. Philadelphia, PA: Jaypee Brothers Medical Publishers (P) Ltd.

5. Dewitt, S. K. (2018). The Echo Notebook. (5th edition). St. Mary's, GA: Self Published.

6. Lilly, L. S. (2003). Pathophysiology of Heart Disease. (3rd. ed) Philadelphia, PA: Lipponcott Williams & Wilkins.

7. Zoghbi, W. A., Adams, D., Bonow, R. O., Enriquez-Sarano, M., Foster, E., Grayburn, P. A…Weissman, N. J. (2017). Recommendations for Noninvasive Evaluaton of Native Valvular Regurgitation. Journal of the American Society of Echocardiography, 30(4), 303-371.

8. Mitchell, C., Rahko, P. S., Blauwet, L. A., Canaday, B., Finstuen, J. Foster, M…Velazquez, E. J. (2019). Guidelines for Performing a Comprehensive Transthoracic Echocardiographic Examination in Adults: Recommendation from the American Society of Echocardiography

9. Zoghbi, W. A., Adams, D., Bonow, R. O., Enriquez-Sarano, M., Foster, E., Grayburn, P. A…Weissman, N. J. (2017). Recommendations for Noninvasive Evaluaton of Native Valvular Regurgitation. Journal of the American Society of Echocardiography, 30(4), 303-371.

10. Dewitt, S. K. (2018). The Echo Notebook. (5th edition). St. Mary's, GA: Self Published.

11. Feigenbaum, H., Armstrong, W. F., Ryan, T. (2005). Feigenbaum's Echocardiography. (6th ed.). Philadelphia, PA: Lippincott Williams & Wilkins.

12. Lang, R. M., Goldstein, S. A., Kronzon, I., Khandheria, B. K., Mor-Avi, V. (2016). ASE's Comprehensive Echocardiography. (2nd edition). Philadelphia, PA: Elsevier Saunders.

Valvular Heart Disease
Infective Endocarditis
Ashlee Davis, BSMI, ACS, RDCS, FASE

Definition

A microbial infection which enters the heart via the bloodstream typically confined to the external lining of a valve, but may affect the lining of the heart, great vessels or intracardiac devices.

Etiology

- An invasion of microorganisms, usually bacterial; the classic manifestation is a vegetation
- Acute infective endocarditis is most often caused by Staphylococcus aureus (common in right sided infection in intravenous drug abusers)
- Subacute infective endocarditis is usually caused by viridans streptococci, enterococci, coagulase-negative staphylococci or gram-negative coccobacilli
- Incidence rate is 5 to 10 per 100,000 in industrial countries.
- High complication rate, 1 year mortality 20 to 40% despite current antibiotic treatments and surgical techniques

History

- Fever of unknown origin
- Positive blood cultures of appropriate organisms such as Streptococcus viridans, Streptococcus bovis, Staphylococcus aureus, Enterococcus species, or HACEK.
- Heart failure (dyspnea, orthopnea, paroxysmal nocturnal dyspnea, fatigue, cough, weight gain)
- Underlying heart disease
- Recent invasive procedure (e.g., dental procedure, IV drug abuse)
- "Flu like" symptoms (e.g., fatigue, chills, sweats, nausea, vomiting, headache, myalgias, arthralgias, anorexia, weight loss, malaise)
- Serologic abnormalities (e.g., positive rheumatoid factor, elevated white blood cell count)
- Chest pain (most common in intravenous drug abuse), abdominal pain, back pain

Physical Examination

- Changing or new valvular regurgitation murmur
- Skin lesions (e.g., petechiae, splinter hemorrhages, Osler nodes, Janeway lesions)
- Embolic event (e.g., CVA, pulmonary embolism)
- Pallor (due to anemia)
- Clubbing
- Splenomegaly

Cardiac Auscultation

- Systolic/diastolic/continuous murmur(s) (85 to 95%)

Electrocardiogram

- Conduction abnormalities (e.g., prolonged PR interval, right bundle branch block) (ominous sign – may indicate abscess formation)
- Left ventricular hypertrophy (suggests significant mitral or aortic regurgitation)
- Myocardial ischemia/infarction (due to emboli to coronary artery)

Chest X-ray/CMR/CT

- Limited role
- May demonstrate signs of heart failure
- Evidence of pulmonary emboli (right heart endocarditis)
- Pulmonary infiltrates (suggests right heart emboli)
- Widening of the aorta (suggests mycotic aneurysm)
- CT/CMR may provide information concerning perivalvular extension, aortic root aneurysm/fistulas, coronary artery involvement

• Treatment

- Prevention (endocarditis prophylaxis, especially for high-risk patients)
- Antimicrobial therapy (4 to 6 weeks)
- Anticoagulation (embolic event)
- Digitalis/Diuretics (heart failure)
- Afterload reduction (heart failure, severe mitral and/or aortic regurgitation)
- Valve debridement/repair or replacement (HF due to significant valvular regurgitation/stenosis/perforation, hemodynamic evidence of increased LVEDP, PHV dehiscence, highly resistant organism, recurrent emboli, persistent vegetation, large (>10mm) vegetation)
- Left sided endocarditis can lead to stroke, distal infection, downstream ischemia, myocardial infarction
- Right sided endocarditis can lead to pulmonary embolism
- Pericardial effusion suggesting purulent pericarditis
- Cardiac conditions associated with the highest risk of adverse outcome from endocarditis for which prophylaxis with dental procedures is recommended
- Prosthetic heart valve or heart valve repair with prosthetic material
- History of infective endocarditis
- Cardiac transplant with abnormal heart valve function

- Certain Congenital heart defects including:
  - Unrepaired or partially repaired cyanotic CHD, including palliative shunts and conduits
  - Completely repaired congenital heart defect with prosthetic material or device, during the first 6 months after the procedure**
  - Repaired CHD with residual defects, such as persisting leaks or abnormal flow, at the site or adjacent to the site of a prosthetic patch or prosthetic device

* Except for the conditions listed above, antibiotic prophylaxis is no longer recommended for any other form of CHD.

** Prophylaxis is recommended because endothelialization of prosthetic material occurs within 6 months after the procedure. Circulation, 2007; 115:1-19

Echocardiographic Presentations of Endocarditis

M-mode

- Severe acute aortic regurgitation may cause premature closure of the mitral valve. C point of mitral valve occurs on or before onset of the QRS complex. Increased left ventricular end-diastolic pressure (LVEDP)

- Severe acute aortic regurgitation may cause premature opening of the aortic valve The aortic valve is open before onset of QRS complex and increased LVEDP.

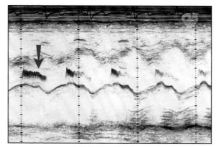

Figure 10.77: **Thickened aortic valve closure line due to vegetation**

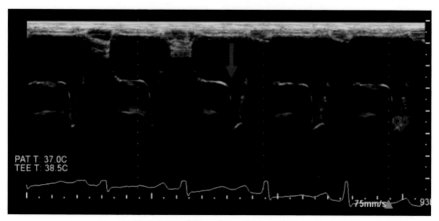

Figure 10.78: **AOV preclosure in severe AR**

Table 10.22: The Role of Echocardiography in Endocarditis
• Identifying predisposing cardiac disease
• Important role in diagnosing vegetations
• Identifying complications
• Assessing hemodynamics
• Evaluating effectiveness of therapy
• Assessing prognosis and risk of complications

2D

- Vegetation defined as an irregularly shaped oscillating mass with independent motion, usually found on the flow side of the cardiac valves, adherent to myocardium, or attached to intracardiac devices.

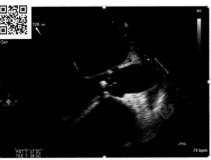

Figure 10.79: **Small aortic valve vegetation**   Figure 10.80: **Mitral valve endocarditis**

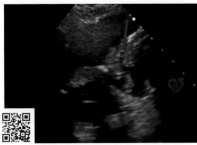
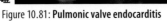
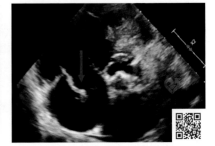

Figure 10.81: **Pulmonic valve endocarditis**   Figure 10.82: **Tricuspid valve endocarditis with flail**

- Vegetations prolapse into the upstream chamber
- Chamber dilatation if regurgitation is significant
- Global and segmental systolic ventricular function usually normal or hyperdynamic unless coronary arteries have been compromised by embolization
- Ruptured chordae tendineae/flail leaflet may result from infection
- Flail leaflets best seen by 2D/3D echocardiography

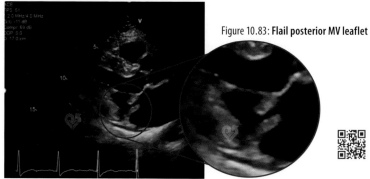

Figure 10.83: **Flail posterior MV leaflet**

- Mitral valve leaflet aneurysm may result from a weakening of the spongiosa layer

- Abscess as defined by thickened area or mass within the myocardium or annular region

- Aneurysm as defined as echolucent space bound by thin tissue

- Fistula seen as a connection between two distinct cardiac blood spaces through nonanatomical channel

- Leaflet perforation may be seen as a defect in body of valve leaflet with evidence of flow through the defect

- Evaluate:
  - Ventricular surface of mitral valve leaflets/chordae tendineae in patients with aortic valve vegetation to rule out "seeding" (metastatic or satellite vegetations)

  - Arterial walls for mycotic aneurysm (especially aortic root)

  - Intracardiac fistula (e.g., aorta to right ventricle, right atrium, left atrium)

  - Pericardial effusion (may suggest intracardiac abscess or purulent pericarditis)

  - Prosthetic valves evaluate for: new or worsening paravalvular regurgitation, valvular dehiscence (rocking motion >15°), and paravalvular complications such as abscess or pseudo aneurysm

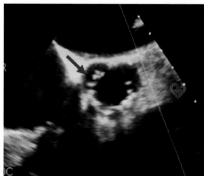

Figure 10.84: **Aortic valve abscess**

- Ring abscess is a serious complication of infective endocarditis; possible echocardiographic findings include:
  - Echo-free cavity in valve annulus

  - Echo-free cavity in adjacent structures including interventricular septum, aortic root and anterior mitral valve leaflet

- Localized echo density in mitral annulus resembling calcification
- Sinus of Valsalva aneurysm
- Aorto septal discontinuity caused by abscess cavity
- Echo report should describe the vegetation: location, size, shape (e.g., globular, polypoid, tubular, frondlike, pedunculated)
- Measure vegetation diameter (small: <5mm; moderate: 5 to 10mm; large: >10mm)
- Important that the sonographer design the study for endocarditis (utilize high frequency transducer, harmonic imaging, zoom feature, B-mode color, cine-loop)

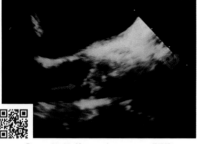

Figure 10.85: **Vegetation seen on TAVR**

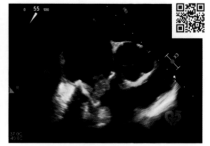

Figure 10.86: **TV ring vegetation**

Doppler

- Evaluate the presence and severity of valvular regurgitation
- When there is severe, acute aortic regurgitation, the mitral valve should be sampled at the leaflet tips with PW Doppler and the deceleration time measured; <140 msec with an increased E/A ratio indicates significant hemodynamic changes due to severe aortic regurgitation (indicates increased LVEDP)

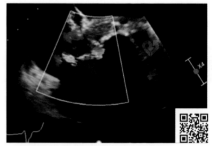

Figure 10.87: **Fistula between aortic valve and RA**

- Diastolic mitral regurgitation is associated with severe, acute aortic regurgitation and indicates increased LVEDP
- Abscess may cause a continuous flow pattern within the site
- A fistula between the aorta and either the left atrium or right atrium will demonstrate continuous, high-velocity flow. High velocity systolic flow may suggest a fistula between the left ventricle and right or left atrium. High velocity diastolic flow suggests a communication between the aorta and left ventricle
- Color flow through the body of a leaflet may suggest valve perforation

- Determine:
  - Valvular obstruction (rare except in mitral bioprosthetic valve endocarditis)
  - SPAP/MPAP/PAEDP/PVR

Transesophageal Echocardiography

- Test of choice in patients with infective endocarditis especially in patients with small vegetations (<5mm), abnormal native valves and prosthetic heart valves
- TEE is useful in examining the aortic and mitral annulus for abscess. The medial, lateral and posterior aspects are well defined, but the anterior portion may be difficult to visualize.
- In aortic valve endocarditis, TEE is excellent in detecting complications such as abscess, mitral valve leaflet perforation, mitral-aortic intervalvular fibrosa aneurysm
- A follow-up study after one week of antimicrobial treatment may be warranted to evaluate vegetation size and density
- TEE can determine the presence, timing and duration of valvular regurgitation
- A multiplane probe with a high frequency transducer with regional expansion of the image is imperative

3D

- Used to define location relative to surrounding anatomy
- 3D color may be useful to define regurgitant jets, perivalvular leak, or fistula.
- Used for communication to surgeons

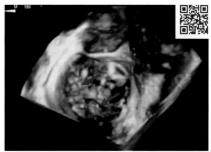

Figure 10.88: **MV vegetations**

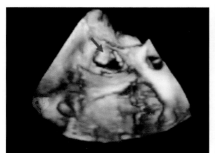

Figure 10.89: **Aortic valve endocarditis**

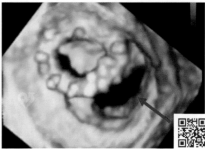

Figure 10.90: **Mitral valve ring dehiscence**

10

Valvular Heart Disease / **Infective Endocarditis**

Major Criteria [4]

- Blood Culture positive for IE (2 separate blood cultures)
- Microorganisms consistent with IE from persistently positive blood cultures, defined as follows:
  - At least 2 positive blood cultures drawn >12 hours apart or all of 3 or a majority of 4 separate blood cultures at least 1 hour apart, Single positive blood culture for Coxiella burnetti or antiphase I IgG antibody titer >1:800
  - Evidence of endocardial involvement
  - Echocardiogram positive for IE, defined as follows:
  - Oscillating intracardiac mass on valve or supporting structures, in the path of regurgitant jets, or on implanted material in the absence or an alternative anatomic explanation; or abscess; or new partial dehiscence of prosthetic valve
  - New valvular regurgitation (worsening or changing of pre-existing murmur not sufficient)

Minor Criteria [4]

- Predisposition, predisposing heart condition or injection drug use
- Fever temperature >38°C
- Vascular phenomena, major arterial emboli, septic pulmonary infarcts, mycotic aneurysm, intracranial hemorrhage, conjunctival hemorrhages, and Janeway's lesions
- Immunologic phenomena: Glumorulonephritis, Osler's nodes, Roth's spots, and rheumatoid factor
- Microbiological evidence: Positive blood culture but does not meet a major criterion as noted above or serological evidence of active infection with organism consistent with IE
- Echocardiographic minor criteria eliminated
- Definite Endocarditis: 2 major +1 minor, or 3 minor criteria
- Possible Endocarditis: 1 major +1 minor, or 3 minor, or findings consistent with infective endocarditis but neither definite nor rejected

Important to Note

- The order of frequency of infection is mitral valve, aortic valve, tricuspid valve and pulmonic valve.
- Other potential sites for infective endocarditis include intracardiac wires (e.g., pacemaker) atrial/ventricular walls, eustachian valve, coarctation of the aorta, patent ductus arteriosus, mural thrombus and mitral annular calcification.
- Tricuspid valve vegetations are generally larger than left heart vegetations.
- Infective endocarditis affects the tricuspid valve 60% of the time in intravenous drug users.

- The sensitivity for diagnosing vegetations by TTE is 70% and by TEE is >95% for native valves. Both are significantly lower in prosthetic valves, dropping to 50% by TTE and 90% by TEE.
- The classic triad for the clinical diagnosis of infective endocarditis is fever, positive blood cultures and new murmur.
- Lambl's excrescence is a normal finding due to aging and may be confused with valve vegetation.
- Vegetations <3mm in size may not be detected by transthoracic echocardiography.
- Vegetations >1cm may indicate a higher morbidity and mortality.
- A tricuspid valve vegetation size of >2cm predicts an increased risk of mortality.
- Sources of error include papilloma, thrombi, myxomatous degeneration, healed (old) vegetations and too small to identify (resolution artifact).
- A vegetation which increases in size or remains static rather than shrinking after therapy may predict a poor prognosis.
- The absence of a vegetation by echocardiography does not rule out the diagnosis of infective endocarditis.
- Infective endocarditis is often associated with patients who have pre-existing valve disease (e.g., mitral stenosis, mitral valve prolapse, bicuspid aortic valve).
- The reason for infection is often evident (e.g., dental, surgical, traumatic).
- Ruptured chordae tendineae, valve excrescences, torn bioprosthetic leaflets, Libman-Sacks vegetations and papillary fibroelastoma may mimic the echocardiographic appearance of infective vegetations.
- Younger patients (<50 years of age), large vegetation (>6.5mm) and increased C-reactive protein (CRP) levels may identify patients at a higher risk for major embolic events during hospitalization.

10

Valvular Heart Disease / **Infective Endocarditis**

Table 10.23: Evaluation for Infective Endocarditis	
• Vegetation	• Intracardiac shunt
• Valve regurgitation	• Premature closure of the mitral valve (acute aortic regurgitation) (increased LVEDP)
• Valve stenosis (rare) (most likely involving prosthetic heart valve)	• Restrictive mitral valve inflow pattern (acute aortic regurgitation) (increased LVEDP)
• Valve ring abscess	• Prosthetic valve dehiscence
• Valve perforation	• Pericardial effusion
• Valve aneurysm	• Heart failure
• Flail leaflet	
• Fistula	

Table 10.24: Definitions of Terms Used in the Duke Criteria [6]

Major Criteria

1. Positive blood culture for IE

   A. Typical microorganism consistent with IE from two separate blood cultures as noted below:

   (i) viridans streptococci, Streptococcus bovis, or HACEK group, or

   (ii) community-acquired Staphylococcus aureus or enterococci, in the absence of a primary focus, or

   B. Microorganisms consistent with IE from persistently positive blood cultures defined as:

   (i) ≥2 positive cultures of blood samples drawn >12 hours apart or

   (ii) all of 3 or a majority of ≥4 separate cultures of blood (with first and last sample drawn ≥1 hour apart)

2. Evidence of endocardial involvement

   A. Positive echocardiogram for IE defined as

   (i) oscillating intracardiac mass on valve or supporting structures, in the path of regurgitant jets, or on implanted material in the absence of an alternative anatomic explanation, or

   (ii) abscess, or

   (iii) new partial dehiscence of prosthetic valve, or

   B. New valvular regurgitation (worsening or changing of preexisting murmur not sufficient)

Minor criteria

1. Predisposition: predisposing heart condition or intravenous drug use

2. Fever: temperature ≥38.0° C (100.4°)

3. Vascular phenomena: major arterial emboli, septic pulmonary infarcts, mycotic aneurysm, intracranial hemorrhage, conjunctival hemorrhages and Janeway lesions

4. Immunologic phenomena: glomerulonephritis, Osler's nodes, Roth spots and rheumatoid factor

5. Microbiological evidence: positive blood culture but does not meet a major criterion as noted above or serological evidence of active infection with organism consistent with IE

6. Echocardiographic findings: consistent with IE but do not meet a major criterion as noted above

Table 10.25: Duke Clinical Criteria for Diagnosis of Infective Endocarditis

Definite Infective Endocarditis

Pathological Criteria

- Micro-organisms: demonstrated by culture or history of a vegetation, in a vegetation that has embolized, or in an intracardiac abscess, or

- Pathological lesions: vegetation or intracardiac abscess present, confirmed by histology showing active endocarditis

Clinical criteria, using specific definitions listed in Table 10.24

- 2 major criteria, or

- 1 major criteria and 1 minor criteria, or 3 minor criteria

- 5 minor criteria

Possible Infective Endocarditis

- Findings consistent with Infective Endocarditis that fall short of "Definite" but not "Rejected"

Rejected

- Firm alternate diagnosis for manifestations of endocarditis, or

- Resolution of manifestations of endocarditis with antibiotic therapy for ≤4 days, or

- No pathological evidence of Infective Endocarditis at surgery or autopsy, after antibiotic therapy for ≤4 days

10

Valvular Heart Disease / **Infective Endocarditis**

References

1. P. Nihoyannopoulos, J. Kisslo. (2018) Echocardiography. Cham, Switzerland. Springer International Publishing.

2. Embil JM, Chan KL. The American Heart Association 2007 endocarditis prophylaxis guidelines: a compromise between science and common sense. Can J Cardiol. 2008;24(9):673−675. doi:10.1016/s0828-282x(08)70664-0

3. W. Armstrong, T. Ryan. (2018) Feigenbaum's Echocardiography. Wolters Kluwer.

4. Definitions of Terms Used in Duke Criteria, J. Am Coll Cardiol 1999, 33; 33:2023-9

5. Zoghbi WA, Adams DB, Bonow RO, Enriquez-Sarano M, Foster E, Grayburn PA, Hahn RT, Han Y, Hung J, Lang RM, Little SH, Shah DJ, Shernan S, Thavendiranathan P, Thomas JD: Recommendations for Noninvasive Evaluation of Native Valvular Regurgitation A Report from the American Society of Echocardiography Developed in Collaboration with the Society for Cardiovascular Magnetic Resonance. J Am Soc Echocardiogr 30:305-371, 2017.

6. J Am Coll Cardiol 1999; 33:2023-9.

10

Valvular Heart Disease / **Infective Endocarditis**

Prosthetic Heart Valves
Carissa Marsiglio, BS, RDCS

Indications
- Valvular stenosis
- Valvular regurgitation
- Native valve endocarditis
- Aortic dissection with severe aortic regurgitation

Complications of Prosthetic Heart Valves
- Calcification/degeneration (most common for bioprosthetic valves)
- Thrombus/thromboembolism (most common for mechanical valves)
- Infective endocarditis (e.g., vegetation, valve ring abscess, fistula)
- Perivalvular leak
- Dehiscence (suggests infective endocarditis, degeneration/disintegration of sewing ring and annulus)
- Stenosis (e.g., degenerative, thrombotic)
- Regurgitation (central/valvular, perivalvular)
- Valve bed abnormalities (e.g., pseudoaneurysm, hematoma)
- Pannus (fibrous ingrowth of tissue, mainly in mechanical valves, which may lead to regurgitation or stenosis, and may induce secondary thrombosis/thromboembolism)
- Ventricular dysfunction
- Hemolysis/anemia (in almost all mechanical valves, common in perivalvular leak)
- Prosthesis-patient mismatch (PPM)
- Left ventricular outflow tract obstruction due to mitral valve replacement (geometric mismatch)
- Bleeding is inherently a complication with mechanical valve prostheses due to the need for blood thinners
- Tissue valves are less durable than mechanical valves. Survival rate to 10 years is 60 to 70%. The durability is worse in young patients (<65 years of age) and in patients with hypertension, diabetes and renal failure.

Bioprosthetic Valves

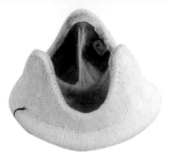

Figure 11.1: **Porcine valve (stented)**

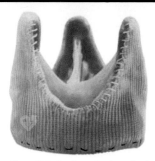

Figure 11.2: **Porcine valve (stentless)**

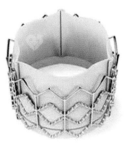

Figure 11.3: **SAPIEN (TAVR)**

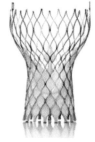

Figure 11.4: **CoreValve (TAVR)**

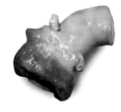

Figure 11.5: **Homograft**

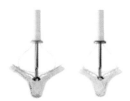

Figure 11.6: **MitraClip**

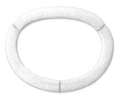

Figure 11.7: **Valve ring**

Stented Porcine

- Carpentier-Edwards
- Medtronic Hancock I, II
- St. Jude Medical Biocor
- Medtronic Mosaic
- Medtronic Intac
- Wessex
- Labcor Synergy

Pericardial

- Carpentier-Edwards
- Ionescu-Shiley
- Hancock
- Sorin Mitroflow
- Bioflo
- Labcor-Santiago

Stentless

- St. Jude Toronto SPV
- Medtronic Freestyle
- Extended Biocor
- Edwards Prima
- CryroLife-O'Brien
- O'Brien-Angell
- Sorin pericarbon

Percutaneous (TAVR, TAVI, TVPR, MitraClip)

- Edwards SAPIEN, SAPIEN-XT
- Medtronic CoreValve
- Medtronic Melody
- MitraClip

Valve Ring

- Carpentier-Edwards
- Duran
- Kay
- Puig-Massna-Shiley

Autograft

- Ross procedure: substituting patient's pulmonary valve into aortic position and then using homograft in pulmonic position

Homograft

- Tissue from a human donor

Mechanical Valves

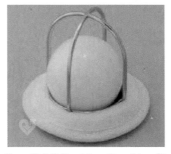

Figure 11.8: **Ball and Cage (Starr-Edwards)**

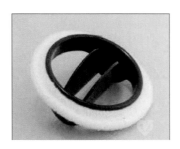

Figure 11.9: **Bileaflet Tilting Disc (St. Jude's)**

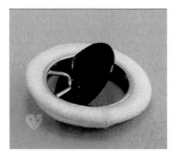

Figure 11.10: **Tilting Disc (Bjork-Shiley)**

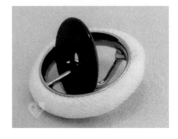

Figure 11.11: **Tilting Disc (Medtronic-Hall)**

All mechanical valves have a sewing ring, moving component and a cage, strut or frame

Ball and cage

- Starr-Edwards (most common)
- Smeloff-Cutter
- Braunwald-Cutter
- Magovern-Surgitool
- Magovern-Cromie
- Harken
- DeBakey-Surgitool
- Hufnagel

Caged disc

- Beall-Surgitool (most common)

Tilting single disc

- Medtronic-Hall
- Bjork-Shiley
- Lillehei-Kaster
- Hall-Kaster
- Wada-Cutter
- Omniscience
- Omnicarbon
- Ultracor

Bileaflet tilting disc

- St. Jude valve (most common)
- Carbomedics
- Duromedics (Hemex)
- Gott-Daggett
- Sorin bicarbon
- On-X
- Edwards Tekna
- Edwards Mira
- Medtronic Advantage

2D

Bioprosthetic Valves

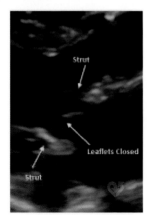

Figure 11.12: **Carpentier Edwards Bioprosthetic MVR during ventricular systole**

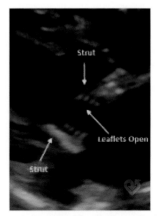

Figure 11.13: **Carpentier Edwards Bioprosthetic MVR during ventricular diastole**

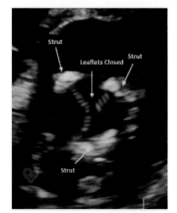

Figure 11.14: **Carpentier Edwards Bioprosthetic SAX MVR during ventricular systole**

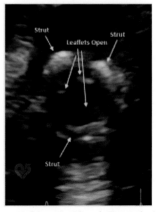

Figure 11.15: **Carpentier Edwards Bioprosthetic SAX MVR during ventricular diastole**

- May identify leaflet thickness, calcification, leaflet motion (restricted motion, flail leaflet), thrombus, dehiscence, vegetation, abscess, geometric mismatch, pericardial effusion, constrictive pericarditis and/or pulmonary embolism
- Any structure visualized above the level of the sewing ring may indicate an abnormality (e.g., flail, vegetation)
- Sewing ring of valve replacement should move in concert with the heart (no excessive rocking motion (dehiscence) should be present)
- Evaluate ventricular dimensions, thickness, global and segmental systolic function

Mechanical Valves

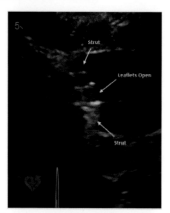

Figure 11.16: **St. Jude Mechanical AVR during ventricular systole**

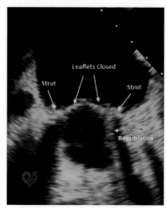

Figure 11.18: **St. Jude Mechanical MVR during ventricular systole (TEE)**

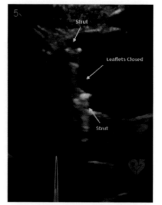

Figure 11.17: **St. Jude Mechanical AVR during ventricular diastole**

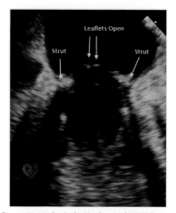

Figure 11.19: **St. Jude Mechanical MVR during ventricular diastole (TEE)**

- Somewhat helpful in evaluating for the complications of mechanical valves, although reverberations/shadowing and shielding from the ultrasound beam by mechanical parts make the diagnosis difficult and can obscure pathology
- Incomplete contact of disc/ball to frame or abnormal tilting of disc/ball is abnormal
- Absence of disc/ball motion may suggest significant thrombus/pannus formation
- Determines the presence of pericardial effusion, constrictive pericarditis and/or pulmonary embolism
- Evaluate ventricular dimensions, thickness, global and segmental systolic function

Doppler

- Evaluate patients soon after surgery (4 to 6 weeks) to obtain baseline Doppler values. This allows for chest wound healing, chest wall edema to resolve, and LV function to recover
- Heart rate, blood pressure and ventricular systolic and diastolic function should be noted
- An average of 3 beats (5 beats with an arrhythmia) should be utilized to obtain the hemodynamic measurements
- All prosthetic valves are inherently stenotic. The degree of obstruction is dependent on the type, size and site of the prosthetic valve.
- For bioprosthetic valves, "normal" (closing volume and leakage volume) regurgitation may be present. A single, central small jet seen only as the valve closes is consistent with normal tissue valve function
- The mechanical valves have normal regurgitation. These regurgitant jets (washings jets) are usually short, narrow and non-turbulent (exception: Medtronic-Hall)

Bioprosthetic/Mechanical Mitral Valve

- Note the transducer position where the optimal Doppler signal was obtained so it may be used for follow-up studies (most often the apical or para-apical position)
- There will be a higher peak velocity, peak pressure gradient, mean pressure gradient and pressure half-time as compared to a normal native mitral valve
- Coarse striations may indicate a flail/torn leaflet (bioprosthetic valves)
- Determine the presence and severity of mitral regurgitation
- Due to shadowing/flow masking/shielding, mitral regurgitation is difficult to assess by transthoracic echocardiography. The following may indicate significant mitral valve prosthetic regurgitation:
- Large flow convergence (PISA)
- Mitral valve peak E velocity of ≥1.9m/s
- Mean gradient of >5mmHg
- Shortened pressure half-time (<130msec)
- Shortened isovolumic relaxation time (<60msec)
- VTIPrMV/VTILVOT of >2.2
- Unexplained pulmonary hypertension at rest or with exercise
- Blunted or frank reversal of the pulmonary vein may indicate significant mitral valve prosthetic regurgitation
- TEE may be required
- Determine SPAP/MPAP/PAEDP/PVR at rest and exercise
- A perivalvular leak is abnormal (moderate or greater may be clinically significant)

Table 11.1: Doppler Parameters of Prosthetic Mitral Valve Function *(ASE Recommendations)* [3]

	Normal	Possible stenosis	Suggests significant stenosis
Peak velocity (m/s)	<1.9	1.9 to 2.5	≥2.5
Mean gradient (mmHg)	≤5	6 to 10	>10
VTI$_{PrMV}$/VTI$_{LVOT}$	<2.2	2.2 to 2.5	>2.5
EOA (cm²)	≥2.0	1 to 2	<1
PHT (msec)	<130	130 to 200	>200

Bioprosthetic/Mechanical Aortic Valve

- Note the transducer position where the optimal Doppler signal was obtained so it may be used for follow-up studies (most often the apical or right parasternal position)
- Ventricular systolic function and significant aortic regurgitation affects the peak velocity and pressure gradients
- A higher peak velocity, peak pressure gradient, mean pressure gradient and acceleration time (AT)/ejection time (ET) ratio will be present as compared to a normal native aortic valve
- Determine the presence and severity of aortic regurgitation
- Determine SPAP/MPAP/PAEDP/PVR at rest and exercise
- A perivalvular leak is abnormal (moderate or greater may be clinically significant)

Table 11.2: Doppler Parameters of Prosthetic Aortic Valve Function in Mechanical and Stented Biologic Valves *(ASE Recommendations)* [3]

Parameter	Normal	Possible Stenosis	Suggests Significant Stenosis
Peak velocity (m/s)*	<3	3 to 4	>4
Mean gradient (mmHg)*	<20	20 to 35	>35
Velocity ratio	≥0.30	0.29 to 0.25	<0.25
EOA (cm²)	>1.2	1.2 to 0.8	<0.8
Contour of the jet velocity	Triangular, early peaking	Triangular to intermediate	Rounded, symmetrical
Acceleration time (msec)	<80	80 to 100	>100

*Assumes normal left ventricular systolic function, may be affected by significant aortic regurgitation

Bioprosthetic/Mechanical Tricuspid Valve

- Tissue valves are most often placed in the tricuspid position to lower the incidence of thrombosis
- Higher peak velocity, peak pressure gradient, mean pressure gradient and pressure half-time may be present as compared to a normal native tricuspid valve
- Determine the presence and severity of tricuspid regurgitation
- Determine SPAP/MPAP/PAEDP/PVR at rest and exercise

- Determine the presence and severity of regurgitation utilizing PISA with conventional as well as off axis views to overcome the artifact of shadowing/flow masking/shielding
- A perivalvular leak is abnormal (moderate or greater may be clinically significant)

Table 11.3: Doppler Parameters of Prosthetic Tricuspid Valve Function *(ASE Recommendations)* [3]	
Consider valve stenosis*	
Peak velocity[†]	>1.7 m/s
Mean gradient[†]	≥6mmHg
Pressure half-time	≥230 msec
EOA and VTI_{PRTV}/VTI_{LVOT}	No data yet available for tricuspid prostheses

* Because of respiratory variation, average ≥5 cycles
† May be increased also with valvular regurgitation

Bioprosthetic/Mechanical Pulmonary Valve

- Tissue valves or homografts are most often placed in the pulmonic position to lower the incidence of thrombosis
- Higher peak velocity, peak pressure gradient, mean pressure gradient and pressure half-time may be present as compared to a normal native tricuspid valve
- Determine the presence and severity of pulmonary regurgitation
- Determine SPAP/MPAP/PAEDP/PVR at rest and exercise
- A perivalvular leak is abnormal (moderate or greater may be clinically significant)

Table 11.4: Findings Suspicious for Prosthetic Pulmonary Valve Stenosis *(ASE Recommendations)* [3]
Peak velocity through the prosthesis >3 m/s or >2 m/s through a homograft*
Increase in peak velocity on serial studies†
Impaired RV function or elevated RV systolic pressure
Cusp or leaflet thickening or immobility
Narrowing of forward color map

* Suspicious but not diagnostic of stenosis   † More reliable parameter

Aortic Homograft

- Difficult to visualize by 2D echocardiography
- Least stenotic prosthetic heart valve
- Durability is still in question
- Undersizing of valve may lead to significant regurgitation
- Perivalvular leaks are generally not present
- Perivalvular abscess is uncommon (no sewing ring)
- A small central holodiastolic jet may be normal. A large, holodiastolic jet seen soon after implantation may suggest undersizing or leaflet trauma and is abnormal

Percutaneous Interventions

Transcatheter Pulmonic Valve Replacement (TPVR)

- Transcatheter pulmonic valve replacement (TPVR) is the minimally invasive delivery of a pulmonic valve through a catheter. More than 6000 patients worldwide have received TPVR for a variety of underlying congenital heart abnormalities. Currently only USFDA approved for placement of a competent valve within an RV-PA conduit, although trials are now underway assessing devices designed for native outflow tracts
- TPVR prostheses include the Edwards SAPIEN XT, and Medtronic Melody valve

Transcatheter Aortic Valve Replacement (TAVR)

- Transcatheter aortic valve replacement (TAVR), (also referred to as transcatheter aortic valve implantation (TAVI)), is the minimally invasive delivery of an aortic valve through a catheter to treat patients with severe symptomatic aortic stenosis. The approach to deliver the valve include transfemoral and transapical. In 2019, the USFDA has expanded indication to include patients with severe aortic valve stenosis at low surgical risk
- TAVR prostheses include the Edwards SAPIEN, SAPIEN XT, and Medtronic CoreValve.

Echocardiography in TAVR

Pre-procedure

- Determines the presence and severity of aortic stenosis
- Determines the anatomic characteristics of the aortic valve (e.g., number of leaflets (bicuspid valve may be a contraindication), mobility, thickness of the cusps, extent/distribution of calcification)
- Evaluation for significant basal septal hypertrophy is important (significant hypertrophy may be a contraindication for it may be a potential cause of prosthesis displacement)
- Evaluate for mitral stenosis
- Determines the presence and severity of aortic regurgitation
- Determines the presence of LV thrombus (important for transapical approach)
- Determines LV/RV global and segmental systolic function
- Aortic annular measurement is critical (undersizing may result in device migration, significant perivalvular regurgitation; oversizing may result in difficulty to vascular access, difficulties crossing the aortic valve)
- Aortic annular measurement is measured using the parasternal long axis view, zoom of the LVOT, on a frozen image during ventricular systole. Measurement is taken at the point of insertion of the aortic valve leaflets, from tissue-blood interface to blood-tissue interface, trailing edge to leading edge, regardless of the degree of aortic valve calcification.

• 3D TEE helpful in distinguishing tricuspid valve aortic valve vs bicuspid aortic valve, defining aortic annulus anatomy, positioning of the catheter during implantation, assessment of valve regurgitation immediately following valve deployment.

Peri-procedure

• Evaluates aortic prosthesis misplacement
• Embolization towards the aorta or left ventricle
• Deployed valve is positioned too high (towards the aorta or too low towards the mitral valve)
• Determines the presence and severity of aortic regurgitation (e.g., central/valvular, perivalvular)
• Determines the presence and severity of mitral regurgitation (e.g., aortic prosthesis may impinge on the mitral valve anterior leaflet)
• Identifies LV dyssynchrony caused by RV pacing
• Identifies damage/distortion of subvalvular mitral apparatus by delivery system
• Evaluates for new segmental wall motion abnormalities (e.g., acute coronary ostial occlusion)
• Determines the presence of pericardial effusion/cardiac tamponade (may suggest LV/RV perforation)
• Determines the presence of aortic dissection/aortic root rupture

Post-implantation

• Follow-up evaluation is similar to surgically implanted prostheses
• Careful determination of LVOT diameter measurement (e.g.; may be measured at inferior aspect of the valve stent)
• Careful determination of the LVOT velocity is important in calculation of effective orifice area (e.g.; flow acceleration may occur at two levels – subvalvular and post-cusp so flow may be measured at the edge of the stent)
• Quantification of aortic regurgitation (prosthesis regurgitation may consist of central/valvular and multiple small perivalvular jets)
• Suggested normal values for TAVR: Mean pressure gradient: <20mmHg; EOA >1.1cm^2, Velocity ratio >0.35

11

Prosthetic Heart Valves / Echocardiography in TAVR / Percutaneous Interventions

Percutaneous Mitral Valve Intervention

- Percutaneous repair is indicated in significate mitral valve regurgitation
- Approaches include indirect annuloplasty-coronary sinus technique (MONARC, CARILLON, PTMA), direct annuloplasty (QuantumCor, Accuinch), leaflet repair (MitraClip™, Mobius), ventricular remodeling (iCoapsys)
- TTE/TEE/3D useful in patient selection, determining the etiology, presence and severity of mitral regurgitation, anatomic suitability for the device, during the procedure (e.g., transeptal puncture, placement of device), detection of complications, assessing residual/recurrence of mitral regurgitation, reversal of LV remodeling (6-month assessment is reasonable)

MitraClip™

USFDA approved for primary or degenerative mitral valve lesions. Utilization for secondary lesions is under investigation. The anterior and the posterior mitral leaflets are percutaneously "clipped" to convert the MV into a double orifice valve analogous to the surgically performed Alfieri stitch. Transesophageal echocardiography (TEE) imaging is integral to the success of the procedure. Its role extends from assessing suitability, procedural guidance, confirming success, and exclusion of complications

Good Candidates:

Primary Mitral Regurgitation	Secondary Mitral Regurgitation
• A_2 or P_2 prolapse	• Central MR jet
• Central MR jet	• Tenting height <11mm
• Flail gap <10mm	• Coaptation length >2mm
• Flail width <15mm	• Pliable valve leaflets
• Sufficient tissue for coaptation	• Sufficient tissue for coaptation
• Mitral valve area >4cm²	

Post-Implantation
MitraClip™

Determine:

- Peak velocity, peak pressure gradient, mean pressure gradient, effective orifice area (e.g.; planimetry of double orifice, PHT, continuity equation)
- Severity of mitral regurgitation (Grade 2 or less expected outcome)

Normal:

- Peak gradient: 8.9 ± 4.0mmHg
- Mean pressure gradient (MPG): 3.6 ± 1.7mmHg
- Pressure half-time (PHT): 98 ± 30 msec
- Mitral valve area (MVA) by PHT: 2.46 ± 0.73cm²
- SPAP: 38.8mmHg ± 12mmHg
- Predictive: MVA <1.94cm² and MPG ≥5mmHg, moderate or greater residual MR, and residual iASD after 6 months associated with adverse outcomes

Prosthesis-Patient Mismatch (PPM)

Prosthesis-Patient Mismatch (PPM) can be considered to be present when the effective prosthetic valve area after insertion into the patient is less than that of a normal human valve. The effective orifice area (EOA) determined by the continuity equation indexed for body surface area (BSA) is the recommended prosthesis parameter to use to identify PPM.

Aortic Valve Prostheses
• Nonsignificant if the indexed EOA is >0.85cm²/m²
• Moderate: indexed EOA between 0.66 and 0.85cm²/m²
• Severe: indexed EOA ≤0.65cm²/m²

Mitral Valve Prostheses
• Nonsignificant if indexed EOA >1.20cm²/m²
• Moderate: indexed EOA 0.91 to 1.20cm²/m²
• Severe: indexed EOA ≤0.90cm²/m²

Evaluation of Prosthetic Valve by TEE

The following general questions should be answered:
• Is there valve dehiscence?
• Is there evidence of torn/flail leaflets, ball/disc variance?
• Are there mass lesions? (e.g., vegetations, thrombi, pannus)
• Is there valve ring abscess/pseudoaneurysm/fistula?
• How much closing volume/leakage, or volume/pathologic valvular regurgitation/perivalvular leak is present?
• Is there valvular stenosis?

Mitral Valve
• Transverse 4-chamber (0°) view is an excellent view to evaluate a mitral valve prosthetic valve
• Due to the artifact of shadowing/flow masking/shielding, TEE is the test of choice in evaluating prosthetic mitral valve regurgitation. To evaluate prosthetic mitral valve regurgitation, the mitral prosthetic valve should be placed in the center of the display screen and there should be one full rotation of the transducer from 0 to 180° with color flow Doppler on to rule out significant mitral regurgitation
• It is easier to evaluate the left ventricular side of a tissue prosthesis as compared to a mechanical prosthesis
• The steps involved in determining the severity of the mitral regurgitation are similar to native valve regurgitation

Aortic Valve

- More difficult to evaluate as compared to the mitral valve due to the distance from the transducer
- The views of choice include 0° (transverse 4-chamber with anterior tilt), 40 to 60° (short-axis) and 120 to 150° (long-axis) and a transgastric long-axis and 5-chamber is helpful
- The posterior aspect of the aortic valve prostheses should be evaluated for abscess
- The anterior portion of the aortic prostheses may be difficult to image due to shadowing/flow masking/shielding by the posterior aortic valve ring
- Aortic regurgitation should be evaluated similar to native valve regurgitation
- Flow convergence (PISA) may be easier to identify as compared to transthoracic approach

Tricuspid Valve

- The views of choice include 0° (transverse 4-chamber), 40 to 60° (short-axis at the base)
- Distance from the probe and shadowing/flow masking/shielding due to the sewing ring make evaluation of the tricuspid valve prostheses difficult

TEE-Miscellaneous

- Helpful in patients who are too unstable to undergo cardiac catheterization
- Surface study is inadequate for diagnosis
- Microcavitations may be present in the area of mechanical valve opening and closing. This phenomenon is generally considered normal.
- Regurgitation jets appear larger as compared to transthoracic
- Intraoperative monitoring for perivalvular leak, valve regurgitation and/or dysfunction
- A small amount of perivalvular regurgitation may be expected immediately after surgery
- Assists in determining annular dimension, device placement, perivalvular/ valvular regurgitation and post-procedure assessment in percutaneous aortic valve replacement (TAVR)

Stress Echocardiography

- May be helpful in eliciting abnormal hemodynamics in a patient with apparent normal resting examination
- Determine peak velocity, peak pressure gradient, mean pressure gradient, effective orifice area, severity of regurgitation and pulmonary artery pressures
- An increase in cardiac output may result in significantly higher pressure gradients which may explain symptoms

- In general, an increase of the mean gradient >15mmHg with exercise suggests significant obstruction for aortic valves, a mean gradient >18mmHg suggests obstruction for mitral valves

Important to Note

- Valve replacement is merely substituting one disease for another.
- The basic principles that hold true for the evaluation of native valve stenosis may be generally applied to prosthetic heart valves.
- In general, obstruction, regurgitation (central/valvular and/or perivalvular), thromboembolism, endocarditis or valve ring abscess are the questions needed to be answered during a routine echocardiographic examination of a prosthetic heart valve.
- To properly evaluate a prosthetic valve, one should know the valve type, valve size, date of implantation, patient body habitus, ventricular function and blood pressure.
- To evaluate prosthetic heart valves the following should be routine: chamber dimension and function, valve type and movement, peak flow velocity, maximum and mean pressure gradients, pressure half-time, effective orifice area by the continuity equation, pulmonary artery pressures, diastolic filling profile, color flow jet length, duration and area, pulmonary vein (mitral regurgitation) or descending thoracic aorta flow (aortic regurgitation) and regurgitant fraction.
- The number of the size of the diameter represents the outer diameter of the valve. The true valve diameter and internal geometric area (IGA) will be smaller than the outer diameter size.
- Smaller valve sizes have higher Doppler velocities especially in high output conditions.
- The pressure half-time method may overestimate the valve area in prosthetic valves due to the empirical number of 220. The continuity equation is recommended to determine the mitral valve effective orifice area.
- Bovine pericardial valves are more prone to sudden failure due to a tear in one of the leaflets than other bioprosthetic valves.
- Valve strands may be seen in 15% of mechanical mitral valves especially with transesophageal echocardiography. They appear as thin, filamentous structures on the left atrial side of the valve. They may be several millimeters in length, chaotic in movement and are associated with an increased risk of stroke.
- The stentless aortic valve may demonstrate a perivalvular lumen and is considered a normal finding if there is no diastolic flow present between the bioprosthesis and the aortic root.
- Pressure recovery may lead to an apparent overestimation of the pressure gradient especially in smaller sized (e.g., 19mm, 21mm) St. Jude's aortic valves.

11

Prosthetic Heart Valves / Stress Echocardiography

• To determine the effective orifice area for aortic prostheses, measurement of the left ventricular outflow tract diameter is preferred. If the LVOT diameter cannot be accurately measured, the external diameter of the valve (which is usually the size of the valve) may be substituted. The LVOT diameter should be recorded on the echo report sheet so that in follow up studies the sonographer can compare LVOT diameter measurement results from study to study.

• Normal regurgitation in prosthetic valves is the combination of the closing volume and the leakage volume. Mechanical valves have a greater normal regurgitant volume as compared to tissue valves.

• Larger valve sizes have a greater regurgitant volume. Normal closure and leakage flow may be distinguished from pathologic regurgitation in that they are low velocity, non-aliased, thin jets with a small jet area.

Table 11.5: Normal Doppler Values for Bioprosthetic Valves

	Peak Velocity (m/s)	Mean Gradient (mmHg)	Pressure Half-time (msec)	Valve Area Mean (cm²)	Range (cm²)
Mitral Valve					
Hancock	1.5 ± 0.3	4.3 ± 2.1	129 ± 31	1.7	1.3 to 2.7
Carpentier-Edwards	1.8 ± 0.2	6.6 ± 2.1	90 ± 25	2.5	1.6 to 3.5
Carpentier-Edwards pericardial		4.4 ± 2			2.6 ± 0.6
Ionescu-Shiley	1.5 ± 0.3	3.0 ± 1.0	93 ± 25	1.7	2.4 ± 0.8
Aortic Valve					
Aortic homograft	1.9 ± 0.4	7.8 ± 2.7		2.2	1.7 to 3.1
Non-stented					
SPV-Toronto	2.2 ± 0.4	3 (2 to 20)			1.8 to 2.3
Hancock	2.4 ± 0.4	11 ± 2		1.8	1.4 to 2.3
Carpentier-Edwards	2.4 ± 0.5	14 ± 6		1.8	1.2 to 3.1
Carpentier-Edwards pericardial	1.5 ± 0.9	4.4 ± 1.8			2.5 ± 0.6
Medtronic (Mosaic) (23mm)	2.3 ± 1.2	12 ± 3			
Tricuspid Valve					
Heterograft	1.3 ± 0.2	3.2 ± 1.1	145 ± 37		

Table 11.6: Normal Doppler Values for Mechanical Valves [1,2]

Mitral Valve	Peak Velocity (m/s)	Mean Gradient (mmHg)	Pressure Half-time (msec)	Valve Area Mean (cm²)	Range (cm²)
Starr-Edwards	1.8 ± 0.4	4.6 ± 2.4	110 ± 27	2.1	1.2 to 2.5
Bjork-Shiley	1.6 ± 0.3	4.1 ± 1.6	90 ± 22	2.4	1.6 to 3.7
St. Jude Medical	1.5 ± 0.3	3.5 ± 1.3	77 ± 17	2.9	1.8 to 4.4
Medtronic-Hall	1.7 ± 0.3	3.1 ± 0.9	89 ± 19	2.4	1.5 to 3.9
Omniscience	1.8 ± 0.3	3.3 ± 0.9	125 ± 29	1.9	1.6 to 3.1
Carpentier-Edwards*	1.4 ± 0.3	3.8 ± 0.4	98 ± 16	2.6	1.8 to 3.8
Duran*	1.3 ± 0.3	3.8 ± 1.1	89 ± 19	2.8	1.9 to 3.9

• Ring

Aortic Valve	Size (mm)	Vmax (m/s)	Mean Gradient (mmHg)	Velocity Ratio	AVA (cm)
Tilting-disk	19	2.1 ± 0.7			
	21	2.8 ± 0.9	16		1.1 ± 0.3
	23	2.6 ± 0.4	14 ± 5		1.3 ± 0.3
	25	2.1 ± 0.3	13 ± 3		1.4 ± 0.4
	27	1.9 ± 0.2	10 ± 3		2.0 ± 0.3
	29	1.9 ± 0.2	7 ± 6		
Bileaflet	19	3.0 (2.0 to 4.5)	20 (10 to 30)	0.37	1.0 ± 0.3
	21	2.7 (2.5 to 3.5)	14 (10 to 30)	0.40	1.3 ± 0.2
	23	2.5 (2.0 to 3.5)	12 (10 to 30)	0.37	1.3 ± 0.3
	25	2.4 (2.0 to 3.5)	12 (5 to 30)	0.42	1.8 ± 0.4
	27	2.2 (2.0 to 3.1)	11 (5 to 20)	0.46	2.4 ± 0.6
	29	2.0 (2.0 to 2.5)	10 (5 to 15)	0.49	2.7 ± 0.3
	31	2.1 (1.5 to 2.5)	10 (5 to 15)	0.49	3.1
Ball-cage		3.1 ± 0.5	24 ± 4	0.32	1.1 ± 0.2

Values shown are mean ± 1 SD or mean (range). Velocity ratio = left ventricular outflow velocity/aortic jet velocity. Data from:

Tricuspid Valve	Vmax (m/s)	Mean Gradient (mmHg)	Pressure Half-time (msec)
Ball and cage	1.3 ± 0.2	3.2 ± 0.8	140 ± 48
St. Jude Medical	1.2 ± 0.3	2.7 ± 1.1	108 ± 32
Bjork-Shiley	1.3	2.2	144
Average*	1.3 ± 0.2	3.1 ± 1.0	140 ± 42

*The average differences between maximum and minimum values due to respiratory variation are:
• Peak velocity: 0.5 ± 0.2 m/s
• Mean pressure gradient: 0.3 ± 0.2mmHg
• Pressure half-time: 81.6 ± 36.9 msec
These differences emphasize the importance of measuring multiple cycles in patients who have tricuspid prostheses.

References

1. Bjork-Shiley, Medtronic Hall; b St. Jude; c Starr-Edwards.

2. Reisner et al: JASE 1:201, 1988; Zabalgoitia et al: Curr Prob Cardiol 5:271, 1992; Sagar et al: JACC 7: 1986; Baumgartner et al: Circ 82:1467, 1990; Chafizadeh et al: Circ 83:213, 1991; Jaffe et al: AJC 63:1466, 1989

3. Zoghbi, JASE 976; 1014; Recommendations for Evaluation of Prosthetic Valves With Echocardiography and Doppler Ultrasound. 9/2009

Pericardial Disease
Christopher J. Kramer, BA, ACS, RDCS, FASE

Pericardial Effusion

Definition
Pericardial effusion is an abnormal accumulation of fluid within the pericardial cavity or between serosal layers. Normal pericardial serous fluid ranges from 15 to 50mL. Pericardial effusions can be classified as transudative, exudative, hemorrhagic or malignant or by their temporal development: acute, subacute and chronic (>3 months).

Etiology
• Idiopathic
• Infections
  - Mycobacterium tuberculosis
  - Bacterial (e.g., Staphylococcus, Streptococcus, pneumococcus, Hemophilus, Neisseria, Chlamydia)
  - Viral (e.g., Coxsackie virus, echovirus, adenovirus, CMV, HIV)
• Malignancies
  - Metastatic (e.g., lung cancer, breast cancer, lymphoma, leukemia, melanoma)
• Iatrogenic
  - Pacemaker, ICD or CRT insertion
  - Post ablation intervention
  - Percutaneous coronary intervention
  - Post-cardiac surgery
  - CPR
• Connective tissue diseases
  - Systemic lupus erythematosus (SLE) (e.g., rheumatoid arthritis, scleroderma)
• Metabolic diseases
  - Hypothyroidism
  - Chronic renal failure
• Other
  - Pericarditis
  - Blunt chest trauma
  - Penetrating chest wall injury
  - Aortic dissection
  - Myocarditis
  - Post myocardial infarction

History

- Chest pain
- Dyspnea (may indicate cardiac tamponade or constrictive pericarditis)
- Fatigue
- Fever, sweats, chills
- Edema
- Tachypnea (may indicate cardiac tamponade)
- Palpitations (due to atrial arrhythmias)
- Odynophagia (suggests large effusion)

Physical Examination

- Quiet, hypodynamic heart with cardiomegaly
- Elevated jugular venous pressure

Complications

- Cardiac tamponade

Cardiac Auscultation

- Distant heart sounds
- Ewart's sign

Electrocardiogram

- Sinus tachycardia
- Low voltage of the QRS complexes throughout ECG
- Electrical alternans (suggests large effusion)
- Supraventricular and/or ventricular arrhythmias

Chest X-ray/CMR/CT

- Normal (suggests no, small or moderate effusions)
- Cardiomegaly with clear lungs (may indicate pericardial effusion)
- Globular shaped heart (water bottle heart) due to pericardial effusion
- CMR/CT allows evaluation of pericardial effusion, type of effusion (e.g., bloody vs exudative), pericardial thickness and confirms echocardiographic signs of cardiac tamponade

Cardiac Catheterization

- Limited role
- Increase and equalization of diastolic intracardiac pressures with a decrease in stroke volume suggests cardiac tamponade

Medical Treatment

- Treat underlying etiology
- NSAIDs, Colchicine, Corticosteroid

Surgical Treatment

- Pericardiocentesis (identify the etiology or to relieve cardiac tamponade)
- Pericardial window
- Pericardiectomy

M-mode/2D

- Echo-free space between the epicardium and the pericardium a(<15 to 35mL)
- Swinging heart (suggests large effusion)
- Loculated effusion (especially post-cardiac surgery/trauma)
- Fibrin strands (may indicate long-standing effusion, or inflammatory, hemorrhagic, malignant etiology)
- Inferior vena cava plethora may indicate increased right atrial pressure
- 3D may provide information concerning fluid location and volume
- To semi-quantitate the amount of pericardial effusion add maximal diastolic diameter of the anterior pericardial effusion and the maximal diastolic diameter of the posterior pericardial effusion then multiply by 100.

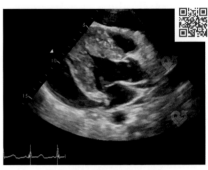

Figure 12.1: **Swinging heart 2D**

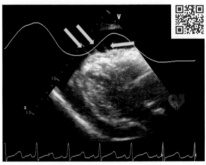

Figure 12.2: **Fibrin strands**

- Semi-quantitate pericardial effusion utilizing prolate ellipse method/Simpson's method of discs/3D volume

PW/CW Doppler

- Respiratory variation of mitral valve and tricuspid valve peak velocities and velocity time integrals suggest cardiac tamponade

Transesophageal Echocardiography

- May improve detection of loculated effusions or hematoma especially post-cardiac surgery or trauma

Differential Diagnosis

- Loculated effusion may mimic a pericardial cyst. Cysts can be differentiated from pericardial effusion because cysts are distinct from the pericardial layer and a discrete pericardial layer surrounding the cyst is usually visible. Pericardial cysts are located typically at the right costophrenic angle

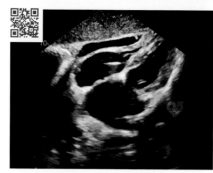

Figure 12.3: **Pericardial cyst**

- TTE can visualize epicardial fat layer, paracardial fat layer (fat deposits in mediastinum outside of parietal pericardium)(sometime difficult by TTE) and pericardial fat layers (sum total of epicardial and paracardial fat layers)

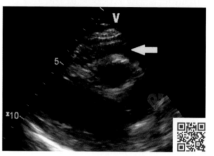

Figure 12.4: **Epicardial fat**

- Epicardial fat is sandwiched in between the epicardium and myocardium and is primarily located anteriorly (7% posteriorly)

- Epicardial fat appears on the echocardiogram as an anterior echo-free space and may be confused with pericardial effusion. It is unusual for effusions to be located only anteriorly unless loculated

- Epicardial fat should be measured on the RV free wall in at least two locations, from the long and short axis, with three consecutive beats, >5mm represents increased epicardial fat

- Epicardial fat has a speckled or granular echo reflectance vs. fluid

- Epicardial fat is more commonly seen in elderly, obese, diabetics, women, dyslipidemia

- The incidence of epicardial fat increases with age (<1% in patients <30 years old and up to 15% in those >80 years old), usually with small deposits

- Epicardial fat is often brighter than myocardium and moves in concert or unison with heart

- If the diagnosis is not apparent, the following should be reported: "Anterior clear space noted, probably adipose tissue but cannot rule out pericardial cyst, tumor, extracardiac mass, thymus gland, foramen of Morgagni, left atrial dilatation, thrombus, massive ascites or loculated effusion. Clinical correlation is suggested."

- Pleural effusion may present as a posterior echo-free space

- A pericardial effusion is anterior to the descending thoracic aorta, while a pleural effusion is posterior to the descending thoracic aorta

- A pericardial effusion does not change with respiration, while a pleural effusion may change with respiration

Important to Note

- When a large effusion is present, the following diagnoses should be deferred until the effusion abates: mitral valve prolapse, tricuspid valve prolapse, aortic valve prolapse, pulmonic valve prolapse, systolic anterior motion of the mitral valve, mid-systolic notching of the pulmonary valve, mid-systolic notching of the aortic valve, paradoxical motion of the ventricular septum, paradoxical motion of the posterior left ventricular wall

- Pericardial effusion often collects first behind the right atrium and may be best visualized in the apical 4-chamber view and the subcostal four-chamber view. Right atrial intracavitary pressure is the lowest in the heart and therefore higher intracavitary pressures in the ventricles and left atrium tends to squeeze the effusion to the area of least resistance which is adjacent to the right atrium

- Pericardial effusion may collect in the oblique sinus located posterior to the LA left atrium. This is best seen in the parasternal long-axis view

- Pericardial effusion may collect in the transverse sinus located posterior to the origin of the great vessels

- Pericardial effusion is common after cardiac surgery

- It is important to note a loculated effusion (especially post-cardiac surgery) since such an effusion can cause hemodynamic compromise (regional cardiac tamponade)

Table 12.1: Pericardial Effusion Severity Scale

Physiologic	A clear space posteriorly is seen only in systole
Small	(<100mL): clear space is detectable in systole and diastole posteriorly only and is <1cm in width
Moderate	(100 to 500mL): clear space is detectable in systole and diastole anteriorly and posteriorly and is 1 to 2cm in width
Large	(>500mL): clear space is detectable in systole and diastole, surrounds the entire heart and is >2cm in width (may result in swinging heart)
Very Large*	Clear space detectable in systole and diastole, surrounds the entire heart, most likely unevenly distributed in pericardial space and recesses, >2.5cm

Clear space is best measured from multiple 2D positions of the left ventricle at end diastole
* severity varies, echocardiography laboratory specific

Pericarditis

Definition

Pericarditis is an inflammation of the pericardium which may result in the visceral pericardium secreting fluid (pericardial effusion). Pericarditis may be acute, subacute, recurrent.

Etiology

- Idiopathic
- Infectious
  - Viral (e.g., echovirus, coxsackievirus, adenovirus, cytomegalovirus, hepatitis B, infectious mononucleosis, HIV/AIDS)
  - Bacterial (e.g., pneumococcus, staphylococcus, streptococcus, mycoplasma, Lyme disease, hemophilus influenzae)
  - Mycobacteria (e.g., mycobacterium tuberculosis)
  - Fungal (e.g., histoplasmosis, coccidiomycosis)
  - Protozoal
- Immune-inflammatory
  - Connective tissue disease (systemic lupus erythematosus, rheumatoid arthritis, scleroderma, mixed)
  - Arteritis (e.g., polyarteritis nodosa, temporal arteritis)
  - Early post-myocardial infarction
  - Late post-myocardial infarction (Dressler syndrome), late post-cardiotomy/ thoracotomy, late post-trauma
  - Drug induced (e.g., procainamide, hydralazine, cyclosporine) anticoagulants
- Neoplastic disease
  - Primary (e.g., mesothelioma, fibrosarcoma, lipoma)
  - Secondary (e.g., breast and lung carcinoma, lymphomas, leukemias)
- Radiation induced (2 to 31% develop constriction)
- Early post-cardiac surgery
- Device and procedure related
  - Coronary angioplasty, implantable defibrillators, pacemakers
- Trauma
  - Blunt and penetrating, post-cardiopulmonary resuscitation
- Congenital
  - Cysts, congenital absence
- Miscellaneous
  - Chronic renal failure, hypothyroidism, amyloidosis, aortic dissection, heart failure, pregnancy, severe pulmonary hypertension, Trisomy 21 (Down syndrome)

History

- Dependent upon etiology
- Positional chest pain (primary symptom) (precordial, sharp, severe, increases in severity with inspiration, coughing or recumbency, decreases or improves with sitting upright, leaning forward)

12

Pericardial Disease / Pericarditis

- Dyspnea (may indicate cardiac tamponade or constrictive pericarditis)
- Cough
- Fever, sweats, chills
- Tachypnea
- Palpitations (due to atrial arrhythmias)

Physical Examination

- Quiet, hypodynamic heart with cardiomegaly suggests pericardial effusion

Complications

- Cardiac tamponade
- Chronic pericarditis may lead to constrictive pericarditis

Cardiac Auscultation

- Pericardial friction rub (cardinal physical sign) (exercise or repeated auscultation with postural changes may be required to elicit)
- Distant heart sounds (suggests pericardial effusion)
- Ewart's sign (suggests large effusion)

Laboratory

- Elevated white blood count
- Elevated cardiac enzymes (e.g., troponin)
- Elevated C-reactive protein/Westergren or ultrasensitive C-reactive protein sedimentation rate (confirmatory finding)
- Elevated erythrocyte sedimentation rate

Electrocardiogram

- Elevated ST segments throughout with upright T waves (hours to days) (classic finding)
- PR segment depression (common finding)
- Sinus tachycardia
- Reduction in QRS voltage throughout ECG
- Supraventricular arrhythmias
- Electrical alternans (suggests large effusion)

Chest X-ray/CMR/CT

- Cardiomegaly with clear lungs (may indicate pericardial effusion)
- Noncalcified pericardial thickening
- Enhancement of the thickened visceral and parietal surfaces of the pericardial sac with contrast
- CT attenuation values of pericardial effusion can help distinguish between exudative and transudative fluid

- Enhancement of thickened pericardium on T1-weighted SE or LGE images confirms active inflammation (94 to 100% sensitive)
- Significant signal in pericardial tissue on T2W images correlates with edema, neovascularization, and/or granulation tissue
- High T1W signal intensity on SE images is suggestive of exudative effusions
- Thickened pericardium without enhancement shows chronic fibrotic pericarditis
- Loss of the normal slippage of the outer pericardium over the epicardial surface during the cardiac cycle by dynamic tagging is consistent with the presence of pericardial adhesions between inflamed visceral and parietal pericardium

Cardiac Catheterization

- Limited role
- Increase and equalization of diastolic intracardiac pressures with a decrease in stroke volume suggests cardiac tamponade
- Square root sign may indicate constrictive pericarditis

Medical Treatment

- Treat underlying etiology (e.g., uremia)
- Exercise restriction
- Analgesia (aspirin, indomethacin, ibuprofen)
- Steroid therapy (e.g., prednisone)
- Immunosuppression therapy for recurrent pericarditis (e.g., colchicine, azathioprine)

Surgical Treatment

- Pericardiocentesis (indicated to identify the etiology or to relieve cardiac tamponade)
- Pericardial window (may do pericardial biopsy)
- Pericardiectomy

M-mode/2D

- Echo-free space between the epicardium and the pericardium (<15 to 35 mL required for echo free space to be detected)
- Swinging heart (suggests large effusion)
- Loculated effusion (especially post-cardiac surgery/trauma)
- Fibrin strands (may indicate long-standing effusion, or inflammatory, hemorrhagic, malignant etiology)
- Inferior vena cava plethora may indicate increased right atrial pressure

12

Pericardial Disease / Pericarditis

PW/CW Doppler

- Respiratory variation of mitral valve and tricuspid valve peak velocities and velocity time integrals suggest cardiac tamponade

Transesophageal Echocardiography

- May improve detection of loculated effusions or hematoma especially post-cardiac surgery or trauma

Differential Diagnosis

- Epicardial fat has a speckled or granular echo reflectance vs. fluid
- Pleural effusion may present as a posterior clear space
- A pericardial effusion is anterior to the descending thoracic aorta, while a pleural effusion is posterior to the descending thoracic aorta
- A pericardial effusion does not change with respiration, while a pleural effusion may change with respiration

Important to Note

- A patient with pericarditis may have no evidence of pericardial effusion by echocardiography (dry pericarditis).
- When a large effusion is present, the following diagnoses should be deferred until the effusion abates: mitral valve prolapse, tricuspid valve prolapse, aortic valve prolapse, pulmonic valve prolapse, systolic anterior motion of the mitral valve, mid-systolic notching of the pulmonary valve, mid-systolic notching of the aortic valve, paradoxical motion of the ventricular septum, paradoxical motion of the posterior left ventricular wall
- The pericardial friction rub may have three components due to early ventricular diastolic filling, atrial systole and ventricular systole
- May see a positive serum antinuclear antibody test (ANA), initial presentation for SLE, young women with acute pericarditis and pericardial effusion (non-specific finding)
- Typical ECG (ST elevation, AVR shows reciprocal ST-segment depression and reciprocal PR segment depression)

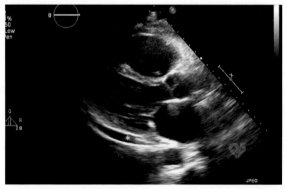

Figure 12.5: **Acute pericarditis demonstrating small pericardial effusion**

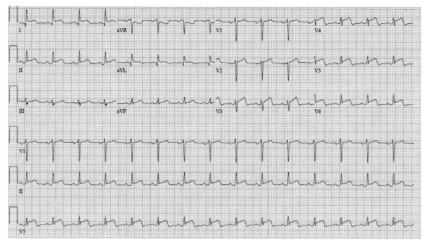

Figure 12.6: **12-lead ECG showing ST elevation**

Cardiac Tamponade

Definition

Life threatening condition caused by an elevation of intrapericardial pressure due to the accumulation of pericardial effusion which results in compression of the cardiac chambers, elevation and equalization of intracardiac pressures, and progressive limitation of ventricular diastolic filling and reduction in stroke volume.

Common Etiologies

• Pericarditis (infection and non-infection)
• Iatrogenic (cardiac invasive procedures and post surgery)
• Malignancy
• Idiopathic
• Infectious
• Immune-inflammatory
• Collagen diseases
• Trauma
• Aortic dissection
• Radiation
• Post-myocardial infarction
• Uremia
• Miscellaneous (renal failure, thyroid disease, amyloidosis)

History

• Symptoms of pericarditis/pericardial effusion

- Dyspnea (most common) (improves with sitting up and leaning forward)
- Chest pain

Physical Examination

- Pulsus paradoxus (hallmark finding) (defined as a drop in systolic blood pressure >10mmHg upon inspiration)
- Total paradoxus (complete absence of a pulse upon inspiration)
- Hypotension
- Narrow pulse pressure due to low systolic pressure
- Sinus tachycardia
- Tachypnea
- Hepatomegaly
- Cold extremities
- Peripheral cyanosis
- Decreased or absent apical impulse
- Ewart's sign
- Beck's triad (elevated venous pressure, hypotension, quiet heart)

Complications

- Hypotension
- Loss of conscientiousness
- Shock
- Death

Cardiac Auscultation

- Diminished heart sounds
- Pericardial friction rub

Electrocardiogram

- Abnormalities associated with pericarditis/pericardial effusion
- Electrical alternans (alternating amplitudes of the QRS complex)
- Total alternans (alternating amplitude of P, QRS and T waves is pathognomic)
- Sinus tachycardia
- Reduced QRS complex in limb leads
- ST-T wave elevation present in all leads except AVR and V1
- Rhythm disturbances (atrial fibrillation, atrial flutter, supraventricular tachycardia)
- Sinus bradycardia (preterminal sign)
- ST segment elevation during pericardiocentesis may indicate needle is in contact with the ventricular epicardium

Chest X-ray/CMR/CT

- May demonstrate normal-sized heart
- Serial chest x-rays may demonstrate increasing heart size
- Cardiomegaly without pulmonary congestion (oligemia)
- Globular shaped heart (water bottle heart)
- Separation of the epicardial and pericardial fat pads

- Systemic venous engorgement with enlargement of the superior vena cava and azygous vein
- CMR/CT provides information concerning localization and quantitation of pericardial fluid, character of the fluid (e.g., bloody, exudative, chylous), chamber collapse (e.g., right atrial collapse) and pericardial thickness

Cardiac Catheterization

- Increase in intrapericardial pressure which is equal to or exceeds intracardiac diastolic pressures
- Increase and equalization of right heart (RA, RV, PA) diastolic and left heart (LA and LV via pulmonary capillary wedge) diastolic pressures (cardiac chambers diastolic pressures separated by <2 to 3mmHg)
- Pericardiocentesis (may include right heart catheterization to monitor pressure changes)

Medical Treatment

- Intravenous volume expansion (e.g., saline, blood, plasma, dextran)
- Isoproterenol
- Vasodilator (e.g., nitroprusside)
- Specific therapy for etiology of pericarditis/pericardial effusion

Surgical Treatment

- Pericardiocentesis (may be performed with echo guidance)
- Pericardial window (created with surgery or by balloon)
- Total/Limited pericardiectomy

M-mode/2D

- Pericardial effusion (circumferential or loculated)
- Pre-systolic collapse of the right atrium (considered present when >30% of the right atrial wall is inverted (collapsed) in late diastole and/or early systole lasting at least one-third of the cardiac cycle (100% sensitive and specific) (starts near the R wave)
- Right ventricular early diastolic collapse or compression (present when inward motion of the right ventricular wall persists at least 0.05 sec after the onset of mitral valve opening) (suggests a 20% decrease in cardiac output) (starts after the end of T wave)

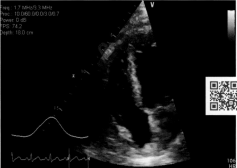

Figure 12.7: **Late diastolic RA collapse**

- Left atrial diastolic collapse in late diastole and/or early systole
- Left ventricular early diastolic collapse or compression
- Dilated inferior vena cava (normal ≤2.1cm) with lack of inferior vena cava collapse is normal collapse (>50%) upon inspiration (IVC plethora) (>90%)
- Dilated hepatic vein(s) (normal 0.5 to 1.1cm) and superior vena cava
- Reduced LV end-diastolic and end-systolic dimensions with "hypertrophied" appearance of myocardium
- RV diastolic diameter increases with inspiration, while LV diastolic diameter decreases (opposite changes during expiration)

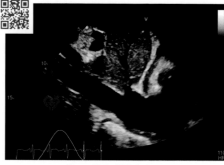

- "Swinging heart" motion pattern
- Inspiratory "bounce" of the interventricular septum toward the left ventricle
- Inspiratory bounce of interatrial septum toward the left atrium

Figure 12.11: **IVC plethora**

- Determine the area of largest pericardial effusion most easily reached percutaneously while avoiding abnormal structures and vital organs for pericardiocentesis
- During pericardiocentesis, identify needle tip using contrast (saline injection) echocardiography

PW/CW Doppler

- Marked respiratory variation of mitral valve decreases with inspiration, and increases with expiration (>30%). Tricuspid valve increases with inspiration, and decreases with expiration (>60%). Peak velocities and velocity time integrals (utilize 25mm/s sweep speed; respirometer)
- Marked respiratory variation of aortic decreases with inspiration, and increases in expiration. Pulmonic increases with inspiration, and decreases in expiration) peak velocities, velocity time integrals and ejections times (utilize 25mm/s sweep speed; respirometer)
- Peak mitral and tricuspid E wave velocities measured on the first beat of corresponding respiratory cycles
- Marked respiratory variation in mitral valve E/A velocity ratio upon inspiration
- Increase in the mitral valve A wave velocity time integral/mitral valve velocity time integral ratio with inspiration
- Marked respiratory variation of the pulmonary vein decreases with inspiration, increase with expiration) peak velocities and velocity time integrals
- Systolic predominance of flow in the superior vena cava
- Right to left shunt through patent foramen ovale

- Increased IVRT with inspiration (>150msec)
- Decreased left ventricular ejection time with inspiration
- Diastolic mitral and/or tricuspid regurgitation
- Antegrade flow into the pulmonary artery during diastole
- Respiratory variation of left ventricular stroke volume (decrease with inspiration; increase with expiration)
- Limitation of right heart filling by hepatic venous Doppler:
    - Normal inspiratory increase in systolic (S wave) and diastolic (D wave) forward flows; systolic is greater than diastolic
    - Normal inspiratory decrease of atrial reversal (AR wave) and systolic reverse (VR wave) flows
    - Marked blunting or reversal of diastolic forward flow in expiration
    - Prominent atrial reversal (AR wave) of flow during expiration
    - Reversal of flow in systole in expiration (less common)
    - Post-pericardiocentesis flow velocities return to normal with little change during respiration. Continued respiratory variation may indicate effusive-constrictive pericarditis

Transesophageal Echocardiography

- May provide information on the pericardium when transthoracic is suboptimal
- May provide guidance during pericardiocentesis in selected cases
- Excellent in detecting loculated effusion or hematoma in patients post-cardiac surgery with decreased cardiac output (regional cardiac tamponade)

Important to Note

- Cardiac tamponade occurs when intrapericardial pressure, which is normally lower than the central veins and right atrium by 3 to 5mmHg, increases due to the accumulation of pericardial effusion to the level of right atrial and right ventricular diastolic pressures and possibly to the level of the left atrium and left ventricular end-diastolic pressures.
- Cardiac tamponade is usually associated with moderate to large effusions but may occur with small, rapidly accumulating effusions.
- Acute cardiac tamponade can occur because of trauma, cardiac rupture, aortic dissection and is associated with a rapid onset of cardiogenic shock.
- Subacute cardiac tamponade occurs when a pericardial effusion develops gradually (i.e., uremia) and the signs and symptoms of cardiac tamponade develop gradually over time.
- Loculated pericardial effusion may result in regional cardiac tamponade by compressing the right heart or left atrium especially within the first two weeks of cardiac surgery or trauma.

12

Pericardial Disease / Cardiac Tamponade

- Low pressure tamponade may occur in patients with pericardial effusion and hypovolemia. This may occur in patients with mildly elevated intrapericardial pressure with severe dehydration, overly vigorous diuresis or massive extrapericardial blood loss.

- Hypertensive cardiac tamponade is a syndrome in which all of the classic clinical and echocardiographic features are present but which occurs with marked elevation in systolic blood pressure.

- Reversed pulsus paradoxus which is a fall in blood pressure with expiration, may be seen in patients on positive pressure respirators and therefore the respiratory variations seen during a cardiac Doppler examination will be reversed.

- Increased respiratory variation in transvalvular flow velocities may be seen in patients with chronic obstructive pulmonary disease, severe tricuspid regurgitation or right ventricular infarction but the lower mitral flow velocity usually occurs later during inspiration.

- In cardiac tamponade, the order in which changes occur are fairly predictable. Changes in tricuspid valve occur first, followed by changes in the mitral valve with right atrial collapse being the next change and right ventricular diastolic collapse occurring last.

- Right atrial collapse has a high sensitivity but a low specificity, occurs when the intrapericardial pressures are ≥4mmHg, is best seen during expiration or apnea, best seen in the mid-portion of the right atrial lateral wall in the apical/subcostal views.

- Right ventricular diastolic collapse/compression has a low sensitivity but a high specificity, occurs when the intrapericardial pressures are ≥10mmHg, is best seen on the right ventricular anterior wall and infundibulum in the parasternal long-axis and short-axis views.

- To determine mitral valve and tricuspid valve respiratory variation percent change: (TV % change will calculate to be a negative value)

% Respiratory Change =

$$\frac{\text{Peak velocity first expiration} - \text{Peak velocity first inspiration}}{\text{Peak velocity first expiration}}$$

Table 12.2: Echocardiographic Findings for Cardiac Tamponade

Pericardial effusion (usually moderate to large)

Respiratory variation of the atrioventricular valves (tricuspid valve followed by mitral valve)

Pre-systolic collapse/inversion of the right atrium

Right ventricular diastolic collapse/compression in early diastole

Inferior vena cava plethora

Abnormal hepatic vein flow with reduced/reversed diastolic flow during expiration

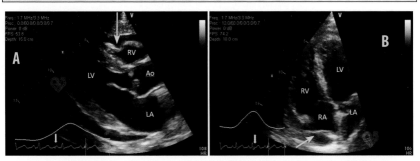

Figure 12.8: A) Early RV diastolic collapse in PLAX view. B) RA collapse in the apical 4-chamber view.

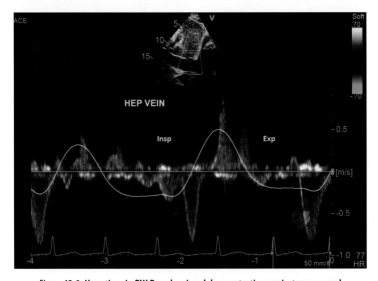

Figure 12.9: Hepatic vein PW Doppler signal demonstrating expiratory reversal

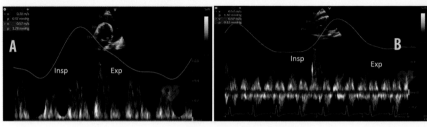

Figure 12.10: **PW Doppler of the mitral valve (A) and tricuspid valve (B) inflow patterns demonstrating respiratory changes during cardiac tamponade**

Constrictive Pericarditis

Definition

A thickened, fibrotic and adherent pericardium restricting diastolic filling and causing ventricular interdependence.

Common Etiologies

• Idiopathic (42 to 61%)
• Post-cardiac surgery (11 to 37%)
• Post-radiation therapy (2 to 31%)
• Infectious (e.g., tuberculosis, bacterial, fungal, parasitic) (3 to 15%)
• Autoimmune (connective tissue) disorders (3 to 7%)
• Miscellaneous causes (1 to 10%)
  - Uremic pericarditis
  - Malignancy/Neoplatic
  - Post-trama
  - Sarcoidosis
  - Drug-induced

History

• Heart failure
• Pericarditis/pericardial effusion
• Mediastinal irradiation

Physical Examination

• Increased jugular venous pressure with prominent x and y descents (hallmark finding: 93%)
• Pulsus paradoxus (uncommon)(exaggerated drop in systolic blood pressure >10mmHg during inspiration)
• Kussmaul's sign (lack of an inspiratory decline in JVP)

- Other findings
  - Profound cachexia
  - Peripheral edema
  - Ascites
  - Pulsatile hepatomegaly
  - Pleural effusion

Cardiac Auscultation

- Diastolic pericardial knock has higher frequency and occurs earlier than S3 (47%)
- Holosystolic/pansystolic functional tricuspid regurgitation murmur

Electrocardiogram

- Nonspecific ST and T wave changes (common)
- Sinus tachycardia (to maintain cardiac output)(common)
- Low voltage QRS complexes throughout ECG (27%)
- Atrial fibrillation (22%)
- If extends to atrial wall, intra-atrial conduction delay and wide, notched, low-amplitude P-wave
- Distinguish patterns between acute pericarditis and myocardial infarction

Chest X-ray/CMR/CT

- Calcification of the pericardium is especially at the apex and posteriorly. Best seen in the lateral view (suggests tuberculosis).
- CMR/CT allows for accurate measurement of the thickness of the pericardium (pathologic >4mm), presence and location of pericardial thickness/calcium and confirms echocardiographic findings (e.g., distorted ventricular contours, septal bounce, inferior vena cava/hepatic vein dilatation)
- CMR late gadolinium enhancement (LGE) of the pericardium

Cardiac Catheterization

- Simultaneous right and left diastolic ventricular pressures where a "dip and plateau" (square root sign) pattern
- Elevated and equalization of the following end-diastolic pressures: right atrial, right ventricular, pulmonary arterial, pulmonary capillary wedge (left atrial) and left ventricle (pressures to within 2 to 3mmHg) are key findings.
- Kussmaul's sign
- Respiratory variation with RV-LV pressure relationship
- Prominent right atrial and left atrial x and y descents (W or W-shaped pattern)
- Mirror-image discordance between RV and peak LV systolic pressures during inspiration (systolic area index)

Medical Treatment

- NSAIDs/Colchicine/Corticosteroids (transient constrictive pericarditis)
- Diuretics

Surgical Treatment

- Pericardiectomy (pericardial stripping) (treatment of choice)

M-mode

- Pericardial thickening with normal left ventricular dimensions, thickness and systolic function may indicate constrictive pericarditis
- Railroad track sign (parallel motion but separated visceral and parietal pericardium)
- Rapid, early and flat diastolic motion of the LV posterior wall endocardium
- Abnormal systolic septal motion (septal notch)
- Premature opening of pulmonary valve
- Abrupt posterior motion of the ventricular septum in early diastole with inspiration (septal shudder and bounce)
- Colormm V_p may be increased (>100cm/s)

2D

- Bright, (gain dependent) thick pericardium (normal 1.2 ± 0.8mm) (>3mm suggests constrictive pericarditis) (may not be equally distributed)
- Lack of "pericardial slide" or adherence of visceral and parietal pericardium or tethering (best seen on RV free wall from apical or subcostal 4-chamber views)
- Interventricular septal bulge to left during inspiration ("septal bounce/shudder/diastolic checking") and expiratory rightward shift
- Interatrial septal bulge towards left atrium with inspiration
- Normal-sized ventricles with normal or mildly dilated atria
- Dilated inferior vena cava (normal ≤2.1cm) and hepatic veins (normal mean diameter 1.5cm) with lack of inspiratory variation (<50%)
- Early, rapid diastolic expansion with sudden cessation of left ventricular filling
- Shadowing (suggests calcific pericardial disease)
- Enlarged liver, spleen, ascites
- Markedly reduced LV strain value
- LV and RV free wall strain less than septal strain values
- Impaired circumferential deformation, torsion and recoil in early diastole

- Differences in longitudinal and circumferential deformation may be useful to distinguish CP from RCM
  - CP = marked abnormal circumferential deformation, torsion and untwisting velocities, but sparing of longitudinal mechanics
  - RCM = abnormal longitudinal mechanics (base) and relative sparing of LV rotation
- Pericardial effusion with hemodynamic compromise suggests constrictive-effusive variant

PW/CW Doppler

- Marked (>25%) respiratory variation of mitral valve (decrease with inspiration, increase with expiration) and tricuspid valve (>40%) (increase with inspiration, decrease with expiration) peak velocities and velocity time integrals (utilize 25mm/s sweep speed; respirometer)
- The consensus for the calculation of percentage respiratory variation in CP for mitral and tricuspid inflow is (expiration – inspiration)/expiration (TV % change will calculate to be a negative value)
- Respiratory variation of the aortic (decrease with inspiration, increase with expiration) and pulmonic (increase with inspiration, decrease in expiration) peak velocities and velocity time integrals
- Increased mitral valve E/A ratio (>1.5) with decreased deceleration time (<160msec)
- Mild decrease in mitral valve deceleration time during inspiration
- Respiratory variation of mitral valve A wave duration
- Increased IVRT with inspiration (>20% as compared to expiration)
- Significant increase in tricuspid regurgitant peak velocity, time velocity integral and duration with inspiration
- Diastolic tricuspid and mitral regurgitation (more common in restrictive cardiomyopathy)
- Marked (>18%) respiratory variation of the peak pulmonary vein D wave (decrease with inspiration, increase with expiration)
- Pulmonary vein S/D ratio of ≥65% with inspiration
- Systolic blunting of pulmonary venous flow throughout respiratory cycle
- Respiratory variation of pulmonary vein A wave peak velocity and duration (decreases with inspiration, increases with expiration)
- Respiratory variation of the mitral annulus TDI e' (sampling of mitral septal annulus recommended)
- Higher mitral e' septal/medial velocity versus e' lateral wall velocity ("annulus reversus")
- Minimal or no respiratory Doppler (S/D) variation seen with SVC flow
- Preserved mitral annulus TDI e' (>8cm/s) in a patient with heart failure ("annulus paradoxus") (sampling of mitral septal annulus recommended)

12

Pericardial Disease / Constrictive Pericarditis

- Normal mitral annular TDI E/e' ratio (<15) in a patient with heart failure ("annulus paradoxus") (sampling of mitral septal annulus recommended)
- Hepatic venous flow:
  - Normal inspiratory increase in systolic and diastolic forward flows; systolic greater than or equal to diastolic
  - Normal inspiratory decrease in atrial and systolic (v wave) reversal
  - Marked decrease or reversal of forward diastolic flow in expiration
  - Blunting of systolic wave with expiration
  - Inspiratory hepatic vein diastolic flow reversals suggest restrictive cardiomyopathy
  - Prominent atrial reversal flow in expiration; systolic flow reversed in expiration (less common)
- Fluid challenge or maneuvers to increase venous return may be helpful in enhancing cardiac Doppler findings

Transesophageal Echocardiography

- May improve the ability to determine pericardial thickness (≥3mm is suggestive) especially at cardiac apex (difficult to evaluate ventricular lateral walls)
- Thickened, hyper-refractile, echo dense pericardium suggests the diagnosis of constrictive pericarditis

Stress Echocardiography

- May demonstrate increase in systolic pulmonary artery pressure
- May demonstrate fixed cardiac output during exercise

Important to Note

- Constrictive pericarditis is a prime example of heart failure due to diastolic dysfunction. The thickened, fibrotic, calcified pericardium envelopes the heart and impairs diastolic filling which leads to an elevation and equilibration of diastolic pressures and impedes systemic and pulmonary venous return.
- Effusive-constrictive pericarditis is the combination of pericardial effusion and constrictive pericarditis. Echocardiography may demonstrate a small to moderate pericardial effusion with strands of solid material between the epicardium and pericardium.
- A patient with a history of pericardial injury (e.g., post-cardiac surgery), right heart failure, preserved global systolic ventricular function, respiratory variation, a normal mitral valve annulus TDI e' (≥8cm), E/e' ratio <15 and hepatic vein flow reversal with expiration may have constrictive pericarditis.
- Exaggerated inspiratory SVC forward flow may be used to distinguish mitral inflow respiratory variations with COPD from CP

Table 12.3: Echocardiographic Findings for Constrictive Pericarditis

Thickened pericardium

Interventricular/interatrial septal bounce

"Bound down" appearance of the ventricular walls with lack of pericardial slide

Inferior vena cava/hepatic vein dilatation

Normal atrial/ventricular dimensions

Restrictive filling pattern with respiratory variation (MV, TV)

Hepatic vein diastolic flow reversal increased with expiration

Normal mitral annular TDI in patient with HF (mitral annulus e' velocity >8cm/s) (E/e' <15) ("annulus paradoxus")

Higher mitral e' septal velocity versus mitral e' lateral wall velocity ("annulus reversus")

LV free wall strain less than LV septal strain

RV free wall strain less than LV septal strain

Hepatic vein expiratory end-diastolic reversal peak velocity / forward flow peak velocity ratio ≥0.8

SVC systolic flow velocity change <20cm/s with respiration

Table 12.4: Separation of Constrictive Pericarditis from Restrictive Cardiomyopathy

	Constriction	Restriction
Atrial size	Normal	Dilated
Respiratory variation of mitral E velocity	Exaggerated (>25%)	Normal
Annular e'	Normal-elevated	Reduced (≤10cm/s)
Pericardial appearance	Thick/bright	Normal
Septal motion	Abnormal	Normal
Septal position	Varies with respiration	Normal
Mitral E/A	Increased (≥2.0)	Increased (≥2.0)
Deceleration time	Short (≤160 msec)	Short (≤160 msec)
Pulmonary hypertension	Rare	Frequent
Left ventricular size/function	Normal	Normal
Mitral/tricuspid regurgitation	Infrequent	Frequent (TR >MR)
Isovolumic relaxation time	Varies with respiration	Stable with respiration

Bold = Recommended

Table 12.5: Algorithm Comparing Constrictive Pericarditis and Restrictive Cardiomyopathy

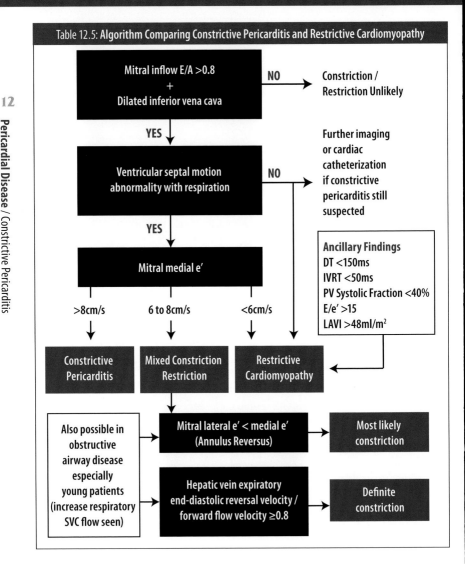

Disease of the Aorta
Danny Rivera, RCS, ACS

Aortic Aneurysm

Definition
• Localized abnormal dilatation of the aorta.

Types
• **Fusiform** – A rather uniform dilatation of the entire circumference of the vessel
• **Saccular** – A weakening in the vessel wall at one point which results in an expansion of a "pouch" with a relatively small neck

Etiology

Thoracic aortic aneurysm
• Genetic/Congenital
  - Marfan syndrome
  - Loeys-Dietz syndrome
  - Ehlers-Danlos syndrome
  - Noonan syndrome
  - Familial
  - Congenital heart disease (e.g.; bicuspid aortic valve, tetralogy of Fallot)

Abdominal
• Atherosclerosis
• Syphilis
• Infection (mycotic)
• Trauma

Degenerative
• Atherosclerosis
• Systemic hypertension
• Mechanical
• Trauma
• Aortic dissection
• Inflammatory
• Takayasu arteritis
• Giant cell arteritis
• Reiter syndrome
• Behscet
• Lupus erythematous
• Idiopathic aortitis
• Infectious
• Syphilis
• Myocobacteria
• HIV
• Staphylococcus

History/Physical Examination

- Asymptomatic
- Atherosclerosis
- Chest pain/Angina
- Back pain
- Cough
- Dyspnea
- Shock

- Superior vena cava syndrome
- Inferior vena cava compression (results in peripheral edema)
- Death due to rupture
- Abdominal systolic bruit
- Decreased lower extremity pulses
- Continuous abdominal bruit

Cardiac Auscultation

- Aortic regurgitation murmur

Electrocardiogram

- Normal
- Evidence of coronary artery disease

Chest X-ray/CMR/CT

- Enlarged aortic shadow
- Egg shell calcification of the ascending aorta (syphilis)
- CMR/CT provides accurate dimension, location, extension and follow-up of aortic aneurysm

Cardiac Catheterization

- Aortography provides information concerning the location, extent and diameter
- Coronary arteriography

Medical Treatment

- Antihypertensive drug regimen (systolic blood pressure below 120mmHg)
- Serial noninvasive evaluation to determine change in aneurysm diameter and extent

- Stabilization of associated atherosclerotic disease (e.g., coronary artery disease)
- Penicillin for patients with syphilitic aortitis

Surgical Treatment

- Resection with graft replacement for symptomatic patients or asymptomatic aneurysm ≥5.5cm; and >5.0cm in patients with bicuspid aortic valve with aortic aneurysm or an aneurysm which demonstrates continued increasing diameter with serial evaluation
- Ross procedure
- Aortic homograft
- Aortic valve repair/replacement
- Endoluminal graft (ELG)

Echocardiographic Views

- Parasternal long-axis view (move up one intercostal space to examine ascending aorta – the first 4cm of the ascending aorta should be visualized)
- Parasternal long-axis view with rotation of the transducer parallel to the sternum
- Parasternal short-axis views
- Apical 2-chamber view with a posterior and medial tilt of the transducer
- Subcostal with examination of the abdominal aorta
- Suprasternal long and short-axis views
- Right parasternal long-axis view
- TEE midesophageal long-axis view of the aorta (130°)
- TEE midesophageal short-axis view (45°) of the ascending aorta
- TEE short-axis views (0°) of the aorta from the diaphragm to the aortic arch

2D

- Dilatation of the aorta (abnormal: men >4.0cm; women >3.8cm)
- Loss of tapering at the sinotubular junction (effacement)
- Systolic expansion of the aortic walls
- Compression of the left atrium
- Measure aorta at the level of the aortic annulus, sinuses of Valsalva, sino-tubular junction and ascending aorta
- Determine the maximum diameter for the following:
  - Aortic annulus dimension: inner edge to inner edge in mid-systole
  - Sinuses of Valsalva: leading edge to leading edge at end diastole
  - Sino-tubular junction: leading edge to leading edge at end diastole
  - Ascending aorta: leading edge to leading edge at end-diastole

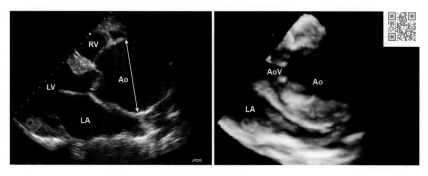

Figure 13.1: Ascending aortic aneurysm on PLAX view in 2D and 3D from the patients, left side perspective

13

Disease of the Aorta / Aortic Aneurysm

Doppler
- Aortic regurgitation (ascending aortic aneurysm)

Transesophageal Echocardiography
- May be useful in defining site, size and extent
- Luminal surface may be investigated for plaque, thrombus formation, debris

Important to Note
- Definition of aneurysm is a segment ≥1.5 x the normal diameter with the intima, media and adventitia layers present.
- Atherosclerotic disease can affect the aorta in a variety of ways: aneurysmal dilatation, atherothrombotic plaque, dissection, intramural hematoma, penetrating ulcer in the aortic plaque or vessel wall, rupture-transection of the aorta, pseudoaneurysm
- Annuloaortic ectasia is an enlargement of the aorta at the sinuses of Valsalva with normal aortic dimensions above the sinotubular junction and is often associated with genetic aortic disease (e.g., Marfan syndrome, Ehlers-Danlos)
- The rate of growth for ascending aortic aneurysms is 0.07mm per year; 1.9mm per year for the descending thoracic aorta
- For ascending aortic aneurysms ≥6.0cm, the risk of rupture, dissection or death is 15%.
- 75% of all aortic aneurysms are located infrarenal. A scan of the abdominal aorta should be included in an echocardiogram.

Table 13.1: The 95% Confidence Intervals for Aortic Root Diameter at Sinuses of Valsalva Based on Body Surface Area (ASE Recommendations) [9]

Aortic Root	Absolute values (cm)		Index values (cm/m^2)	
	Men	Women	Men	Women
Annulus	2.6 ± 0.3	2.3 ± 0.2	1.3 ± 0.1	1.3 ± 0.1
Sinuses of Valsalva	3.4 ± 0.3	3.0 ± 0.3	1.7 ± 0.2	1.8 ± 0.2
Sinotubular junction	2.9 ± 0.3	2.6 ± 0.3	1.5 ± 0.2	1.5 ± 0.2
Proximal ascending aorta	3.0 ± 0.4	2.7 ± 0.4	1.5 ± 0.2	1.6 ± 0.3

- The 95% confidence intervals for aortic root diameter at sinuses of Valsalva based on body surface area (m^2) [9]
  - A: Children and adolescents
  - B: Adults 20 to 39 years old
  - C: Adults 40 years and older

Aortic Dissection

Definition

A tear in the aortic intima through which a column of blood enters the aortic wall, destroying the media and stripping the intima from the adventitia.

Types

DeBakey Classification

- **Type 2:** (5%) Ascending aorta is involved with dissection stopping proximal to brachiocephalic artery
- **Type 3:** (25%) Dissection confined to the descending thoracic aorta and commonly extends into the abdominal aorta
- **Type 1:** (70%) Ascending, transverse and descending aorta are involved (in other words, types 2 and 3)*

*__Remember:__
Type 2 + Type 3 = Type 1

Stanford Duke Classification

- **Type A:** All dissections which involve the ascending aorta (DeBakey's Types 1 and 2)
- **Type B:** All dissections that do not include the ascending aorta (DeBakey's Type 3)

Etiology

- Systemic hypertension
- Atherosclerosis

Genetic

- Bicuspid aortic valve (nine times more frequently associated with dissection than trileaflet aortic valve)
- Marfan syndrome
- Ehlers-Danlos syndrome
- Loeys-Dietz syndrome

Congenital

- Aortic coarctation
- Turner syndrome
- Tetralogy of Fallot

Trauma

- Catheter or stent
- Intraaortic balloon pump
- Motor vehicle accident

Miscellaneous

- Giant cell arteritis
- Takayasu arteritis
- Behcet disease
- Syphilis
- Pregnancy
- Cocaine
- Aging
- Strenuous physical exertion
- Discontinuation of beta blockers
- Renal disease

History/Physical Examination

- Systemic hypertension
- Congenital heart disease (e.g., bicuspid aortic valve)
- Severe ("tearing") chest pain which radiates to the back/abdomen (90%)
- Myocardial ischemia/infarction (10%)
- Heart failure (dyspnea, orthopnea, paroxysmal nocturnal dyspnea, fatigue, cough, weight gain) (7%)
- Neurological symptoms (e.g., syncope (13%), cerebral vascular accident (6%))
- Pulse deficit(s)
- Elevated jugular venous pressure
- Brisk arterial pulse
- Pericardial friction rub

Complications

- Occlusion of major systemic arteries (e.g., carotid, coronary, renal)
- Heart failure
- Cardiogenic shock
- Death due to hemopericardium/rupture

Cardiac Auscultation

- New murmur of aortic regurgitation (50%)

Electrocardiogram

- Lack of ECG changes with severe chest pain
- Left ventricular hypertrophy (25%)
- Myocardial ischemia/infarction (usually inferior wall)

Chest X-ray/CMR/CT

- Widening of the aortic silhouette (90%)
- Cardiomegaly (e.g., pericardial effusion)
- Pleural effusion is usually left (20%)
- CT (with contrast) provides information concerning intimal flap, the two lumens, aortic branches, thrombus in the false lumen, pericardial effusion
- CMR provides information concerning the extent of the dissection and branch vessel involvement, pericardial effusion, entry/exit points, intramural hematoma

Cardiac Catheterization

- Angiogram may allow visualization of true and false aortic lumens, compromised arteries, segmental and global left and right ventricular systolic function, aortic regurgitation and mitral regurgitation

Medical Treatment

- Treatment of systemic hypertension
- Careful evaluation/follow-up of high risk patient's (e.g., Marfan's, Ehlers-Danlos)
- Medical therapy may be sole measure for dissections confined to the descending thoracic aorta
- Morphine
- Sodium nitroprusside
- Intravenous Propranolol/labetalol

Surgical Treatment

- Transection of ascending aorta, intimal tear is resected, both ends of aorta are oversown and a Dacron graft is used to reconnect the two sections of the aorta
- Endoluminal graft (ELG)
- Stent(s)

2D

- Entire aorta requires visualization by combining multiple windows with on-axis and off-axis views including left parasternal, right parasternal, apical, subcostal and suprasternal
- Dilated aorta
- The presence of an intimal flap which is seen as a thin, mobile, linear structure (should be demonstrated in more than one view and motion of intimal flap should not be parallel to the motion of any other cardiac or aortic root structure)
- Demonstration of the true and false lumen with expansion of true lumen and compression of false lumen during ventricular systole
- Spontaneous echo contrast ("smoke") and/or thrombus may be visualized in the false lumen
- Aortic valve leaflet prolapse (dehiscence)
- Compression of cardiac structures (e.g., left atrium)
- Pericardial effusion (a potentially serious finding that may indicate rupture of the dissection)
- Cardiac tamponade is the most common cause of sudden death (60%)
- Left ventricular hypertrophy (e.g., systemic hypertension)
  - Normal IVSd and LVPWd: men 0.6 to 1.0cm; women 0.6cm to 0.9cm)
- Left ventricular volume overload pattern (e.g., significant aortic regurgitation)
- Pleural effusion (usually left)
- Determine:
  - Whether dissection is DeBakey type 1, 2 or 3
  - Involvement of coronary arteries, aortic arch vessels, abdominal aorta and branches

13

Disease of the Aorta / Aortic Dissection

- Identify true lumen vs false lumen: true lumen will demonstrate systolic expansion, little or no spontaneous echo contrast, systolic jets directed away from the lumen, forward flow during systole
- False lumen expands in diastole, spontaneous echo contrast is present, partial or complete thrombosis with reversed, delayed or absence of blood flow
- Presence of segmental wall motion abnormalities
- Right and left ventricular global and segmental systolic function
• Postoperatively evaluate presence and location of persistent intimal flaps, recurring aortic disease, pseudoaneurysm formation, blood flow to major organs, adequacy of aortic valve repair and replacement. Evaluate for infective endocarditis, global and segmental right and left ventricular systolic function

Doppler

• Forward flow may be visualized in the true lumen during ventricular systole with reverse, delayed or no flow in the false lumen
• Reversal of flow may be seen in the false lumen during ventricular diastole
• Absence of flow in the false lumen throughout the cardiac cycle may indicate false lumen thrombosis
• Determine:
- Presence and severity of aortic regurgitation
- Presence and severity of mitral regurgitation
- Presence of cardiac tamponade (e.g., respiratory variation)

Transesophageal Echocardiography

• May improve identification of intimal flap and true and false lumens
• May improve identification of aortic intramural hematoma or penetrating aortic ulcer (a precursor to aortic dissection)
• An aortic wall thickness of >15mm may suggest thrombosis of false lumen
• Improves identification of the complications of aortic dissection including annular dilatation, disruption of the aortic valve leaflets, coronary artery involvement (usually right coronary artery), pericardial effusion, aortic rupture and cardiac tamponade
• Intraoperative pre-operative use of TEE includes identification of:
- Intimal tear
- Entrance tear, additional tears, and exit tear
- True and false lumens
- Optimal site for aortic cannulation
- Aortic annular size
- Aortic rupture
- Branch vessel involvement

SCHOOL OF CARDIAC AND VASCULAR ULTRASOUND 329

- Aortic regurgitation
- Aortic valve dehiscence (prolapse)
- Sizing of allograft replacement
- Wall motion abnormalities
- Global left ventricular systolic function
- Mitral regurgitation due to wall motion abnormalities
- Pericardial effusion
- Pleural effusion

Post-operative

Determine:

• Competency of proximal and distal anastomosis
• Adequacy of aortic valve repair/replacement
• Presence and severity of mitral regurgitation
• Left/right ventricular global and segmental systolic function

Important to Note

• Acute aortic syndrome includes aortic dissection, intramural hematoma (IMH), penetrating aortic ulcer (PAU) atherosclerotic plaque rupture, and aneurysm rupture
• Intramural hematoma represents 5 to 10% of aortic dissections
• Surgical repair is best choice for DeBakey type I, II
• It is important to differentiate the true lumen from the false lumen. The true lumen is usually smaller in diameter, expands in systole, has a more regular shape (e.g., ovoid, circular), is located on the inner (anterior) side of the aorta, is not filled with spontaneous echo contrast or thrombus, contrast agents (e.g., Definity, Optison, and Lumason) opacify the true lumen first and PW Doppler signals are easily obtained, and normal flow pattern present in true lumen with color flow Doppler on.

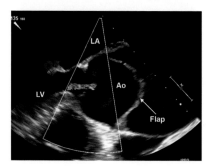 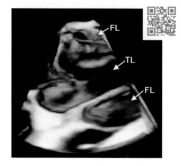

Figure 13.2: **(left)** Mid esophageal long axis view in 2D showing dissection flap of a type A dissection and aortic regurgitation. **(right)** 3D of aortic dissection showing true and false lumen (TL, FL).

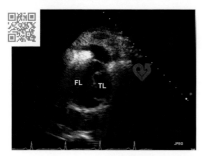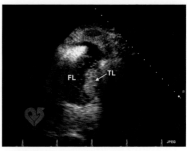

Figure 13.3: **Hi SAX 2D views above aortic valve showing true and false lumen with and without echo contrast of type A dissection.**

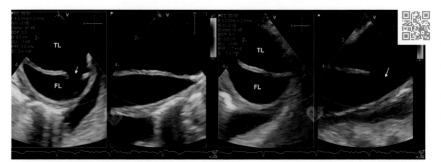

Figure 13.4: **TEE images of abdominal aorta showing type B dissection and point of entry (PoE).**

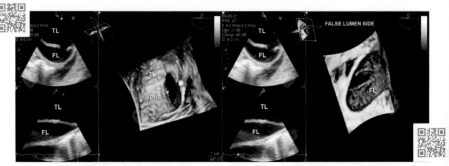

Figure 13.5: **3D TEE images of abdominal aortic dissection showing true lumen**

Figure 13.6: **3D TEE images of abdominal aortic dissection showing false lumen and point of entry (PoE)**

Sinus of Valsalva Aneurysm

Definition

Dilatation of the aortic sinus of Valsalva, a rare cardiac anomaly; may be acquired or congenital; may present as ruptured or unruptured.

Etiology

Congenital usually affects single sinus only (most common)

Acquired
- Marfan syndrome
- Ehlers-Danlos syndrome
- Takayasu arteritis
- Atherosclerosis
- Trauma
- Infective endocarditis
- Fungal infection
- Syphilis
- Tuberculosis
- Senile type (all three sinuses are dilated)
- Iatrogenic (e.g., surgical repair of ventricular septal defect, post-aortic valve replacement)

Associated Conditions
- Aortic regurgitation usually due to aortic valve prolapse (50%)
- Ventricular septal defect (40%)
- Bicuspid aortic valve (15 to 20%)
- Pulmonary stenosis (usually subvalvular)
- Atrial septal defect
- Coarctation of the aorta
- Patent ductus arteriosus

History/Physical Examination
- Asymptomatic (unruptured)
- Dyspnea (ruptured)
- Sudden onset of chest pain (ruptured)
- Heart failure (ruptured)
- Infective endocarditis (ruptured)
- Sudden death (ruptured)

Cardiac Auscultation

Continuous murmur accentuated in diastole may indicate rupture
(a continuous murmur is also associated with patent ductus arteriosus,
aortopulmonary window, coronary artery fistula, ventricular septal defect)

Electrocardiogram
- Normal (unruptured)
- AV conduction defects

Chest X-ray/CMR/CT

- Normal (unruptured)
- Cardiomegaly
- Heart failure

Cardiac Catheterization

- Retrograde thoracic aortography
- Left to right shunt at ventricular or atrial level
- Coronary arteriography

Treatment

- Resection of the aneurysmal sac at its base, repair of the aneurysmal opening and repair of any ventricular septal defect or aortic regurgitation
- Aortic valve repair/replacement (aortic regurgitation)
- Ross procedure

2D

- Parasternal short-axis view of the aortic valve is the best view to visualize the aneurysm
- Abnormal dilatation of one or more of the sinuses; the right sinus is most often affected
- Right coronary cusp – 69% (protrudes into right ventricular outflow tract and/or right atrium)
- Non-coronary cusp – 26% (protrudes into right atrium)
- Left coronary cusp – 5% (protrudes into left atrium)
- Ruptured aneurysm often appears as a finger like projection ("windsock") appearance with echo dropout at the tip of the aneurysm. It may be difficult to differentiate from ventricular septal aneurysm.
- Ventricular septal aneurysm is located below the aortic annulus and demonstrates flow primarily during ventricular systole)
- Systolic-diastolic expansion of aneurysm
- Aortic valve prolapse
- Thrombosis of aneurysm (rare)
- Agitated saline contrast may demonstrate negative contrast effect in the receiving chamber
- Pericardial effusion/cardiac tamponade (hemopericardium)
- Right atrial dilatation (suggests rupture of right- or non-coronary)
- Right ventricular volume overload (rupture of right- or non-coronary)
- Left ventricular volume overload pattern (rupture of left sinus type)
- Dissection of right sinus of Valsalva aneurysm into the interventricular septum (rare)
- Determine left/right ventricular global and segmental systolic function
- Post-operative to confirm complete repair

Doppler

- Swirling flow pattern may be visualized within an unruptured sinus of Valsalva aneurysm
- Ruptured aneurysm will demonstrate high-velocity systolic and diastolic (continuous) turbulent (mosaic) flow pattern into the receiving chamber
- Determine:
  - Shunt direction
  - Peak pressure gradient and mean pressure gradient (CW Doppler)
  - Presence of ventricular septal defect is common
  - Presence and severity of aortic regurgitation is common
  - Presence and severity of tricuspid regurgitation. Commonly seen in ruptured right sinus of Valsalva aneurysm.
  - Presence and severity of right ventricular outflow tract obstruction
- Postoperative evaluation to confirm complete repair and the presence and severity of residual aortic regurgitation

Transesophageal Echocardiography

- May improve delineation of aneurysm

Important to Note

- The most common location for sinus of Valsalva aneurysm to rupture is into the right atrium.
- Sinus of Valsalva aneurysm has a higher incidence in Far Eastern countries than in Western countries.
- Congenital aneurysm has a 4:1 male predominance.
- Sinus of Valsalva aneurysm may be multiple.

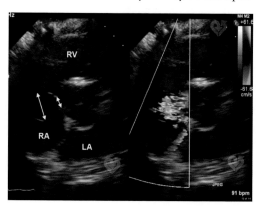

Figure 13.7: Transthoracic SAX view at the level of the aorta showing sinus of Valsalva aneurysm with and without color Doppler.

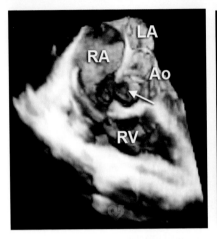
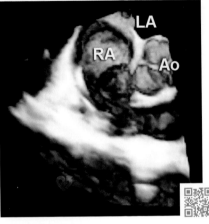

Figure 13.8: **TEE 3D images showing the entry of the sinus of Valsalva aneurysm and its size.**

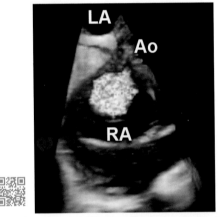

Figure 13.9: **3D TEE image with color Doppler showing the sinus of Valsalva aneurysm filled with flow.**

Supravalvular Aortic Stenosis (SAS)

Definition

Narrowing of the ascending aorta.

Types

- **Hourglass** – An abnormal thickening of the medial layer of the aorta that is associated with Williams syndrome. (most common type)
- **Membranous** – A thin membrane just above the valve with one or multiple openings causing obstruction to flow.
- **Hypoplastic ("strand")** – An under-developed aorta, usually associated with hypoplastic left heart syndrome

- **Coarctation** – a narrowing of the descending thoracic aorta just proximal or just distal to the ductus arteriosus; make sure to evaluate for a bicuspid aortic valve which had been seen in 50% to 80% of coarctations

2D/Cardiac Doppler

- Parasternal long-axis with movement of transducer one intercostal space upward is useful
- Suprasternal long-axis is useful
- Hourglass appearance of supravalvular area of the aorta (hourglass type)
- Membrane located in supravalvular area of the aorta (apical 5-chamber/apical long-axis view may be useful)
- Thickened/sclerotic aortic valve leaflets
- Dilatation of the proximal coronary arteries
- Ostial stenosis of the coronary artery
- Concentric left ventricular hypertrophy
- Determine peak velocity, peak pressure gradient and mean pressure gradient across obstruction

References

1. Weyman, A. E. (1994). Principles and Practice of Echocardiography. Pennsylvania: Lea & Febiger.

2. Lang, R.M., Goldstein, S.A., Kronzon, I., & Khandheria, B. K. (2011). Dynamic Echocardiography. Missouri: Saunders Elsevier.

3. Matthew, J. P., Nicoara, A., Ayoub, C. M., & Swaminathan, M. (2018). Clinical Manual and Review of Transesophageal Echocardiography. New York: Mc Graw Hill Education.

4. Nihoyannopoulos, P. & Kisslo, J. (Eds). (2018). Echocardiography. Switzerland: Springer.

5. Mavroudis, C. & Backer, C. L. (2003). Pediatric Cardiac Surgery. Pennsylvania: Mosby.

6. J Am Soc Echocardiogr 2015;28:119-82

7. Echocardiography in aortic diseases: EAE recommendations for clinical practice. Eur J Echocardiogr. 2011 Aug;12(8):642.

8. Diagnostic goals in aortic dissection. Value of transthoracic and transesophageal echocardiography. Herz 1993 Feb;18(1):77-8.

9. Lang RM, Badano, LP, et al. Recommendations for chamber quantification: a report from the American Society of Echocardiography's Guidelines and Standards Committee and the Chamber Quantification. J Am Soc Echocardiogr 2015 Jan;28(1):1-39.

13

Disease of the Aorta / Supravalvular Aortic Stenosis (SAS)

Cardiac Tumors
Dennis Atherton, RDCS, FASE

- Extremely rare (primary .06%, secondary 1.2%) [1]
- Primary Benign (most common, 80% of all cardiac tumors)
- Secondary metastatic (most common malignant)

Primary Benign

- **Myxoma** – Most common benign cardiac tumor in adults is (50%)
- **Papillary Fibroelastoma** – Most common cardiac valve tumor (15%)
- **Lipoma** – (15%)
- **Rhadomyoma** – Most common benign cardiac tumor in children/newborns (8%)
- **Fibroma** – Second most common pediatric cardiac tumor (4%)
- **Hemangioma** – (2%)
- **Teratoma** – (1%)
- **Paragangliomas** – may also be malignant

Myxoma

Definition

A benign primary cardiac tumor that is usually attached by a stalk (pedunculated) to the left side of the interatrial septum (80%) [2] allowing it to be somewhat mobile. Rarely are they multicentric, friable or located in the venticles. Large myxomas may obstruct blood flow or prolapse into the mitral or tricuspid annulus and mimic stenosis. Growth rate is approximately 1.8cm per year.

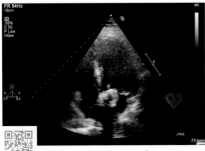
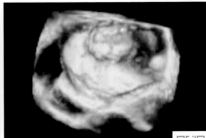

Figure 14.1: **Myxoma 2D**   Figure 14.2: **Myxoma 3D**

History/Physical Examination

- Symptoms are dyspnea (positional), dizziness, syncope, palpitations, chest pain, fever, weight loss, joint pain, clubbing, malaise, TIA/CVA, Raynauds, heart failure.
- Familial (10%) – Carney syndrome and usually found in younger patients
- 65% of cardiac myxomas are found in women.

Complications

- Arrhythmias
- Embolization (Pulmonary emboli or systemic)
- Infection of tumor
- Edema
- Sudden death

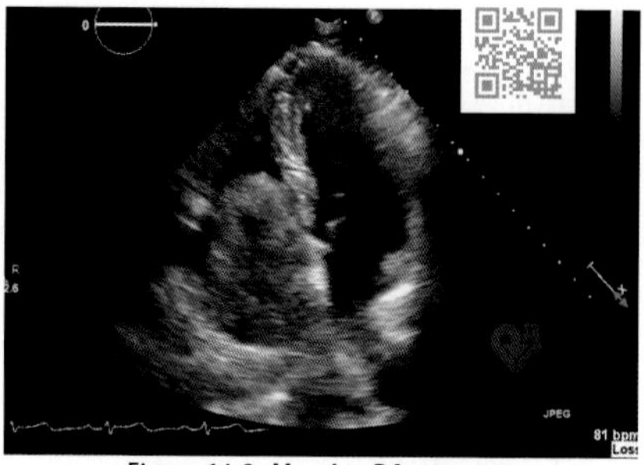

Electrocardiogram

Atrial fibrillation / flutter

Figure 14.3: **Massive RA myxoma**

Chest Xray/CMR/CCT/PET

- Cardiomegaly
- Left or right atrial enlargement
- Pulmonary edema
- Unusual intracardiac calcification
- CMR identification and clues to type of tumor
- CCT can identify tumor and is usually more readily available
- PET primarily used for identification of suspected metastatic tumors

Treatment

- Prompt complete surgical excision. Recurrence possible if not completely excised.
- Dacron patch may be needed for Interatrial excision
- Mitral repair or replacement may be necessary
- Serial echos to rule out recurrence (2 to 5% and usually within 48 months)

Echocardiography

- Most often found in the atria, attached to the septum
- Dramatic motion and may prolapse into the ventricle
- Globular, finely speckled mass with well defined edges and pedunculated (point of attachment may be best visualized utilizing the apical and subcostal 4-chamber views)
- Areas of tumor calcification may be visualized
- Left atrial dilation
- Utilize multiple imaging on-axis and off-axis windows, varied gain settings, B-mode color, harmonic imaging, zoom, contrast and 3D to detect sessile or small myxomas

- Describe the chamber location(s), size, shape, point of attachment, pattern of reflectivity and motion characteristics of the myxoma
- Evaluate first generation relatives of patients with possible familial myxomas
- Determine the length and width of the myxoma
- If able contrast for perfusion information such as vascular channels or a myxoma blush [3]
- Serial echocardiograms to rule out recurrence
- Guides to help differentiate a myxoma from thrombus: myxomas are usually mobile, with sharp demarcated borders, have a mottled appearance, have a point of attachment, normal atrial dimensions and normal atrioventricular valve. A thrombus has an irregular surface, layered, immobile, broad based, located near the posterior wall of the left atrium, with dilated left atrium and abnormal atrioventricular valve.
- Highly mobile myxomas with broad bases may represent an increased risk for embolization
- Extensive intra-myxoma hemorrhage may be associated with precipitous symptomatic deterioration.
- Myxomas can reoccur (3% recurrence rate) and extend into surrounding tissue
- Myxomas may have some low-grade malignant features
- Rarely, 2D echocardiography may not detect a highly vascularized myxoma

Papillary Fibroelastoma

- May also be referred to as cardiac papilloma, papillary fibroma, papillary endocardial tumor, giant Lambl's excrescence, papilloelastoma, fibro-papilloma
- Papillary fibroelastoma is the most common valvular tumor of the heart [4,5]
- Aortic Valve is a most common location (45%)
- Microscopically they resemble a sea anemone
- Occurs with equal frequency in both sets as usually found in patients older than 60 years of age. (Though there have been reported in patients 9 months to 92 years of age)
- Clinically associated with dyspnea, cyanosis, peripheral/pulmonary emboli, cerebral vascular accident transient ischemic attack, visual changes, transient paresis, aphasia, paradoxical embolization, angina, myocardial infarction, heart failure, atrioventricular conduction disturbance and sudden death.
- Left sided papillary fibroelastomas are more often associated with symptoms then one is located in the right heart
- If papillary fibroelastoma is located in the left or right atrium, cardiac auscultation may contact a low frequency sound occurring after S2 consistent with a tumor plop
- There is a known association of left ventricular fibroelastoma with aortic stenosis

- Found attached by a small pedicle on the mid portion of the endocardial surfaces of the atrioventricular valves (85% are valvular), either side of the semilunar valves, in the left ventricular outflow tract, or rarely on the papillary muscles, chordae tendineae, Chiari network, atrial endocardium or ventricular endocardium and may be multiple
- Most common location for aortic valve is the arterial side, ventricular side for the atrioventricular valves
- Rarely exceeds 1cm in diameter (range 0.2 to 4.6) gelatinous in appearance ("cluster of grapes"), consisting of multiple papillary fronds attached to the endocardium by a small stalk.
- Asymptomatic patients with a small left sided, non mobile type may not require surgical resection
- Anticoagulation therapy may be indicated due to the fact that the papillary fibroelastoma can form the nidus for platelet and fibrin aggregation and lead to systemic emboli
- Surgical resection should be considered for patients with large (>1.0cm), mobile type, young patients
- There have been no reported recurrence of papillary fibroelastoma
- Aortic valve location and tumor mobility predictors of cardiac death related to papillary fibroelastoma

Echo/Doppler

- Appear on 2D echocardiography as small, mobile, pedunculated echo dense mass and may be multiple
- The echocardiogram appearance of the papillary fibroelastoma they mimic the appearance of the vegetation clinical information may be required or Lambl's discretion says Lambl's excrescences are usually smaller and broader base with origination from the valve margin
- Doppler may demonstrate no valvular abnormalities, significant regurgitation or stenosis
- TEE Maybe more helpful in identifying and characterizing then TTE during surgical removal

Lipoma

- Circumscribed, encapsulated tumor which is usually solitary, intramuscular, subendocardial, sub epicardial, epicardial or rarely may involve the current valves
- Most are sessile or polypoid with 1/2 originating in the subendocardium, in the sun epicardium, 1/4 in the Epicardium and 1/4 completely intramuscular
- Most frequently located in the left ventricle, right atrium or interatrial septum
- Occur at all ages equal frequency of both sexes
- They may be massive in size, confused with the coma one attached to and atrioventricular valve while the encapsulated and Lipoma maybe quite small

14

Cardiac Tumors / Primary Benign / Lipoma

- Patient is usually asymptomatic although maybe associated with conduction disturbances
- Intra-pericardial lipomas May cause pericardial Effusion
- Surgical excision may be indicated

Lipomatous Hypertrophy of the Interatrial Septum

- A nonencapsulated hyperplasia or of adipose tissue in the anterior atrial septum and may not be a true tumor

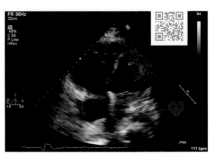

- Has been associated with older age, older age, obesity, diabetes, supraventricular rhythm and conduction disturbances, recurrent pericardial effusions, arterial embolization, pulmonary emboli and sudden cardiac death (rare)

- No specific treatment\
surgical excision (e.g., superior vena cava obstruction; clinically significant arrhythmias)

Figure 14.4: **Lipomatous hypertrophy**

Echo front/Doppler Findings

- Subcostal and apical 4-chamber views are helpful thickened intra-atrial septum (1.5 to 3cm but may be as thick as 7 to 8cm; normal thickness of the intra-atrial septum is less than 1.0cm)
- Dumbbell appearance with sparing of the fossa ovalis
- Lack of encapsulation distinguishes lipomatous hypertrophy from lipoma
- May extend to right atrial wall
- TEE may be helpful in identifying thin fossa ovalis to establish diagnosis, location, extension (e.g., right atrium) sessile behavior and fatty nature

Fibroma

- Usually ventricular, intramural and solitary

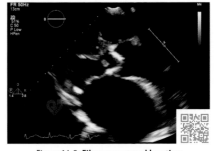

- Has been reported in patients whose age range between 2 to 57 years although three quarters of all fibromas occur in the pediatric population (second most common benign tumor in the pediatric population)[6]

Figure 14.5: **Fibroma unusual location**

- May occur in any cardiac chamber but most commonly found embedded in the myocardium of the anterior wall of the left ventricle, intraventricular septum or right ventricle
- May be large (3 to 10cm)

- Most common clinical symptoms include heart failure 21% sudden death 14%; usually infants, ventricular tachycardia at 13%, atypical chest pain 3.5%, symptoms of ventricular outflow tract obstruction
- Total /partial resection may be indicated (difficult due to size)
- Cardiac transplantation has been used in a young patient with a nonresectable 130g left ventricular fibroma

Echo/Doppler
- Apical front/subcostal views may be the best used to identify
- May appear highly refractile by 2D echocardiography

Rhabdomyoma
- Most common tumor found in children (associated with Tuberous Sclerosis) although may be found in adults [7]
- Most cases present in the first year of life 80%
- Associated with Pringles disease tuberous sclerosis 30 to 50% of cases
- Occur equally in the right and left ventricles were infrequently in the atria 30% and may be multiple 90% are multiple
- Most often involve the ventricular myocardium and may project into the cardiac cavity or may be pedunculated
- Range in size from a few millimeters to a few centimeters
- Symptoms include, arrhythmia, AV block, pericardial effusion, sudden death
- May cause obstruction to outflow or inflow
- May spontaneously disappear 50%
- Treatment includes antiarrhythmic drugs, surgical resection
- There are no reported cases of recurrence

Echo Front/Doppler Findings
- 2D echo findings characteristically demonstrate echo dense multiple nodular masses in several chambers or may appear as a single intramural echodense mass of the interventricular septum or ventricular free wall
- Continuous-wave Doppler may be used to evaluate for the presence and severity of outflow and/or inflow obstruction
- May be detected during a fetal echocardiographic examination (case reported at 30 weeks gestation and removed at 20 months of age)

Primary Malignant Intracardiac
- Angiosarcoma usually involves right atrium (28%)
- Rhabdomyosarcoma often infiltrate ventricular myocardium (11%)
- Fibrosarcoma extensive infiltration of the heart is common (8%)
- Osteosarcoma usually located in the left atrium (7%)

14

Cardiac Tumors / Primary Malignant Intracardiac / Rhabdomyoma

- Malignant fibrous histiocytoma 6% usually located in the left atrium originating from the left atrial posterior wall
- Lymphoma 6% usually located in the right atrium with pericardial effusion
- Leimyosarcoma 5% usually located in the left atrium
- Myxosarcoma 3% usually located in left atrium
- Pericardial mesothelioma – can cause tamponade and constriction
- Primary Lymphoma –HIV/Aids

Sarcomas

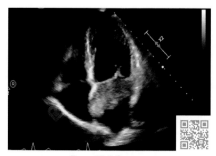

- Almost all primary with malignant cardiac tumors are sarcomas second in the overall frequency to myxomas [8]
- Affects men more often than women 65 to 75%

Figure 14.6: **Sarcoma**

- Clinical presentation includes obstructive symptoms, arrhythmias, chest pain, death

Angiosarcomas

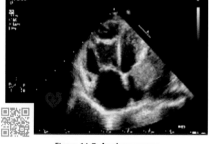

- Most often occur in the right atrium 80% or pericardium
- Present with chest pain, continuous murmur, right heart failure, pericardial effusion front/tamponade/constriction, vena caval obstruction
- May compromise inflow portions of the ventricles

Figure 14.7: **Angiosarcomas**

- Tumor excision, radiation and chemotherapy are palliative measures since course is rapid mean survival of 10 months

Echo Front/Doppler Findings

- 2D echocardiography may demonstrate large mural mass that often extends to the pericardium, vena cava or tricuspid valve
- Doppler may demonstrate flow obstruction (e.g. tricuspid valve)
- TEE may help and differentiation from benign tumors (myxomas arise from the intra-atrial septum wall malignant tumors extend into adjacent structures such as the vena cava or pulmonary vein)

Rhabdomyosarcomas

- Second most common primary sarcoma of the heart
- 25% of tumors occurring patients younger than 20 years of age

- May be found in any cardiac chamber and may be multiple
- May cause inflow tract

Secondary Tumors (metastatic)

- 20 to 40 times more common than primary tumor
- Cardiac metastasis occurring approximately 5% of patients who died of malignant tumors
- Often present with pericardial effusion
- Most common tumors which metastasized to the heart are: Melanoma is common, 50 to 65%, bronchiogenic carcinoma, breast cancer, lymphoma, adenocarcinoma of the colon or stomach, renal cell carcinoma, laryngeal carcinoma, pancreatic cancer and mcinous adenocarcinoma of the cecum front/ovary.
- Renal cell carcinomas may extend from the inferior vena cava to the right atrium and right ventricle
- Occurs most often in patients over 50 years of age, with equal incidence between sexes
- Clinical presentation includes neoplastic disease with cardiac symptoms such as cardiac enlargement, tachycardia,, arrhythmias or heart failure

Echo/Doppler

- Pericardial effusion, wall thickening or protrusion of the tumor mass into a cardiac chamber (vena cava, pulmonary vein) are the most common echocardiographic findings

Pericardial Cyst

- Most common benign tumor of the pericardium 1 per 100,000 [9]
- May range in size from 2 to 16cm
- Symptoms include chest pain, dyspnea, cough or paroxysmal arrhythmia
- Occur most often in the third or fourth decade of life with equal distribution between men and women

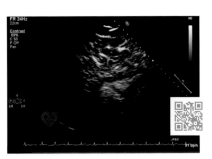

Figure 14.8: **Pericardial cyst**

- Right costophrenic location is most common 70%, may located in the left costophrenic angle 10 to 40% or occasionally may be found along the upper mediastinum, or left cardiac border hila or left cardiac border
- May resemble other tumors of the pericardium such as hemangioma, lymph angioma, lipoma or retrosternal hernia, pericardial fat pad, eveneration of the diaphragm
- Chest x-ray demonstrates a round, sharply demarcated mass

- Treatment includes needle aspiration to determine contents; surgical removal is effective
- Echo front/Doppler findings
- 2D echo demonstrates cyst as an ovoid echo-free space adjacent to a cardiac chamber may be multiple
- Must be distinguished from a loculated pericardial effusion, dilated coronary sinus, ventricular pseudoaneurysm
- Determine location, size, shape, consistency of the cyst

Extracardiac Tumors

- Mediastinal cyst, hematoma, teratoma, thymoma, diaphragmatic hernia, pancreatic cyst
- May appear as displacement of the heart, compression of the cardiac chambers, superior vena cava obstruction, cardiac tamponade, constrictive pericarditis, pulmonary stenosis, tricuspid stenosis

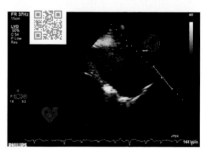

Carcinoid heart disease

Figure 14.9: **Extracardiac tumor compressing**

Definition

The result of the metastasizing carcinoid tumor, usually located in the appendix or ileum but may also occur in the bronchus, biliary tract, pancreas, testis and ovary. Ileal carcinoids often metastasized to the liver and produce the carcinoid syndrome. Carcinoids contain a high concentration of 5 hydroxytriptamine (5–HT) (serotonin) and excreted as 5 hydroxyindoleacetic (5-HIAA) in the urine. Diagnosis is made by documenting more than 30 mg of 5 hydroxyindole acetic acid a serotonin metabolite) in a 24-hour collection

The Carcinoid Syndrome Consists of:

- Cutaneous flushing
- Intestinal hypermobility from/diarrhea liver metastasis
- Bronchial constriction pulmonary carcinoid
- Heart failure (dyspnea, orthopnea, paroxysmal nocturnal dyspnea, fatigue, cough, weight gain)
- Cardiac lesions (e.g endocardial plaques composed of fibrous tissue)
- Death

Cardiac Lesions

- 50% of patients with carcinoid tumors have cardiac involvement [10]
- Half of all test and carcinoid patients are due to heart failure secondary to severe tricuspid regurgitation

- Carcinoid affects the right heart more than the left heart
- Glistening, white–yellowish deposit is most often found on the tricuspid valve the pulmonic valve but may also be found in the vena cava, right atrium, right ventricle and less frequently on the left heart valves and cardiac chamber walls

Cardiac Clinical Manifestation

- Dyspnea most common in patients with carcinoid heart disease
- Harsh, holosystolic murmur at lower left sternal border with inspiratory accentuation tricuspid regurgitation
- Right sided S3
- Right heart failure (e.g. jugular venous distention, hepatomegaly, peripheral edema, ascites, anasarca)
- Pulmonic valve murmurs (stenosis and/or regurgitation)

Medical Treatment

- Somatostatin/Ocreotide (decrease his tumor size, serotonin levels)
- Relief of carcinoid syndrome symptoms diarrhea flushing
- Ketanserin
- Corticosteroids
- Antihistamine
- H1 and H2 blockers-Diphenhydramine
- Aprotinin
- Digitalis/diuretics right heart failure

Surgical Treatment

- Surgical remover of tumor if not metastasized
- Valve replacement bioprosthetic valve to avoid anticoagulation
- Balloon valvuloplasty for tricuspid valve and/or pulmonic valve stenosis

2D Imaging

- Thickened, retracted and increased rigidity of the tricuspid and/or pulmonic valve leaflets
- Total fixation of the leaflets in the partially open position
- Right atrial dilatation/right ventricular dilatation
- Right ventricular volume overload right ventricular dilatation with paradoxical septal motion
- D shaped left ventricle during ventricular diastole due to right ventricular volume overload best visualized in the parasternal short axis of the LV
- Increased right atrial wall/anterior atrial septal thickness best visualized by TEE
- Tumor may be embedded in the myocardium

- Plaque deposition may be seen in the coronary sinus, vena cava, pulmonary artery, coronary artery
- Left heart involvement is rare 5 to 10% of cases, right to left shunting, bronchial tumors, pulmonary metastasis
- Mitral involvement possible usually milder than right heart involvement
- Pericardial effusion 14%
- Liver metastasis may be visualized from subcostal views
- Evaluate right ventricular systolic function

Doppler

- Tricuspid regurgitation most common finding, often severe
- Hepatic vein systolic flow reversal due to significant tricuspid regurgitation
- Dagger shaped tricuspid regurgitation velocity signal indicating a rapid equilibration of right atrial right ventricular systolic pressures
- Tricuspid stenosis which is usually mild
- Pulmonary regurgitation 81%
- Valvular pulmonic stenosis with varying degrees of severity the severity may be underestimated due to severe tricuspid regurgitation
- Mild to moderate mitral regurgitation with left heart involvement

Important to Note

- Tricuspid valve damage is the most common cardiac pathological feature 97% of the cases
- A Doppler gradient >10mmHg may be an indication for pulmonic valve replacement and/or removal

References

1. Tumors of the heart. A 20-year experience with a review of 12,485 consecutive autopsies. Lam KY, Dickens P, Chan ACArch Pathol Lab Med. 1993;117(10):1027.

2. Cardiac myxomas: 24 years of experience in 49 patients. Keeling IM, Oberwalder P, Anelli-Monti M, Schuchlenz H, Demel U, Tilz GP, Rehak P, Rigler B Eur J Cardiothorac Surg. 2002;22(6):971.

3. Eur Heart J Cardiovasc Imaging. 2016 Feb; 17(2): 216. Published online 2015 Nov 17. doi: 10.1093/ehjci/jev300

4. Tumors and tumor-like lesions of the heart valves. Shi-Min Yuan, Hua Jing, and Jacob Lavee Shi-Min Yuan

5. FH Edwards, D Hale, A Cohen, L Thompson, AT Pezzella, R Virmani Primary cardiac valve tumors. Ann Thorac Surg, 52 (1991), pp. 1127-1131

6. Burke A, Tavora F. The 2015 WHO classification of tumors of the heart and pericardium. J Thorac Oncol. 2016;11:441–452. doi: 10.1016/j.jtho.2015.11.009.

7. Bass, J.L., Breningstall, G.N., and Swaiman, K.F. Echocardiographic incidence of cardiac rhabdomyoma in tuberous sclerosis. Am J Cardiol. 1985; 55: 1379–1382

8. Colucci, W.S. and Braunwald, E. Primary tumors of the heart. in: E. Braunwald (Ed.) Heart disease. WB Saunders, Philadelphia; 1980: 1501–1516

9. Patel J, Park C, Michaels J, Rosen S, Kort S. Pericardial cyst: case reports and a literature review. Echocardiography. 2004;21(3):269-272.

10. Pellikka PA, Tajik AJ, Khandheria BK, et al. Carcinoid heart disease. Clinical and echocardiographic spectrum in 74 patients. Circulation 1993; 87:1188.

Congenital Heart Disease
Rob McDonald, RCS, RDCS, RCCS, ACS, FASE

Note: Majority of the textbook demonstrates two-dimensional images using the American Society of Echocardiography (ASE) standard imaging planes, however the Congenital Heart section will contain images that meet ASE Pediatric Echocardiography standard imaging planes. [1]

Atrial Septal Defect (ASD)

Definition

An abnormal opening in the interatrial septum.

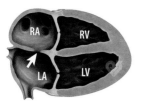
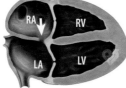
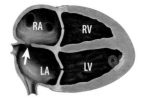

Figure 15.1: **Ostium secundum**   Figure 15.2: **Ostium primum**   Figure 15.3: **Sinus venosus**

Types

• **Ostium secundum** – Located in the mid-portion of the interatrial septum and associated with "hemodynamic" mitral valve prolapse. 67% of ostium secundum ASD's occur in women. (75%)

• **Ostium primum** – Defect located at the inferior portion of the interatrial septum (associated with a cleft mitral valve) (15%)

• **Sinus venosus** – Defect located in the posterior and superior portion of the interatrial septum near the entrance of the superior vena cava or inferior and posterior near the entrance of the inferior vena cava. Associated with partial anomalous pulmonary venous return. (4%)

• **Coronary sinus** – Roof of the coronary sinus is partially or completely absent creating a left to right shunt from the left atrium to the coronary sinus and then into the right atrium. Associated with persistent left superior vena cava which may connect to the coronary sinus or left atrium. (<1%)

• **Common atrium** – Characterized by absence or virtual absence of the interatrial septum. Strong association with the Ellis-van Creveld syndrome, situs abnormalities. (rare)

Shunt

- Predominantly left-to-right with a brief reversal of the shunt during atrial relaxation (early ventricular systole)

History

- Asymptomatic until middle to late adult years (common)
- Dyspnea upon exertion (common after age 30)
- Orthopnea (decreased pulmonary compliance)
- Right heart failure (e.g., jugular venous distention, hepatomegaly, peripheral edema, ascites, anasarca)

Physical Examination

- Skeletal malformations (e.g., Holt-Oram)
- Cyanosis with or without exercise (pulmonary hypertension) (ominous sign)

Complications

- Heart failure
- Pulmonary hypertension
- Eisenmenger's syndrome
- Atrial arrhythmias
- Cerebral vascular accident (paradoxical embolization)
- Infective endocarditis (rare)
- Migraine headaches
- Decompression sickness (e.g., scuba diving)

Cardiac Auscultation

- Fixed splitting of S2 due to delayed emptying of the right ventricle (pathognomic)
- Increased flow across the pulmonary valve causes an ejection-type murmur (may not vary in intensity with respiration)
- Holosystolic murmur at cardiac apex (associated with cleft mitral valve)
- Holosystolic murmur due to tricuspid regurgitation
- Right heart S3, S4
- Increased P2 (indicates pulmonary hypertension)
- High pitched diastolic murmur due to pulmonary regurgitation (Graham-Steell murmur)

Electrocardiogram

- May be normal
- Incomplete/complete right bundle branch block (90%)
- Right atrial enlargement
- Atrial arrhythmias (atrial fibrillation common over the age of 50)
- Right ventricular hypertrophy may indicate pulmonary hypertension

Chest X-ray/CMR/CT

- Cardiomegaly (enlargement of the right atrium, right ventricle and main pulmonary artery and branches)
- Prominent pulmonary vasculature ("shunt vascularity")
- CMR provides information concerning about dimension and location of the defect, Qp/Qs ratio, ventricular function and may be useful when complex anatomy is present (e.g., anomalous pulmonary venous return)

Cardiac Catheterization

- Coronary arteriography in middle age/older patients
- Determines pulmonary artery pressures/vascular resistance

Treatment

- Digitalis/Diuretics (right/left heart failure without pulmonary hypertension)
- Surgical closure with pericardial or Dacron patch if Qp/Qs is ≥1.5:1 (not possible in patients with Eisenmenger's syndrome)
- Antiarrhythmic
- Transcatheter closure (TEE or intracardiac guidance)
- Mitral valve repair and/or replacement (cleft mitral valve)

Ostium secundum

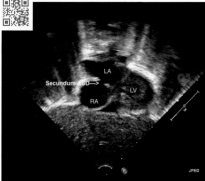

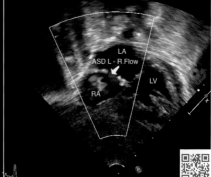

Figure 15.4: Subcostal 4-chamber view demonstrating a secundum atrial septal defect (ASD); left atrium (LA), right atrium (RA), left ventricle (LV).

Figure 15.5: Subcostal 4-chamber view demonstrating a left to right across the secundum atrial septal defect (ASD); left atrium (LA), right atrium (RA), left ventricle (LV).

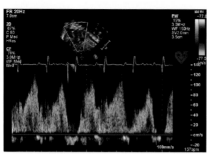

Figure 15.6: Pulse-wave Doppler demonstrating a left to right shunt with flow velocities of 100cm/sec across a secundum atrial septal defect.

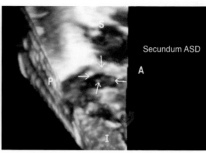

Figure 15.7: 3D echocardiogram demonstrating a secundum atrial septal defect (ASD) orifice (arrows).

Ostium Primum

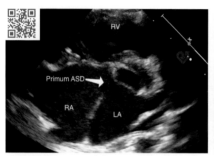

Figure 15.8: Parasternal short-axis view demonstrating a primum atrial septal defect (ASD); left atrium (LA), right atrium (RA), right ventricle (RV).

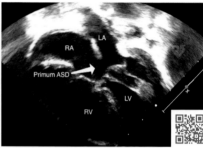

Figure 15.9: Apical 4-chamber view demonstrating a primum atrial septal defect (ASD); left atrium (LA), right atrium (RA), right ventricle (RV), left ventricle (LV).

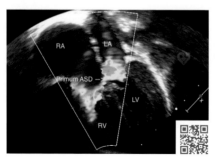

Figure 15.10: Apical 4-chamber view demonstrating a primum atrial septal defect (ASD); left atrium (LA), right atrium (RA), right ventricle (RV), left ventricle (LV).

Sinus Venosus

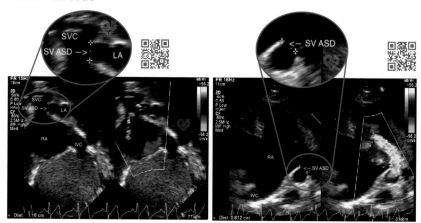

Figure 15.11: **Subcostal long-axis view of the superior vena cava (SVC) and inferior vena cava (IVC) demonstrating a sinus venous (SV) atrial septal defect (ASD) and a left to right shunt by color flow Doppler; left atrium (LA), right atrium (RA).**

Figure 15.12: **Right parasternal view of the superior vena cava (SVC) demonstrating a sinus venous (SV) atrial septal defect (ASD) and a left to right shunt by color flow Doppler; inferior vena cava (IVC), right atrium (RA).**

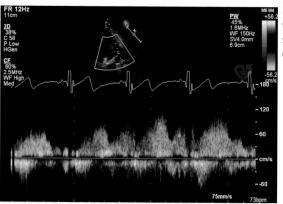

Figure 15.13: **Pulse-wave Doppler with flow velocities of 100cm/sec across the sinus venous ASD defect flow Doppler.**

Common Atrium (Rare)

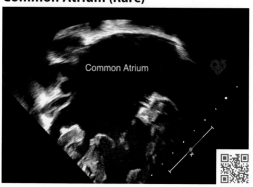

Figure 15.14: **Apical 4-chamber view demonstrating a common atrium.**

15

Congenital Heart Disease / Atrial Septal Defect (ASD)

2D

- Subcostal approach (e.g., 4-chamber, bicaval) is recommended to best visualize the interatrial septum (parasternal short-axis view of the aortic valve, off-axis 4-chamber, or right parasternal views should be attempted)
- Right ventricular volume overload pattern (right ventricular dilatation with paradoxical septal motion)
- Flattened interventricular septum ("pancaking") during ventricular diastole due to right ventricular volume overload
- Right atrial dilatation (normal RA volume: men 25 ± 7mL/m^2; women 21 ± 6mL/m^2)
- Left atrium is usually normal (unless there is a cleft mitral valve or left heart failure)
- Pulmonary artery and pulmonary branch dilatation
- T-artifact (increased echogenicity at the edge of the interatrial septum) as seen from the apical 4-chamber view
- Cleft mitral valve (primum ASD)
- Mitral valve prolapse (ostium secundum)
- Partial anomalous pulmonary venous return (sinus venosus)
- Measure the defect in two orthogonal views (>10mm is considered a large defect)
- Determine:
  - Presence, type, hemodynamic effect and associated defects
  - Dimension of the defect and compare it to the entire interatrial septal length (<20mm is ideal for interventional closure; >25mm is difficult)
  - RV wall thickness, dimension(s), systolic function
  - RVOT diameter (normal 1.7 to 2.7cm and may be increased in large ASD) and compare to LVOT diameter (normal 1.8 to 2.4cm and may be decreased in large ASD)
  - Tricuspid valve annulus diameter (normal 2.2 ± 0.3cm) and compare it to the mitral valve annulus diameter (normal range 2.3 ± 0.5cm) in the apical 4-chamber view

Doppler

- Subcostal approach (4-chamber, bicaval) is recommended to best visualize the interatrial septum (parasternal short-axis view of the aortic valve, off-axis 4-chamber view and right parasternal view of the interatrial septum should also be attempted)
- PW and color flow Doppler demonstrate a left-to-right shunt across the ASD (decrease velocity scale and wall filter)
- Note turbulent flow in the pulmonary artery due to increased blood flow to the lungs

- Determine:
  - Presence and severity of tricuspid and pulmonary regurgitation due to annular stretching from increased right-sided volume
  - Presence and severity of mitral regurgitation if a cleft mitral valve is present
  - Presence and severity of pulmonary stenosis if present
  - Presence of partial anomalous pulmonary venous return (associated with sinus venosus ASD)
  - RVOT VTI (increased in large ASD) and compare to LVOT VTI (decreased in large ASD)
  - Qp/Qs (hemodynamic significant shunt 1.5:1 or greater)
  - SPAP/MPAP/PAEDP/PVR at rest and exercise
  - Width of the ASD by color flow Doppler
  - Left atrial pressure
  - Right/left ventricular systolic and diastolic function

Transesophageal Echocardiography

- Helpful in patients with patent foramen ovale, atrial septal aneurysm, sinus venosus defect, small/fenestrated secundum ASD, cleft mitral valve and in the evaluation of partial anomalous pulmonary venous return (most common is right upper pulmonary vein to the superior vena cava)
- Approaches include mid-esophageal position with imaging angle at 90 to 110° (sinus venosus or ostium secundum) and 0 to 30° for ostium primum defects
- Useful during transcatheter closure of an ASD especially when measuring the diameter of the defect, minimal edge width at each side of the defect, confirmation of the lack of a residual shunt after placement of the device using saline contrast and visualizing a 2 to 4mm thick layer of echo dense material one-month post-procedure

Saline Contrast Technique

- An injection of 5 to 10mL of agitated saline into a left arm vein or leg vein may be used to determine the presence of an ASD and persistent left superior vena cava
- Contrast entering the coronary sinus before entering the right atrium may indicate a persistent left superior vena cava
- Look for contrast crossing the defect into the left atrium or the negative contrast effect due to the left-to-right shunt within three cardiac cycles (may be aided by having the patient cough or Valsalva) The apical and subcostal 4-chamber views are preferred.
- Late appearance (4 to 8 beats after appearance in the right atrium) of saline contrast into the left atrium after a peripheral injection suggests the presence of pulmonary arteriovenous fistula

Post-operative

- Atrial septum may appear thick depending on the type of surgery performed
- Evaluate transcatheter device placement for residual shunts and thrombus
- Flat or paradoxical septal motion may persist (a normal finding after cardiac surgery)
- Right ventricular dilatation may persist, but overtime will return to normal.
- Evaluate mitral valve repair and/or replacement if present
- Determine:
    - Presence and severity of a residual shunt with Doppler
    - SPAP/MPAP/PAEDP/PVR at rest and exercise

Patent Foramen Ovale

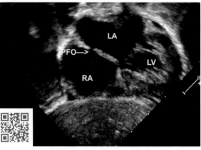 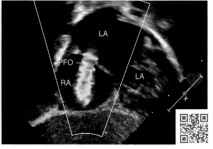

Figure 15.15: **Subcostal 4-chamber view demonstrating a patent foramen ovale (PFO); left atrium (LA), right atrium (RA), left ventricle (LV).**

Figure 15.16: **Subcostal 4-chamber view demonstrating a patent foramen ovale (PFO) by color flow Doppler; left atrium (LA), right atrium (RA), left ventricle (LV).**

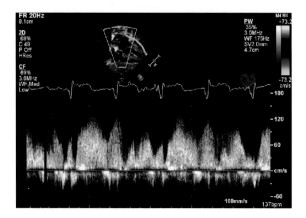

Figure 15.17: **Pulse-wave Doppler demonstrating a left to right shunt with flow velocities of 120cm/sec across the patent foramen ovale.**

Atrial Septal Aneurysm

- An abnormal bulging (>1.5cm in length and excursion) from midline of the interatrial septum may be detected by 2D echocardiography
- The aneurysm is a potential site for either: 1) a shunt and/or 2) a source of embolism

• Perform a saline contrast examination to rule out atrial septal defect peaking in late ventricular systole (peak velocity usually 1.5 m/s) and then peaking again with atrial systole. A slight flow reversal will be seen in early ventricular systole.

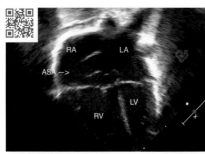

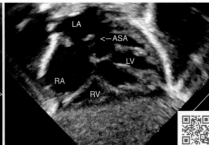

Figure 15.18: **Apical 4-chamber view of an atrial septal aneurysm (ASA) bowing left to right, right atrium (RA), left atrium (LA), right ventricle (RV), left ventricle (LV).**

Figure 15.19: **Subcostal 4-chamber view of an atrial septal aneurysm (ASA) bowing right to left, right atrium (RA), left atrium (LA), right ventricle (RV), left ventricle (LV).**

Important to Note

• After bicuspid aortic valve, atrial septal defects are the second most common congenital lesion found in adolescents and adults (22% of adult congenital heart defects).

• Atrial septal defects may range in size from a small fenestrated atrial septal defect (a few millimeters) to the largest defect (common atrium).

• ASD's have a female preponderance (2:1) and are sometimes familial.

• Lutembacher syndrome is the combination of rheumatic mitral stenosis with atrial septal defect.

• Holt-Oram syndrome is characterized by skeletal abnormalities of the hand and arms (upper limbs) and ostium secundum ASD.

• The normal atrial septal defect pattern as detected by pulsed wave Doppler is flow starting at early to mid-ventricular systole, peaking

Ventricular Septal Defect (VSD)

Definition

An abnormal opening in the interventricular septum.

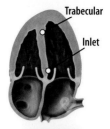

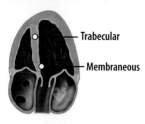

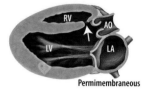

Perimembraneous

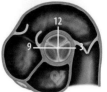

9-12 Perimembraneous
12-3 Outlet

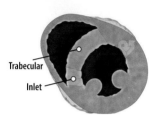

Types

- **Perimembranous** (most common in adults) (80% of all VSD's in adults) (can be associated with aortic regurgitation)
- **Trabecular** (muscular) (second most common in adults; 5 to 20%) (may be multiple)
- **Inlet** (atrioventricular canal, posterior) (8%) (associated with atrioventricular septal defects)
- **Outlet** (supracristal, subpulmonic, doubly committed) (5 to 8%) (common in the Asian population; 30% of all adult VSD's in Asian population) (strong association with aortic regurgitation with aortic valve prolapse)
- **Malalignment** (tetralogy of Fallot, truncus arteriosus)

Shunt

- Left-to-right

History

- Asymptomatic (young patient and/or small shunt)
- Heart failure (dyspnea, orthopnea, paroxysmal nocturnal dyspnea, fatigue, cough, weight gain)
- Infective endocarditis

Physical Examination

- Asthenic habitus (large shunt)
- Signs/symptoms of aortic regurgitation
- Signs/symptoms of mitral regurgitation

- Eisenmenger's syndrome (cyanosis, clubbing, tricuspid regurgitation, pulmonary regurgitation)

Cardiac Auscultation

- Holosystolic murmur, heard best along the left sternal border (often associated with a systolic thrill)
- S3 (large shunt or left ventricular failure)
- Holodiastolic murmur of aortic regurgitation secondary to prolapse of right aortic valve cusp
- Holosystolic murmur of mitral regurgitation, tricuspid regurgitation
- Holodiastolic regurgitation of pulmonary regurgitation (Graham-Steell murmur due to pulmonary hypertension)

Electrocardiogram

- Normal (If shunt is small)
- Left atrial enlargement
- Left ventricular hypertrophy with large shunts
- Biventricular hypertrophy
- Right bundle branch block, right axis deviation and RVH with adults with PAH (pulmonary artery hypertension)

Chest X-ray/CMR/CT

- Normal (small shunt)
- Cardiomegaly (due to left atrial, left ventricular and pulmonary artery enlargement)
- Right ventricular enlargement and/or enlargement of the main pulmonary artery and/or reduced pulmonary vasculature in patients with pulmonary hypertension or infundibular stenosis
- CMR provides information concerning dimension and location of the defect(s), Qp/Qs ratio, ventricular function and may be useful when complex anatomy is present (e.g., tetralogy of Fallot)

Cardiac Catheterization

- Determines pulmonary artery pressures, pulmonary vascular resistance
- Coronary arteriography

Medical Treatment

- Afterload reduction (e.g., hydralazine, nitrates, ACE inhibitors)
- Digitalis/diuretics
- Endocarditis prophylaxis (VSD with unrepaired congenital heart disease or VSD repaired with prosthetic material or device in the preceding six months)

Surgical Treatment

- Surgical patch when Qp/Qs is ≥1.5:1, aortic regurgitation is present, left heart dilatation, reduced left ventricular global systolic function, pulmonary artery systolic pressure >50mmHg and/or progressive/recurrent infective endocarditis is present
- Transcatheter device closure (e.g., Rashkind umbrella; Amplatzer)

2D

- Requires multiple windows and views for complete evaluation
- Left atrial dilatation (normal LA volume: ≤34mL/m²)
- Left ventricular dilatation
- Left ventricular volume overload pattern (left ventricular dilatation with hyperkinesis)
- Main pulmonary artery and pulmonary branch dilatation
- Right ventricular hypertrophy (suggests pulmonary hypertension)
- Evaluate for the presence of aortic valve prolapse, tricuspid valve pouch (ventricular septal aneurysm), infective endocarditis and infective endarteritis
- Determine global and segmental left/right ventricular systolic/diastolic function

Perimembranous

- Parasternal long-axis view of the right ventricular inflow tract (may require medial tilt)
- Parasternal short-axis view aortic valve (10 to 12 o'clock position)
- Apical 5-chamber view
- Subcostal 5-chamber view
- Tricuspid pouch (ventricular septal aneurysm) may be noted (parasternal short-axis of the aortic valve view; right ventricular inflow tract view)

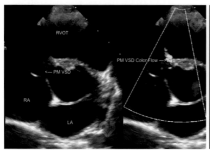

Figure 15.20: **Parasternal short-axis view demonstrating a perimembranous (PM) ventricular septal defect (VSD) with a left to right shunt across the defect; right ventricular outflow tract, right atrium (RA), left atrium (LA).**

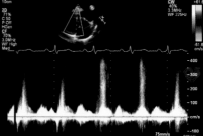

Figure 15.21: **Continuous-wave Doppler demonstrating a flow velocity of 4.5 m/sec across a perimembranous AVSD.**

Trabecular (Muscular)

- Parasternal long-axis view
- Parasternal short-axis view of the left ventricle at the level of the papillary muscles
- Parasternal short-axis view of the left ventricle at the cardiac apex (apical VSD's)
- Apical 4-chamber (T artifact may be visualized)
- Apical 5-chamber view (T artifact may be seen)
- Subcostal 4-chamber, 5-chamber and short-axis views

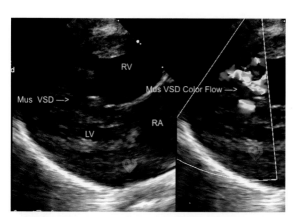

Figure 15.22: **Parasternal long-axis view of the right ventricular inflow tract demonstrating a muscular (Mus) ventricular septal defect (VSD) with a left to right shunt with color flow Doppler; right ventricle (RV), left ventricle (LV, right atrium (RA).**

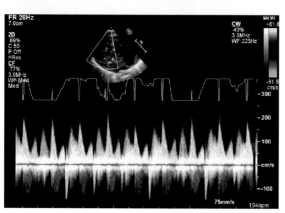

Figure 15.23: **Continuous-wave Doppler with flow velocities of 200cm/sec across the muscular ventricle septal. The low flow velocities would represent high right ventricular systolic pressures and a large defect.**

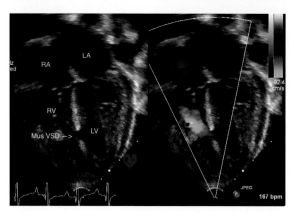

Figure 15.24: **Parasternal long-axis view of the right ventricular inflow tract demonstrating a muscular (Mus) ventricular septal defect (VSD) with a left to right shunt with color flow Doppler; right ventricle (RV), left ventricle (LV, right atrium (RA).**

Outlet

• Parasternal long-axis view with clockwise rotation of transducer with superior tilt
• Parasternal short-axis view of the aortic valve (12 to 2 o'clock)
• Subcostal 5-chamber with superior tilt
• Subcostal short-axis view of the aortic valve

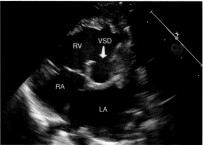

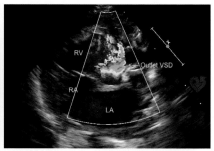

Figure 15.25: **Parasternal short-axis view demonstrating an outlet ventricular septal defect (VSD)(arrow); right atrium (RA), left atrium (LA), right ventricle (RV).**

Figure 15.26: **Color flow Doppler demonstrating a left to right shunt across the outlet ventricular septal defect (VSD); right atrium (RA), left atrium (LA), right ventricle (RV), left ventricle (LV).**

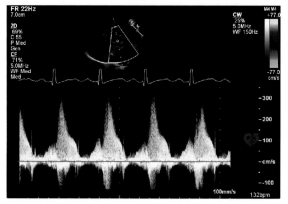

Figure 15.27: **Continuous-wave Doppler of a flow velocity of 3.0 m/sec across the outlet AVSD.**

Inlet

- Parasternal short-axis view of the mitral valve
- Parasternal short-axis view of the left ventricle
- Apical 4-chamber at the level of the atrioventricular valves (posterior tilt)
- Subcostal 4-chamber (posterior tilt)
- Subcostal short-axis views of the mitral valve and left ventricle
- Evaluate for partial and complete atrioventricular septal defect

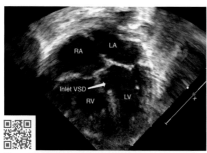

Figure 15.28: **Apical 4-chamber view demonstrating an inlet ventricular septal defect (VSD); right atrium (RA), left atrium (LA), right ventricle (RV), left ventricle (LV).**

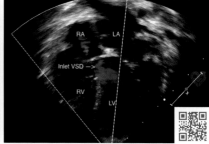

Figure 15.29: **Apical 4-chamber demonstrating a low velocity left to right shunt across an inlet ventricular septal defect (VSD); right atrium (RA), left atrium (LA), right ventricle (RV), left ventricle (LV).**

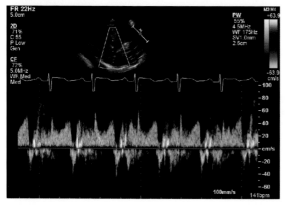

Figure 15.30: **Pulse-wave Doppler demonstrating a flow velocity of 60cm/sec across an inlet AVSD.**

Doppler

- Color flow Doppler is extremely helpful demonstrating a high-velocity turbulent (mosaic) systolic left to right shunt flow (may require an increase in velocity scale and wall filter)
- A low peak systolic velocity across the (AVSD) may represent poor Doppler beam angulation, systemic hypotension, increased right ventricular systolic/ systolic pulmonary artery pressures or a large defect
- Right to left shunting during isovolumic relaxation, early diastole and in patients with pulmonary hypertension

15

Congenital Heart Disease / Ventricular Septal Defect (VSD)

• Evaluate the presence and severity of:
  - Aortic/Mitral/Tricuspid regurgitation
  - Right ventricular outflow tract obstruction
• Determine:
  - Qp/Qs (hemodynamic significant shunt ≥1.5:1)
  - SPAP/MPAP/PAEDP/PVR at rest and exercise

Postoperative

Determine:

• Presence and severity of a residual shunt
• Left atrial and left ventricular dimensions and global and segmental systolic function
• SPAP/MPAP/PAEDP/PVR at rest and exercise

Important to Note

• Ventricular septal defect is the most common congenital heart defect found in children but represents only 10% of cases of congenital heart disease in the adult due to spontaneous closure.

• Left atrial dilatation, left ventricular dilatation and/or aortic regurgitation may be indication to close defect.

Atrioventricular Septal Defect (AVSD)

Definition

Abnormalities of the structures derived from the embryologic endocardial cushions, including a variety of anomalies of the atrial and ventricular septa and the adjacent parts of the mitral valve and tricuspid valve resulting in right heart volume overload. Also referred to as atrioventricular canal defect, endocardial cushion defect.

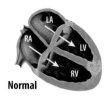

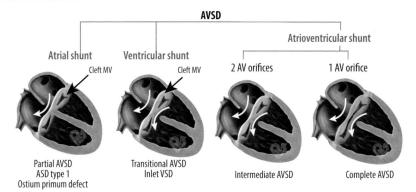

Figure 15.31: **Types of Atrioventricular Septal Defect**

Types[5]

- **Partial:** ostium primum atrial septal defect, cleft anterior mitral valve
- **Transitional:** ostium primum atrial septal defect, cleft anterior mitral valve, inlet ventricular septal defect (small)
- **Intermediate:** ostium primum atrial septal defect, inlet ventricular septal defect (large), common atrioventricular valve annulus with a separated tongue tissue into the two orifices
- **Complete:** ostium primum atrial septal defect, inlet type ventricular septal defect (large), common atrioventricular valve with five leaflets (can be associated with tetralogy of Fallot)

History/Physical Examination

- Trisomy 21 (Down's syndrome) (40% of trisomy 21 has a complete atrioventricular septal defect followed by a ventricular septal defect of 32%)
- Heart failure (dyspnea, orthopnea, paroxysmal nocturnal dyspnea, fatigue, cough, weight gain)
- Cyanosis
- Eisenmenger's syndrome

Cardiac Auscultation

- Holosystolic murmur at the cardiac apex (mitral regurgitation)
- Holosystolic murmur at left sternal border (tricuspid regurgitation)
- Murmurs may not be heard with Trisomy 21 due to pulmonary vascular resistance has not dropped yet

Electrocardiogram

- Incomplete right bundle branch block
- Atrioventricular block
- Atrial arrhythmias
- Biventricular hypertrophy
- Heart block (post-surgical repair)

Chest X-ray/CMR/CT

- Cardiomegaly with increased pulmonary vascular markings
- CMR provides information concerning dimension and location of the defects, ventricular function and may be useful when complex anatomy is present (e.g., tetralogy of Fallot)

Cardiac Catheterization

- Determines pulmonary artery pressures, pulmonary vascular resistance
- Coronary arteriography

15

Congenital Heart Disease / Atrioventricular Septal Defect (AVSD)

Treatment

- Close the atrial and/or ventricular septal defects with patch material and repair the atrioventricular valves

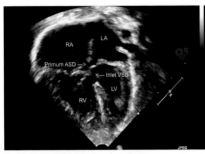

Figure 15.32: **Apical 4-chamber view** demonstrating a complete atrioventricular septal defect; right atrium (RA), left atrium (LA), right ventricle (RV), left ventricle (LV).

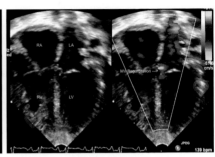

Figure 15.33: **Apical 4-chamber view** demonstrating a complete atrioventricular septal defect with mild left atrioventricular valve regurgitation; right atrium (RA), left atrium (LA), right ventricle (RV), left ventricle (LV).

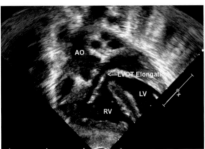

Figure 15.34: **Modified apical 5-chamber view** demonstration left ventricular outflow tract (LVOT) elongation; aorta (AO), right ventricle (RV), left ventricle (LV).

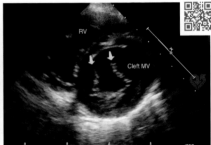

Figure 15.35: **Parasternal short-axis view** demonstration a cleft mitral valve (MV); right ventricle (RV).

2D

- Apical 4-chamber view reveals that both atrioventricular valves are inserted at the same level in primum atrial septal defect
- Posterior angulation of the probe reveals the inlet ventricular septal defect when present
- Apical 5-chamber view reveals elongation of the left ventricular outflow tract
- Subcostal view reveals the atrial septal defect/inlet ventricular septal defect
- Short-axis view of the mitral valve reveals valve morphology (e.g., cleft mitral valve, number of valve leaflets)
- Right ventricular volume overload pattern (right ventricular dilatation with paradoxical septal motion)

- Evaluate for associated lesions (10%) (e.g., subaortic stenosis which may be caused by abnormal chordal insertions across outflow tract, (4 to 7%) double orifice mitral valve (5%), coarctation, patent ductus arteriosus, tetralogy of Fallot)
- Determine:
  - Location and size of atrial and ventricular septal defect(s)
  - Leaflet number, papillary muscle size, number and position, and chordal insertion
  - Right and left ventricular dimensions (left/right ventricles may be underdeveloped called an unbalanced atrioventricular septal defect with right or left dominant)
  - Left ventricular volume (<20mL/m² or RV/LV ratio 2:1 or greater may indicate inadequate left ventricular development)

Doppler

Determine:

- Presence and severity of atrioventricular valve regurgitation
- Location and size of shunts (atrial septal defect, ventricular septal defect(s), left ventricle to right atrial, right ventricle to left atrial)
- Right/Left ventricular systolic and diastolic function
- SPAP/MPAP/PAEDP/PVR at rest and exercise

Transesophageal Echocardiography

- May better define chordal and papillary muscle arrangement
- Useful in evaluating postoperative repair of atrial septal defect, cleft mitral valve, ventricular septal defect(s), iatrogenic atrioventricular stenosis, presence and severity of subaortic stenosis, tricuspid regurgitation and mitral regurgitation.
- Mitral valve is well visualized in upper transgastric position at 0 and 90° planes

Postoperative

- Evaluate septal defect repairs for residual shunting
- Evaluate for the presence and severity of atrioventricular regurgitation
- Evaluate for the presence and severity of iatrogenic atrioventricular stenosis
- Evaluate for subaortic stenosis
- Revaluate right/left ventricular systolic and diastolic function
- Determine:
  - RVSP/SPAP in patients with residual ventricular septal defect shunting
  - SPAP/MPAP/PAEDP/PVR at rest and exercise

Important to Note

- Right atrial dilatation and/or right ventricular dilatation may be an indication to close defects

Patent Ductus Arteriosus

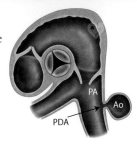

Definition

Persistent patency of the fetal vessel that connects the pulmonary artery with the aorta.

Etiology

- Prematurity (60% of all births in infants whose gestation is <28 weeks)
- Maternal rubella
- High altitude

Pathology

- Closure begins within a few hours of birth and is completely sealed within two to three weeks

Shunt

- Left to right (may be right to left or bidirectional)

History

- Exercise intolerance (initial symptom in 32% of adult cases)
- Heart failure (dyspnea, orthopnea, paroxysmal nocturnal dyspnea, fatigue, cough, weight gain)
- Infective endocarditis/endarteritis (common in the second and third decade affecting the pulmonary end of the ductal channel)
- Pulmonary hypertension
- Eisenmenger's syndrome

Physical Examination

- Widened pulse pressure
- Cyanosis (may be localized to lower extremities) (pulmonary hypertension)

Cardiac Auscultation

- Continuous, high pitched machinery like murmur with peak intensity occurring in late ventricular systole best heard in the pulmonic area or throughout the precordium
- Absence of classic machinery type murmur may indicate pulmonary hypertension

Electrocardiogram

- Normal (small shunt)
- Left atrial enlargement
- Left ventricular hypertrophy
- Atrial fibrillation
- P pulmonale (pulmonary hypertension)

Chest X-ray/CMR/CT

- Normal (small shunt)
- Left heart prominence
- Pulmonary shunt vascularity
- Prominent central pulmonary arteries/pruning of the peripheral pulmonary vessels (pulmonary hypertension)
- Calcification of the ductus (older adult)
- CT may provide information concerning visualization of entire length of the patent ductus, presence of calcification

Cardiac Catheterization

- Determines pulmonary artery pressures, pulmonary vascular resistance
- Coronary arteriography

Treatment

- Thoracotomy incision with ligation, division or placement of a clip on the ductus
- Transcatheter closure (e.g., coil, synthetic plug, occluder) via the femoral vein
- Indomethacin (newborns)
- Nonsteroidal anti-inflammatory drugs such as an ibuprofen (Advil. Infant Mortrin) or indomethacin (premature infants)

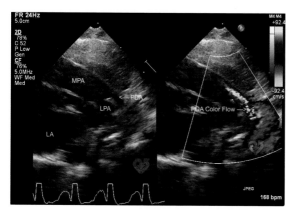

Figure 15.36: **Parasternal long-axis view of the right ventricular outflow tract demonstrating a left to right shunt across a patent ductus arteriosus; right atrium (RA), left atrium (LA), right ventricle (RV), left ventricle (LV).**

2D

- Conventional parasternal short-axis view at the cardiac base with pulmonary artery bifurcation visualization, high left parasternal short-axis view at the cardiac base (ductal view) and suprasternal notch views may provide direct visualization
- Left atrial dilatation (normal LA volume: $\leq 34 \text{mL/m}^2$)
- LA/Ao ratio >1.4:1.0
- Left ventricular dilatation
- Left ventricular volume overload (left ventricular dilatation with hyperkinesis)

15

Congenital Heart Disease / Patent Ductus Arteriosus

- Dilated pulmonary artery (normal 1.5 to 2.1cm)
- Evidence of pulmonary hypertension
- Measure the length and diameter of the ductus for transcatheter closure

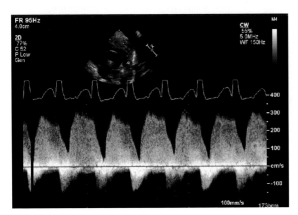

Figure 15.37: **Parasternal short-axis view demonstrating a 3.1 m/second flow velocity across the patent ductus arteriosus.**

Doppler

- Parasternal short-axis view at the cardiac base with visualization of the pulmonary bifurcation, high parasternal short-axis view at the cardiac base and suprasternal notch views may allow direct color flow Doppler visualization
- PW (turbulence with aliasing) and color flow (mosaic pattern) demonstrate a left-to-right shunt
- Flow reversal in the descending thoracic aorta/abdominal aorta
- Increased peak velocity and VTI across mitral valve
- Decreased peak velocity and VTI across tricuspid valve
- Increased peak velocity and VTI across left ventricular outflow tract/aortic valve
- Decreased peak velocity and VTI across right ventricular outflow tract/ pulmonic valve
- A right to left shunt will be colored blue (flow away from the transducer)
- Determine:
    - Qp/Qs (hemodynamic significant shunt ≥1.5:1)
    - SPAP/MPAP/PAEDP/PVR at rest and exercise

Transesophageal Echocardiography

- Midesophageal position with at an angle of between 60 to 80º may allow visualization of the ductus

Post-operative

- For transcatheter closure:
  - Evaluate position of coil or device
  - Evaluate for the degree of residual shunting (small shunt is acceptable)

Important to Note

- Flow within a ductus may be left to right, right to left or bidirectional.
- Brief right to left shunting may occur in the absence of a significant elevation of pulmonary artery pressures due to the time lag between right and left ventricular contraction.
- Left atrial dilatation and/or left ventricular dilatation may be an indication to close.

Ebstein's Anomaly

Definition

- A congenital malformation of the tricuspid valve in which attachments of one, two, or all three leaflets are displaced downward from the annulus to the right ventricular wall.

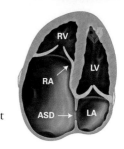

- The portion of the right ventricle above the displaced leaflet(s) is composed of atrial tissue; referred to as right ventricular dysplasia or the "atrialized" portion of the right ventricle.

Associated Anomalies

- Atrial septal defect (75% with a right-to-left shunt)
- Patent foramen ovale
- Ventricular septal defect
- Pulmonic stenosis (valvular) or "Functional" pulmonary atresia

History/Physical Examination

- Dyspnea
- Right heart failure (e.g., jugular venous distention, hepatomegaly, peripheral edema, ascites, anasarca)
- Palpitations (especially if associated with accessory bypass tracts)
- Cyanosis (intermittent) (due to right to left shunt across atrial septal defect and/or patent foramen ovale)

Cardiac Auscultation

- Tricuspid regurgitation murmur
- Diastolic rumble due to increased flow across tricuspid valve

Electrocardiogram

- Wolff-Parkinson-White type B (25 to 30%)
- Atrial and/or ventricular arrhythmias

Chest X-ray/CMR/CT

- Cardiomegaly due to right atrial enlargement
- Reduced vascularity without pulmonary enlargement
- CMR may provide information concerning valvular regurgitation, right ventricular volume and function

Cardiac Catheterization

- Zucker catheter demonstrates simultaneous right ventricular electrocardiogram and right atrial pressure tracing (pathognomic finding)

Treatment

- Preoperative echo index may be useful in determining candidates for valve excision or replacement
- Catheter ablation for supraventricular arrhythmias
- Closure of atrial septal defect
- Annuloplasty for tricuspid regurgitation
- Tricuspid valve repair (Cone procedure) and/or replacement
- Glenn shunt (in the presence of "Functional pulmonary atresia)
- Maze procedure
- Cardiac transplantation

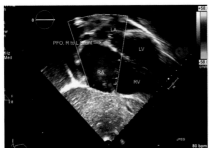

Figure 15.38: **Subcostal 4-chamber view of an patent foramen ovale (PFO) with right to left shunt; right atrium (RA), left atrium (LA), right ventricle (RV), left ventricle (LV).**

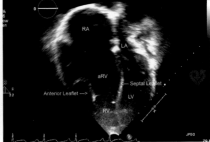

Figure 15.39: **Apical 4-chamber view demonstration Ebstein's anomaly; atrialized/ functional right ventricle (aRA), left atrium (LA), right ventricle (RV), left ventricle (LV).**

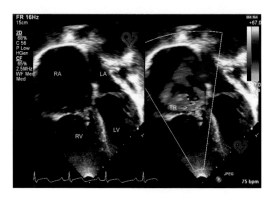

Figure 15.40: **Apical 4-chamber view demonstration Ebstein's anomaly with moderate tricuspid regurgitation (TR); right ventricle (RA), left atrium (LA), right ventricle (RV), left ventricle (LV).**

2D

- The apical 4-chamber view reveals the extent of the tricuspid valve displacement; Ebstein's is diagnosed when the level of the mitral valve annulus to the displaced tricuspid septal leaflet measures ≥20mm or ≥8mm/m^2

- Parasternal long-axis view of the right ventricular inflow tract allows evaluation of posterior tricuspid valve leaflet involvement

- Right atrial dilatation (normal RA volume: men 25 ± 7mL/m^2; women 21 ± 6mL/m^2)

- "Thin" right ventricular free wall with poor systolic function

- "Small" and D-shaped (compressed) left ventricle

- Bulging of the interatrial septum leftward

- Aneurysmal right ventricular outflow tract (RVOT/aortic root ratio of ≥2:1 is considered an indication of an aneurysmal RVOT)

- Anterior tricuspid valve prolapse (rare), diastolic doming and/or eccentric closure

- Delayed closure of the tricuspid valve as compared with the mitral valve ≥80 msec (M-mode)

- Determine:

  - Ratio of the mitral valve-apex distance to the tricuspid valve-apex distance measured in the apical 4-chamber view (normal ratio 1 to 1.2:1; Ebstein's range from 1.8 to 3.2:1)

  - Degree of adherence of the anterior leaflet of the tricuspid valve leaflet to the right ventricular free wall

  - True size and systolic function of the functional right ventricle (an atrialized/functional right ventricle ratio >0.5 indicates poor right ventricular systolic function)

  - Right ventricular cavity ratio (a ratio of functional to total right ventricular cavity of <35% indicates a poorer prognosis)

  - Presence and size of an atrial septal defect and/or patent foramen ovale (agitated saline contrast may be required)

  - Right ventricular and left ventricular global systolic function

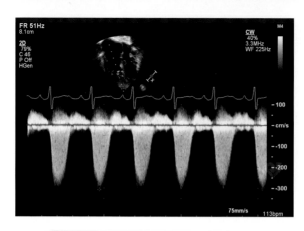

Figure 15.41: **Tricuspid regurgitation with a flow velocity of 3.1 m/sec in an Ebstein's anomaly.**

Doppler

Determine:

- Presence and severity of the coexisting tricuspid regurgitation (usually moderate to severe)
- Presence and severity of coexisting tricuspid stenosis (usually mild)
- Presence of an atrial septal defect (predominantly right-to-left shunt)
- Presence of a patent foramen ovale (predominantly right-to-left shunt) (decrease color velocity scale, wall filter)
- Presence and severity of pulmonary regurgitation
- Presence and severity of valvular pulmonic stenosis/atresia
- Presence and severity of associated defects (e.g., ventricular septal defect)
- SPAP using the tricuspid regurgitation method (usually low)
- Qp/Qs in patients with patent foramen ovale and/or atrial septal defect (hemodynamic significant shunt ≥1.5:1)
- Peak velocity across the pulmonic valve may be low (83 ± 14cm/s)

Two peaks of flow (late diastole and ventricular systole) across the pulmonic valve may be present (PW/CW Doppler)

Transesophageal Echocardiography

- May improve delineation of septal and posterior tricuspid valve leaflets displacement, chordal attachments and atrial septal defect and/or patent foramen ovale and associated defects (e.g., ventricular septal defect)

Post-operative

Determine:

- Mobility of the tricuspid valve
- Length of the functional right ventricle
- Presence and severity of the tricuspid regurgitation

- Presence and severity of iatrogenic tricuspid stenosis
- Peak velocity across the pulmonic valve (usually increased post-surgery)
- Assess Glenn procedure if there is "Functional" pulmonary atresia
- LV/RV systolic and diastolic function

Valvular Pulmonic Stenosis

Definition

An obstruction of blood flow from the right ventricle to the main pulmonary artery during ventricular systole.

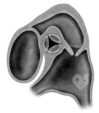
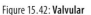
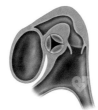
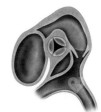

Figure 15.42: **Valvular**   Figure 15.43: **Subvalvular**   Figure 15.44: **Supravalvular**

Etiology

- Congenital (most common cause) (most commonly due to fusion of the valve cusps)
- Carcinoid (most common cause of acquired valvular pulmonary stenosis)
- Rheumatic
- Infective endocarditis (rare)
- Complex congenital lesions (e.g., tetralogy of Fallot, complete atrioventricular defect)
- Syndromes (e.g., Noonan's)

History

- Asymptomatic (mild to moderate pulmonic stenosis)
- Dyspnea upon exertion

Physical Examination

- Jugular venous pulse with marked atrial "a" wave
- Systolic thrill at left parasternal border
- Cyanosis (severe pulmonic stenosis with right to left shunt across a patent foramen ovale/atrial septal defect)
- Right heart failure (e.g., jugular venous distention, hepatomegaly, peripheral edema, ascites, anasarca)
- Habitus of Noonan's syndrome (small stature, shield chest, web neck)

Cardiac Auscultation

- The murmur of valvular pulmonic stenosis is described as a harsh systolic ejection crescendo-decrescendo murmur heard best in the second left intercostal space which can radiate into the lung fields

Electrocardiogram

- Normal (mild pulmonic stenosis)
- Right ventricular hypertrophy

Chest X-ray/CMR/CT

- Normal (mild to moderate pulmonic stenosis)
- Cardiomegaly due to right atrial enlargement and right ventricular hypertrophy
- Post-stenotic dilatation of the main pulmonary artery
- Decreased to normal pulmonary vasculature
- CMR/CT provides information concerning the distal pulmonary artery branches and ventricular function

Cardiac Catheterization

- Recommended when the cardiac Doppler peak velocity is >3 m/s
- Determines transvalvular peak to peak gradient (because of the pulse pressure of the pulmonary circuit and activation of time of the right ventricular contraction, the catheterization peak to peak gradient compares well with the Doppler peak instantaneous gradient)

- Percutaneous balloon valvuloplasty (recommended in symptomatic patients with a peak to peak gradient of >30mmHg; in asymptomatic patients with peak to peak gradients of 40mmHg))
- Coronary arteriography

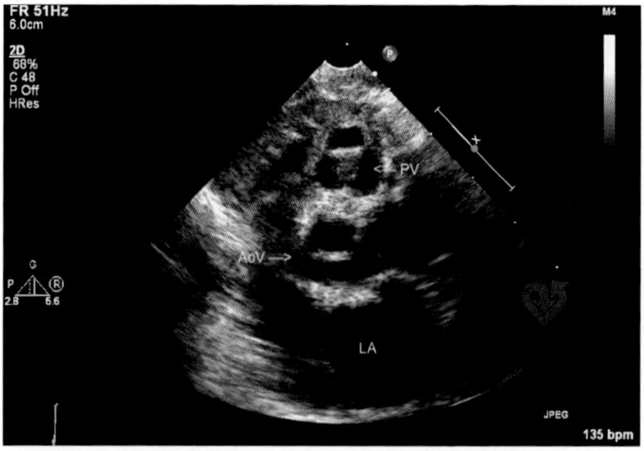

Figure 15.45: **Parasternal short-axis view of the critical pulmonary stenosis in a cross-sectional view of the trip-leaflet pulmonary valve; pulmonary valve (PV), aortic valve (AoV), left atrium (LA).**

Medical Treatment

Treatment for heart failure

Surgical Treatment

- Valvuloplasty
- Valve replacement (indicated for valves that are dysplastic, calcified, severely regurgitant or valves with endocarditis)

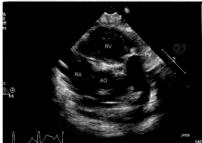

Figure 15.46: **Parasternal short-axis view of a thick pulmonary valve; right atrium (RA), pulmonary valve (PV), aorta (AO).**

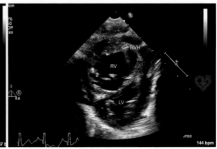

Figure 15.47: **Parasternal short-axis at the level of the left ventricle and right ventricle demonstrating right ventricular hypertrophy; right ventricle (RV), left ventricle (LV).**

2D

- Thickened pulmonic valve leaflets (may be unicuspid, bicuspid (20%), tricuspid, quadricuspid or dysplastic)
- Systolic "doming" of the pulmonary valve leaflets
- Diastolic "doming" (pulmonic valve prolapse)
- Right ventricular hypertrophy (possible asymmetric septal hypertrophy)
- Right atrial dilatation will vary depending of the degree of tricuspid regurgitation (normal RA volume: men $25 \pm 7\text{mL/m}^2$; women $21 \pm 6\text{mL/m}^2$)
- Post-stenotic dilatation of the main and left pulmonary arteries
- D-shaped left ventricle due to flattening of the interventricular septum during ventricular systole
- Calcification of the pulmonic valve (rare)
- Determine:
  - Right ventricular dimensions, thickness and global and segmental systolic/diastolic function
  - Presence of associated abnormalities (e.g., atrial septal defect, ventricular septal defect, "double chambered" right ventricle)
  - Suitability for percutaneous balloon valvuloplasty by measuring pulmonic valve annulus and determining the thickness of the pulmonic valve

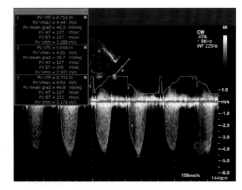

Figure 15.48: **Continuous wave Doppler of pulmonic stenosis**

PW Doppler

- Sample the entire right ventricular outflow tract because subinfundibular, infundibular, main and pulmonary branch stenosis are possible, either as a part of valvular pulmonic stenosis or as separate entities

• Increased velocity across the pulmonic valve (>1 m/s) in valvular pulmonic stenosis

CW Doppler

• Left parasternal, modified apical 5-chamber, subcostal approaches may be the most useful
• Determine:
  - Peak instantaneous pressure gradient
  - Mean transvalvular pressure gradient
  - Velocity ratio (RVOT$_{VTI}$ ÷ Pulmonic valve$_{VTI}$)
  - Pulmonic valve area utilizing the continuity equation
  - Presence and severity of infundibular obstruction which appears as dagger shaped, late peaking systolic gradient indicating a dynamic obstruction
  - Presence and severity of pulmonary regurgitation
  - SPAP/MPAP/PAEDP/PVR at rest and exercise
  - Postoperatively the peak instantaneous pressure gradient and determine the presence and severity of infundibular stenosis

Table 15.1: Pulmonary Valve Stenosis Severity *(ASE Recommendations)*			
	Mild	**Moderate**	**Severe**
Peak velocity (m/s)	<3	3 to 4	>4
Peak gradient (mmHg)	<36	36 to 64	>64

Baumgartner H, Hung J, Bermejo J, Chambers JB, Evangelista A, Griffin, BP, Iung B. Echocardiographic Assessment of Valve Stenosis: EAE/ASE Recommendations for Clinical Practice. J Am Soc Echocardiogr 2008;22(1):1-23. doi:10.1016/j.echo.2008.11.029

Color Flow Doppler

• May aid in determining the direction of the stenotic jet, (usually central) thus aiding in the CW Doppler interrogation of the stenotic valve

• Flow convergence (PISA) may be useful in quantitating the severity

• Determine:
  - Presence and severity of coexisting pulmonary regurgitation and tricuspid regurgitation

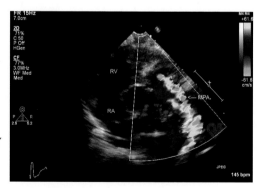

Figure 15.49: **Parasternal short-axis view at the base demonstrating turbulence of blood flow across the pulmonary valve.**

  - Presence and direction of shunting in patients with patent foramen ovale and/or atrial septal defect and/or ventricular septal defect

Transesophageal Echocardiography

May improve assessment of the pulmonary valve and right ventricular outflow tract (midesophageal window using 0 to 90º; deep transgastric window at 90º and/or anterior angulation of transgastric 4-chamber view)

Post-operative

Evaluate transvalvular peak velocity, peak and mean gradient, degree of pulmonary regurgitation, degree of right ventricular dilatation (hypertrophy), right ventricular global/segmental systolic and diastolic function

Table 15.2: Echocardiographic and Doppler Parameters Useful in Grading Pulmonary Regurgitation Severity			
Parameter	Mild	Moderate	Severe
Pulmonic valve	Normal	Normal or abnormal	
RV size	Normal	Normal or dilated	Dilated [†]
Jet size, color Doppler[‡]	Thin (usually <10mm in length) with a narrow origin	Intermediate	Broad origin; variable depth of penetration
Ratio of PR jet width/pulmonary annulus			>0.7 [§]
Jet density and contour (CW)	Soft	Dense	Dense; early termination of diastolic flow
Deceleration time of the PR spectral Doppler signal			Short, <260 msec
Pressure half-time of PR jet			<100 msec [jj]
PR index[{]		<0.77	<0.77
Diastolic flow reversal in the main or Prominent branch PAs (PW)			Prominent
Pulmonic systolic flow (VTI) compared to systemic flow (LVOT VTI) by PW[#]	Slightly increased	Intermediate	Greatly increase
RF**	<20%	20% - 40%	>40%

PW, Pulsed wave Doppler.
* Unless there are other reasons for RV enlargement.
† Exception: acute PR.
‡ At a Nyquist limit of 50-70cm/sec.
§ Identifies a CMR-derived PR fraction $40%.

{ Defined as the duration of the PR signal divided by the total duration of diastole, with this cutoff identifying a CMR-derived PR fraction >25%.
jj Not reliable in the presence of high RV end diastolic pressure.
Cutoff values for RVol and fraction are not well validated.
§ Steep deceleration is not specific for severe PR.
**RF data primarily derived from CMR with limited application with echocardiography.

Zoghbi WA, MD, Adams D, Bonow RO MD, Enriquez-Sarano M, Elyse Foster E, Grayburn PA, Hahn RT, Han Y, Hung J, Lang RM, Little SH, MD, Shah DJ, Shernan S, Thavendiranathan P, Thomas JD, Weissman NJ. Recommendations for Noninvasive Evaluation of Native Valvular Regurgitation: A Report from the American Society of Echocardiography Developed in Collaboration with the Society for Cardiovascular Magnetic Resonance. J Am Soc Echocardiogr 2017;30(4):303-371.

Important to Note

- The congenital stenotic pulmonary valve may be trileaflet, bicuspid, unicuspid or dysplastic.
- In the presence of a right ventricular outflow tract obstruction, the systolic pulmonary artery pressure may be calculated using tricuspid regurgitation:

SPAPmmHg =
4 x tricuspid regurgitation peak velocity[2]
+ right atrial pressure - pulmonary valve transvalvular gradient

- Pregnancy is not well tolerated when moderate to severe pulmonary valve stenosis is present and correction is recommended before conception.
- Evaluation for the presence of tetralogy of Fallot should be included in the exam.

Tetralogy of Fallot

Definition

- The combination of four defects: 1) large, overriding aorta, 2) malalignment ventricular septal defect*, 3) pulmonary stenosis* and 4) right ventricular hypertrophy.

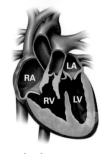
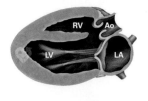

- The pulmonary stenosis may be valvular, subvalvular (infundibular), supravalvular, atretic, or any combination.

* Important components of tetralogy

History

- Childhood exercise intolerance/squatting
- "Tet" spells (episodic faintness and increased cyanosis)
- Palliative repair (e.g., Blalock-Taussig, Central, Potts)
- Heart failure

Physical Examination

- Central cyanosis (most common cyanotic lesion in the adult population)
- Clubbing

Shunt

- Due to the obstruction at the pulmonary level, blood shunts right-to-left out to the aorta

Complications

- Progressive right ventricular outflow tract stenosis
- Hypoxic ("tet") spells
- Anemia
- Polycythemia
- Coagulopathies
- Brain abscess
- Cerebral vascular accident
- Infective endocarditis
- Acquired aortic valve disease
- Arrhythmias

Cardiac Auscultation

- Loud systolic ejection murmur at middle/upper left sternal border (outflow tract obstruction)
- Systolic murmur along left sternal border (ventricular septal defect)
- Pulmonary regurgitation (common in postoperative patients)
- Aortic regurgitation murmur
- Continuous murmur (arterial collateral channels)

Electrocardiogram

- Right ventricular hypertrophy (moderate to severe pulmonic stenosis)
- Biventricular hypertrophy (mild pulmonic stenosis)

Chest X-ray/CMR/CT

- "Boot-shaped" heart (coeur en sabot) (severe pulmonic stenosis)
- Cardiomegaly (right atrial enlargement and right ventricular hypertrophy)
- Right-sided aortic arch (25%)
- CMR may provide information concerning ventricular volumes, anatomy of the right ventricular outflow tract, aorta, aortopulmonary collaterals, valvular regurgitation

Cardiac Catheterization

- Pressure gradient between right ventricular infundibulum and main pulmonary artery
- Coronary arteriography to determine anomalous origins of left coronary artery, coronary artery disease

Medical Treatment

- Treat hypoxic spells (e.g., oxygen, morphine)
- Propranolol to prevent hypoxic spells
- Treat anemia/polycythemia
- Implantable cardioverter defibrillator

Surgical Treatment

- Blalock-Taussig shunt (palliative)
- Central (palliative)(rare)
- Potts (palliative)(rare)
- Close ventricular septal defect
- Repair pulmonary stenosis (pulmonary valvotomy/valvectomy/transannular patch/percutaneous valve replacement)
- Excision of right ventricular outflow tract bundles when present via a right ventriculotomy

- Rastelli procedure (tetralogy with pulmonary atresia; anomalous coronary artery crossing the RVOT)
- Repair associated malformations (e.g., atrial septal defect, aortopulmonary collaterals)

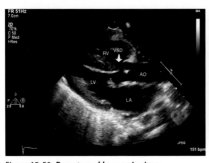

Figure 15.50: **Parasternal long-axis view demonstrating an overriding aorta with malalignment ventricular septal defect (VSD); right atrium (RA), left atrium (LA), right ventricle (RV), left ventricle (LV).**

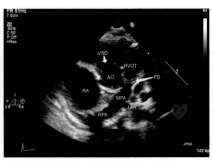

Figure 15.51: **Parasternal short-axis view demonstrating right ventricular hypertrophy; right ventricle (RV), left ventricle (LV).**

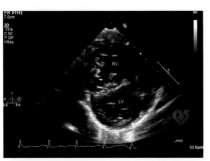

Figure 15.52: **Parasternal short-axis view demonstrating pulmonary stenosis with a small pulmonary artery system; ventricular septal defect (VSD), right ventricular outflow tract (RVOT), pulmonary stenosis (PS), main pulmonary artery (MPA), left pulmonary artery (LPA), right pulmonary artery (RPA), right atrium (RA).**

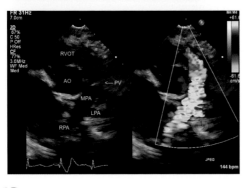

Figure 15.53: **Parasternal short-axis view demonstrating pulmonary stenosis with a small pulmonary artery system and turbulences of flow by color Doppler; ventricular septal defect (VSD), right ventricular outflow tract (RVOT), pulmonary stenosis (PS), main pulmonary artery (MPA), left pulmonary artery (LPA), right pulmonary artery (RPA), right atrium (RA).**

2D

- Parasternal long-axis view demonstrates overriding aorta, ventricular septal defect and right ventricular hypertrophy
- Examine aortic arch position to rule out right aortic arch (25%)

- Parasternal short-axis view of the aortic valve demonstrates small pulmonic annulus, right ventricular outflow tract obstruction and size of the main pulmonary artery and pulmonary artery branches, dilated aorta and ventricular septal defect
- Determine:
  - Right ventricular dimension, thickness and systolic function
  - Size of the main pulmonary artery/pulmonary artery branches (important for surgical planning)
  - Presence of associated anomalies (e.g., atrial septal defect 23% (pentalogy of Fallot), right sided aortic arch 25%; anomalous coronary distribution (37%), coronary fistula (rare), absence of pulmonary valve 3%, additional ventricular septal defects 3 to 15%, complete atrioventricular canal, anomalous bundles of the right ventricle. [1]

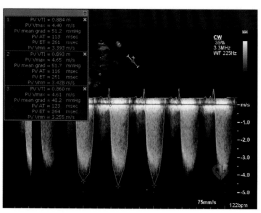

Figure 15.54: **Continuous-wave Doppler demonstrating severe pulmonary stenosis with a flow velocity of 4.6 m/sec and a mean gradient of 52mmHg.**

Doppler

- Localize the region of RVOT stenosis with PW Doppler
- Determine:
  - Maximum instantaneous pressure gradient and mean pressure gradient across the right ventricular outflow tract with CW Doppler
  - Velocity and direction of shunt across the ventricular septal defect (usually low velocity and predominantly right to left)
  - Presence of associated anomalies (e.g., atrial septal defect, coexisting ventricular septal defects)
  - Presence and severity of coexisting aortic regurgitation
  - Presence and severity of coexisting pulmonic regurgitation

Transesophageal Echocardiography

- Angles between 80 and 130° will aid in the evaluation of the site and degree of obstruction of the right ventricular outflow tract, malaligned ventricular septal defect and aortic override.

- Evaluate the descending thoracic aorta for aortic to pulmonary arterial collaterals
- Deep transgastric position with angles between 30 and 60° allows visualization of the underside (ventricular) side of ventricular septal defect patch

Post-surgical

Evaluate:
- Ventricular septal defect repair (residual shunt present in 10 to 25%)
- Degree of residual right ventricular outflow tract obstruction (mild obstruction between 25 to 40mmHg present in 70 to 80%)
- Right ventricle to pulmonary artery conduit for stenosis at the proximal and distal anastomosis site, pseudointimal peel
- Aneurysmal bulging of right ventricular outflow tract in patients with transannular patch for relief of right ventricular outflow tract obstruction

Determine:
- Presence and severity of aortic regurgitation
- Presence and severity of pulmonary regurgitation (often severe) especially in patients with transvalvular repair
- Right ventricular dimensions, thickness and global systolic function and diastolic function
- Dimension of the aorta
- Reoperation may be necessary in 7% due to persistent RVOT obstruction

Congenitally Corrected Transposition of the Great Arteries

Definition

Characterized by inverted ventricles and their attached outflow valves are reversed (l (levo)-transposition of the great arteries). The aorta is usually anterior to and left of the pulmonary artery. Also called congenitally corrected-transposition, ventricular inversion.

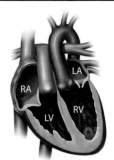

History/Physical Examination

- Asymptomatic (childhood and young adulthood)
- Dyspnea upon exertion
- Sudden death
- Pulmonary venous congestion (due to anatomic right ventricular failure) (middle age)
- Cyanosis

Cardiac Auscultation

- Systolic ejection murmur at left upper sternal border (pulmonic stenosis)
- Left sided (systemic) atrioventricular valve regurgitation radiates to left sternal border

Electrocardiogram

- Variable degrees of AV block (prolonged P-R interval to complete heart block) (75%)
- Absence of left precordial Q waves in leads II, V5 and V6
- Atrial arrhythmias

Chest X-ray/CMR/CT

- Positional abnormality (dextrocardia 20%)
- Cardiomegaly (due to ventricular septal defect, severe left sided tricuspid valve regurgitation)
- Straight left upper cardiac border
- "Waterfall" appearance due to abnormal pulmonary artery position
- CMR/CT provides information concerning the systemic right ventricular volumes and function

Cardiac Catheterization

- Coronary arteriography to evaluate presence of anomalous coronary arteries, coronary artery disease

Medical/Surgical Treatment

- Treatment of heart failure
- Antiarrhythmic
- Pacemaker implantation for AV conduction abnormalities
- Repair of associated lesions (e.g., ventricular septal defect, pulmonic stenosis)
- Double switch procedure (Mustard procedure combined with arterial switch procedure)
- Tricuspid valve repair/replacement

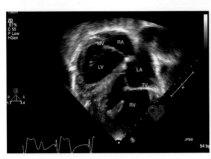

Figure 15.55: **Apical 4-chamber demonstrating corrected transposition of the great arteries (ventricular inversion); mitral valve (MV), tricuspid valve (TV), right atrium (RA), left atrium (LA), right ventricle (RV), left ventricle (LV).**

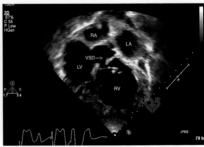

Figure 15.56: **Apical 4-chamber demonstrating corrected transposition of the great arteries (ventricular inversion) with a ventricular septal defect (VSD); mitral valve (MV), tricuspid valve (TV), right atrium (RA), left atrium (LA), right ventricle (RV), left ventricle (LV).**

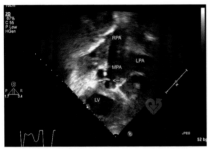

Figure 15.57: **Apical 4-chamber view tilting anterior to the first vessel coming off the left ventricle (LV); pulmonary valve (PV), main pulmonary artery (MPA), left pulmonary artery (LPA), right pulmonary artery (RPA), right atrium (RA).**

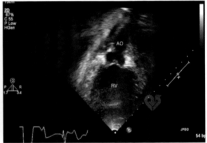

Figure 15.58: **Apical 4-chamber view tilting more anterior to the second vessel coming off the right ventricle (RV); aorta (AO).**

2D

- Segmental approach required (cardiac malposition (dextrocardia) is common)
- Apical 4-chamber view confirms the diagnosis by demonstrating the abnormally inferiorly placed left atrioventricular valve (tricuspid valve) in the left-sided morphologic right ventricle
- Parasternal short-axis view at the cardiac base usually demonstrates aorta leftward, anterior and superior to the pulmonic valve
- Malalignment of interatrial septum and interventricular septum, dextrocardia best seen in subcostal 4-chamber view
- Interventricular septum may be difficult to image in the parasternal long-axis view because its orientation is perpendicular to the frontal plane
- Right ventricular dilatation (normal Basal RV diameter 25 to 41mm) with decreased systolic function with increasing age

- Evaluate:
  - Abnormalities of the left sided tricuspid valve (90%) (e.g., Ebstein's anomaly, deficient valve tissue, thickened valve leaflets, tricuspid valve ring)
  - Ventricular septal defect (70%) (usually perimembranous)
  - Pulmonary stenosis (40%)
- Determine the left-sided right ventricular (systemic) volumes and ejection fraction by the Simpson's method of discs

Doppler

Determine:

- Presence and severity of left sided tricuspid (systemic) valve regurgitation
- Presence and degree of shunting of ventricular septal defect
- Presence and severity of pulmonary stenosis

d-Transposition of the Great Arteries

Definition

The aorta is connected to the right ventricle. It should normally be connected to the left ventricle. The pulmonary artery is connected to the left ventricle when it should normally be connected to the right ventricle.

History/Physical Examination

- Cyanosis
- Tachypnea
- Dyspnea
- Failure to thrive and congestive heart failure in newborn period.
- Right ventricular lift

Cardiac Auscultation

- Loud, single S2
- Systolic murmur at left sternal board (ventricular septal defect)
- Systolic ejection murmur at left upper sternal boarder (pulmonary stenosis)
- Diastolic flow murmur at apex

Electrocardiogram

- Right axis deviation
- Right or combined ventricular hypertrophy (combined in the presence of ventricular septal defect)

Chest X-ray/CMR/CT

- Oval (egg-shaped) cardiac silhouette with narrowed superior mediastinum
- Increased pulmonary vascularity
- Mild cardiomegaly

Cardiac Catheterization

- Perform balloon septostomy
- Evaluated pulmonary artery pressures

- Evaluated presence, number, location of ventricular septal defects by ventriculography if indicated
- Evaluate coronary artery anatomy

Medical/Surgical Treatment

- Prostaglandin E1
- Treatment of congestive heart failure

Surgical Treatment

- Balloon septostomy (Rashkind procedure), if there is a small atrial septal defect/patent foreman ovale
- Arterial switch (Jatene repair), the great arteries are switched with reimplantation of the coronary arteries (current practice)
- Atrial switch, a baffle directing the correct blood flow through the atriums (Mustard/Senning procedure)
- Rastelli repair (associated with d-transposition of the great arteries with ventricular septal defect and pulmonary stenosis)

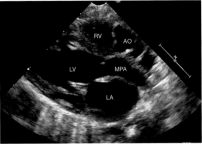

Figure 15.59: Parasternal long-axis view demonstrating d-transposition of the great arteries; main pulmonary artery (MPA), aorta (AO), left atrium (LA), right ventricle (RV), left ventricle (LV).

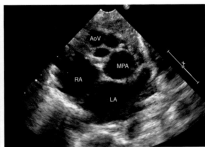

Figure 15.60: Parasternal short-axis view demonstrating d-transposition of the great arteries with aortic valve (AoV) anterior and to the right of the main pulmonary artery (MPA); left atrium (LA), right atrium (RA).

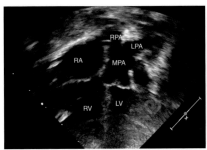

Figure 15.61: Apical 5-chamber demonstrating d-transposition of the great arteries with the main pulmonary artery (MPA) coming off the left ventricle (LV); , right ventricle (RV), right atrium (RA), right pulmonary artery (RPA), left pulmonary artery (LPA).

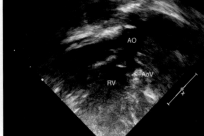

Figure 15.62: Apical view titling more anteriorly to demonstrate the aorta (AO) coming off the right ventricle (RV) in d-transposition of the great arteries; aortic valve (AoV).

2D

- Parasternal long-axis view helps make the diagnosis by demonstrating that both vessels are seen in the same imaging plane. The pulmonary artery comes off the left ventricular and abruptly bends posteriorly in this view. The aorta is more superior and courses anteriorly
- Parasternal short-axis view demonstrates both great arteries with the aorta anterior and to the right of the pulmonary artery
- Evaluate the coronary arteries
- Evaluate for shunt lesions (patent ductus arteriosus, foramen ovale, atrial septal defect, ventricular septal defect)
- Evaluate for left ventricular outflow tract obstruction
- Evaluate the semilunar valves (bicuspid aortic or pulmonic valves)
- Assess ventricular function and wall thickness

Doppler

Determine:

- Presence and severity of any left ventricular outflow tract obstruction
- Presence and degree of shunting of patent foramen ovale, atrial septal defect, patent ductus arteriosus, and ventricular septal defect
- Presence and severity of pulmonary and aortic stenosis

Transesophageal Echocardiography

May improve delineation of associated lesions such as size and location of shunt lesions, presence and severity of semilunar valve stenosis and post-operative repair

Post-operative

- Arterial switch (Jatene procedure)
- The transposed great arteries are transected and brought over to their normal position. The coronary arteries are excised and re-implanted into the new neo-aorta sinuses. Closure of any shunt lesions. The pulmonary artery and its branches are brought forward (LeCompte maneuver) and the distal aorta is moved posteriorly.
- Evaluate the aorta and pulmonary arteries (main and branch pulmonary arteries)
- Assess the re-implanted coronary arteries
- Assess for any residual shunt lesions (patent ductus arteriosus, atrial septal defect, and ventricular septal defect)
- Assess for ventricular function, wall thickness and regional wall motion abnormalities
- Determine the presence and severity of neo-aortic valve insufficiency

15

Congenital Heart Disease / d-Transposition of the Great Arteries

15

Congenital Heart Disease / Other Congenital Heart Defects / Anomalous Origin of the Left Coronary Artery from the Pulmonary Artery

Atrial Switch (Mustard/Senning Procedure)

- A baffle is created using synthetic material (Mustard) or the patient's own tissue (Senning) to direct the correct blood flow through the atriums into the ventricles.
- Parasternal long- and short-axis views to demonstrate the flattening of the interventricular septum, right and left ventricular function and wall thickness
- Apical 4-chamber view to visualize the systemic (pulmonary veins to right heart) and pulmonary (inferior and superior vena cava to the left heart) venous channels
- Assess for left ventricular outflow tract obstruction
- Assess for baffle leaks and obstruction
- Assess the presence and severity of any atrioventricular valve regurgitation

Rastelli Procedure

- Removal of any obstructive right ventricular muscle and there is a large intra-ventricular baffle put into place closing the ventricular septal defect and redirecting left ventricular outflow anteriorly to the aortic valve. A valved homograft conduit is utilized to achieve right ventricular to pulmonary artery continuity.
- Assess for any residual shunts (ventricular septal defect)
- Assess for any left ventricular outflow tract obstruction across the ventricular septal defect
- Assess for any conduit insufficiency and stenosis
- Assess right and left ventricular function and wall thickness

Other Congenital Heart Defects

Anomalous Origin of the Left Coronary Artery from the Pulmonary Artery

Definition

The left coronary artery arises abnormally from the pulmonary artery.

Echo/Doppler

- Left ventricular dilatation with global and segmental left ventricular systolic dysfunction

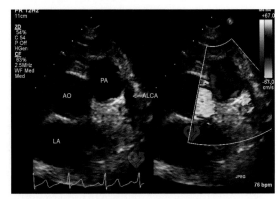

Figure 15.63: **Parasternal short-axis view demonstrating anomalous left coronary artery coming off anterior of the pulmonary artery (PA); aorta (AO), left atrium (LA).**

- Dilated right coronary artery best seen in the parasternal short-axis view of the aortic valve
- Mitral regurgitation
- Left to right shunt entering the pulmonary artery distal to the pulmonary valve

Cor Triatriatum

Definition

A membrane which divides the body of the left atrium.

Echo/Doppler

- Best views include parasternal/apical long-axis, apical 4-chamber and subcostal 4-chamber

Image courtesy of David B. Adams

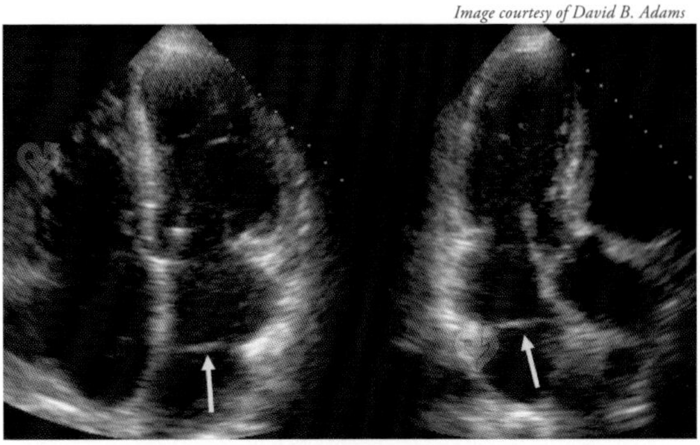

Figure 15.64: **Apical 4-chamber (left image) and apical LAX (right image) showing a membrane in the LA (arrows).**

- Membrane may be seen in the left atrium moving towards the mitral valve in diastole and away during ventricular systole
- Upper left atrial chamber receives the pulmonary veins and the lower left atrial chamber contains the left atrial appendage and the foramen ovale
- Associated defects include atrial septal defect (70 to 80%), persistent left superior vena cava, atrioventricular septal defect, aortic coarctation and anomalous pulmonary venous return
- Doppler may demonstrate turbulent flow, increased velocities and pressure gradient across the membrane
- Color flow Doppler is helpful in differentiating mitral supravalvular ring from cor triatriatum with the mosaic jet originating in the body of the left atrium while in supravalvular ring the mosaic jet forms downstream close to the left ventricle

Mitral Valve Supravalvular Stenosing Ring

Definition

A membrane located at the level of the mitral valve annulus.

Echo/Doppler

- A thin band of echoes located just above the mitral valve or within the funnel of the mitral valve leaflets

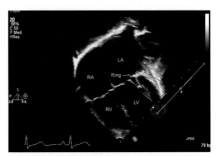

Figure 15.65: **Apical 4-chamber view demonstration a mitral valve ring; right atrium (RA), left atrium (LA), right ventricle (RV), left ventricle (LV).**

- Mitral valve leaflets may appear thick and myxomatous
- Motion of the ring may be detected with the ring moving towards the mitral valve orifice in diastole and away from the leaflets during ventricular systole
- Associated with atrial septal defect, persistent left superior vena cava to the coronary sinus, aortic coarctation, ventricular septal defect and Shone's syndrome
- Doppler may demonstrate turbulent flow, increased velocities and pressure gradient similar to that which is seen in mitral valve stenosis

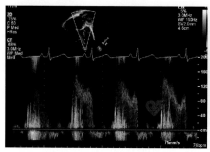

Figure 15.66: Continuous-wave Doppler demonstration a flow velocity of 160cm/sec across the mitral valve ring.

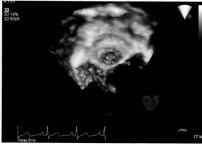

Figure 15.67: 3D echocardiogram showing the mitral valve ring.

Double Orifice Mitral Valve

Definition

A condition in which an accessory mitral valve orifice is present. Double orifice mitral valve may be created by the MitraClip in the cath lab or surgically by the Alfieri operation.

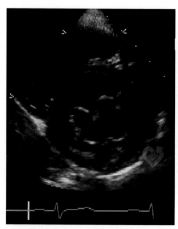

Figure 15.68: Parasternal short-axis view of a congenital double orifice mitral valve MV

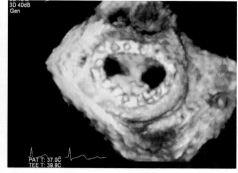

Figure 15.69: 3D TEE image of the MV from the surgeon's view (LA). Note the double MV orifice created by an Alfieri stitch. An annuloplasty ring was also implanted.

Echo/Doppler

- Parasternal/subcostal short-axis of the mitral valve are the best views to identify the two mitral valve orifices
- Parasternal short-axis of the left ventricle at the level of the papillary muscles allows the visualization of abnormalities (e.g., abnormal papillary muscle rotation, single papillary muscle)
- Associated defects include AV septal defect, ventricular septal defect, Ebstein's anomaly, ttralogy of Fallot and aortic coarctation
- Doppler may demonstrate flow, stenosis and/or regurgitation, through both orifices

Noncompaction of Ventricular Myocardium (Hypertrabeculation)

Definition

Noncompaction of the myocardium without an associated cardiac anomaly is a rare congenital disorder.

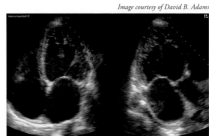

Image courtesy of David B. Adams

Echo/Doppler

- Multiple prominent ventricular trabeculations and deep intratrabecular recesses (especially mid-lateral, mid-inferior, apical) ("spongy" appearance of myocardium)

Figure 15.70: **Apical 4-chamber and LAX in a patient with LV Noncompaction. Note the spongy appearance of the apical myocardium.**

- Dilated ventricle(s)
- Depressed global systolic ventricular function
- Diastolic dysfunction
- Multiple deep intratrabecular recesses communicating with the ventricular cavity as visualized on color flow Doppler (decrease color velocity scale, wall filter) (multiple views may be required including PSAX LV, PSAX cardiac apex, apical 4-chamber, apical long axis)
- Proposed echocardiographic criteria: Thickness of the noncompacted layer (NC) to compacted layer (C) are best measured in the short axis views at the mid and apical levels at end-systole with a ratio of >2 diagnostic (NC/C)
- Contrast agents may be useful (e.g., Optison, Definity)

Parachute Mitral Valve

Definition

A congenital abnormality in which there is only one papillary muscle in the left ventricle and the chordae of the two mitral valve leaflets insert into this single papillary muscle.

15

Congenital Heart Disease / Other Congenital Heart Defects / Noncompaction of Ventricular Myocardium (Hypertrabeculation)

Echo/Doppler

- Single LV papillary muscle (usually posteromedial papillary muscle) best seen in the parasternal short-axis view of the left ventricle at the level of the papillary muscles

- Additional papillary muscle (usually small), may be present but receive no chordae tendineae

- Mitral valve leaflets and chordae are normal

- Doppler findings will be similar to mitral stenosis

Images courtesy of David B. Adams

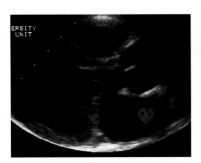 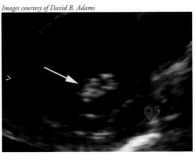

Figure 15.71: **Parasternal long-axis view in a patient with a parachute MV. Note the tethering of the MV leaflets in diastole.**

Figure 15.72: **Parasternal short-axis view at the level of the papillary muscles. Note the single pap muscle (arrow).**

Persistent Left Superior Vena Cava (PLSVC)

Definition

The left horn of the sinus venosus persists and may drain to the coronary sinus, left atrium or left pulmonary vein.

Echo/Doppler

- The persistent left superior vena cava may be imaged from the suprasternal long-axis view with a leftward tilt

Images courtesy of David B. Adams

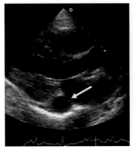 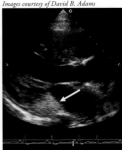

Figure 15.73: **Parasternal long-axis level in a patient with a PLSVC and a dilated coronary sinus (arrow).**

Figure 15.74: **Parasternal long-axis level in a patient with a PLSVC showing saline contrast in the dilated coronary sinus (arrow).**

- Pulsed wave/color flow Doppler will demonstrate a low velocity, biphasic flow pattern away from the transducer in the persistent left superior vena cava

- Dilated coronary sinus best seen in the parasternal long-axis view and apical 4-chamber view with a posterior tilt

- Agitated contrast saline injected into a left arm vein demonstrates contrast in the coronary sinus before arriving into the right atrium

Syndromes and Genetic Abnormalities

Ehlers-Danlos Syndrome (EDS)

Definition

A heterogeneous group of connective tissue disorders with simple mendelian inheritance. The cardinal manifestations of EDS are hyperextensible ("stretchy") skin, hypermobile joints and easy bruising.

Image courtesy of David B. Adams

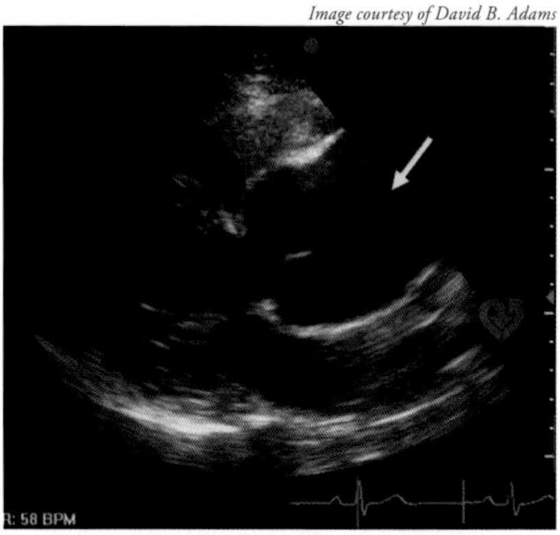

Figure 15.75: **Parasternal long-axis view in a patient with Ehlers-Danlos showing a dilated aortic root (arrow).**

Echo/Doppler

• Aortic root dilatation (annuloaortic ectasia)

• Sinus of Valsalva aneurysm

• Aortic aneurysm (unruptured, ruptured)/dissection

• Dilatation of the proximal innominate artery

• Valvular prolapse (e.g.; mitral valve, aortic valve)

• Valvular regurgitation (e.g.; mitral regurgitation, aortic regurgitation)

• Evaluate for additional congenital defects (e.g.; ASD, VSD, Tetralogy of Fallot, bicuspid aortic valve)

Friedreich's Ataxia

Definition

Cardiac abnormalities are a characteristic feature of the autosomal recessively inherited spinocerebellar degeneration known as Friedreich's ataxia (FA), which is the most common hereditary ataxia.

Echo/Doppler

• Concentric increase in left ventricular wall thickness (most common 68%) (may resemble hypertrophic cardiomyopathy)

• Globally decreased left ventricular systolic function, ejection fraction, fractional shortening (7%)

• Increased left atrial dimension

• Increased right ventricular mass (uncommon)

• Asymmetrical septal thickening (uncommon)

• Dilated cardiomyopathy (uncommon)

Holt-Oram (Heart-Hand) Syndrome

Definition

An autosomal dominant syndrome characterized by skeletal abnormalities and congenital cardiac defects.

Echo/Doppler

- Atrial septal defect (ostium secundum)
- Dilatation of right ventricle, right atrium, paradoxical motion of the ventricular septum consistent with right ventricular volume overload
- Ventricular septal defect (trabecular type)
- Complex congenital heart disease/vascular malformations
- Nonobstructive cardiomyopathy
- Mitral valve prolapse (10 to 20% of patients)

Kawasaki Disease

Definition

- Febrile illness of unknown etiology resulting in vasculitis.
- Also referred to as mucocutaneous lymph node syndrome.

Echo/Doppler

- Coronary artery aneurysm (usually proximal) (may be filled with thrombus)
- Left ventricular global and segmental systolic dysfunction
- Myocardial infarction
- Pericardial effusion (30%)
- Mitral regurgitation (30%)
- Aortic regurgitation (uncommon)
- Transesophageal echocardiography may be useful

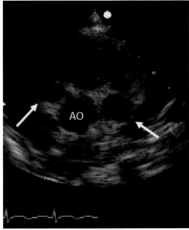

Figure 15.76: **Parasternal short-axis view at the AV level showing dilated proximal right and left coronaries (arrows).**

Loeys-Dietz Syndrome (Aortic Aneurysm Syndrome)

- Autosomal dominant aortic aneurysm syndrome characterized by the triad of arterial tortuosity and aneurysms, hypertolerism and cleft palate caused by heterozygous mutations in the genes encoding transforming growth factor beta receptors
- Aggressive arterial aneurysms (mean age of death 26 years of age)
- Vascular disease may be widespread
- Increased pregnancy related complications

Marfan syndrome

Definition

A hereditary condition of connective tissue, bones, muscles, ligaments and skeletal structures.

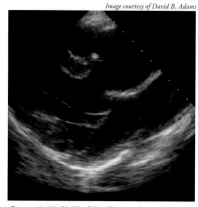

Image courtesy of David B. Adams

Figure 15.77: **PLAX of Marfan syndrome patient**

Echo/Doppler

- Proximal aortic dilatation (aortic annulus, sinuses of Valsalva, ascending aorta)
- Aortic dissection (most common cause of death)
- Multivalvular prolapse (especially mitral valve prolapse)
- Dilated mitral annulus
- Mitral annular calcification
- Left atrial compression
- Left ventricular volume overload pattern (left ventricular dilatation with hyperkinesis)
- Aortic and/or mitral regurgitation
- Coronary artery dissection
- Prophylactic repair of ascending aortic aneurysm in Marfan's has been recommended when the aortic diameter reaches 5.0cm or increase in diameter ≥0.5mm

Noonan's Syndrome

Definition

- Noonan's syndrome is inherited in an autosomal dominant manner and is characterized by congenital heart disease, short stature, abnormal facies and the somatic features of Turner's syndrome but a normal karyotype.
- Congenital heart defects are common in this genetic condition.

Echo/Doppler

- Valvular pulmonic stenosis (40%) with thickened, dysplastic pulmonary valve cusps
- Secundum atrial septal defect (33%)
- Ventricular septal defect (10%)
- Patent ductus arteriosus (10%)
- Localized anterior septal hypertrophy
- Diffuse right ventricular hypertrophy
- Left ventricular hypertrophy
- Partial atrioventricular canal with left ventricular outflow obstruction
- Constrictive pericarditis
- Dilatation of the ascending aorta

Scimitar Syndrome

Definition

Partial or total anomalous pulmonary venous connection of the right lung into the inferior vena cava (rare).

"Scimitar" refers to the appearance of the anomalous right pulmonary vein on chest radiography. The silhouette resembles an ancient curved scimitar sword along the right border of the heart.

Echo/Doppler

- Partial or total anomalous pulmonary venous connection of the right lung into the inferior vena cava
- Sinus venosus atrial septal defect
- Dextrocardia

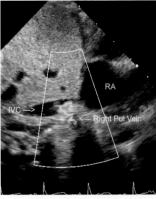

Figure 15.78: **Subcostal long-axis view of the inferior vena cava (IVC) with the right pulmonary vein draining into the IVC in a Scimitar syndrome patient.**

Shone's Syndrome

Definition

A combination of left ventricular inflow tract and left ventricular outflow tract obstructions.

Echo/Doppler

- Supravalvular mitral valve ring, parachute mitral valve
- Subaortic stenosis
- Bicuspid aortic valve
- Aortic coarctation

References

1. Lai WW, Geva T, Shirali GS, Frommelt PC, Humes RA, Brookmm, Pignatelli PH, Rychik J. Guidelines and Standards for Performance of a Pediatric Echocardiogram: A Report from the Task Force of the Pediatric Council of the American Society of Echocardiography. J Am S oc Echocardiogr 2006;19:1413-1430.

2. Menillo AM, Pearson-Shaver AL. Atrial septal defect. https://www.ncbi.nlm.nih.gov/books/NBK535440/

3. Reller MD, Strickland MJ, Riehle-Colarusso T, Mahle WT, Correa A. Prevalence of Congenital Heart Defects in Metropolitan Atlanta, 1998-2005. J Pediatr 2008;153:807-13.

4. Suchoń E, Podolec P, Płazak W, Tomkiewicz-Pajak L, Pieculewicz M, Mura A, Tracz W. Atrial septal defect associated with mitral valve prolapse—prevalence and clinical significance. Przegl Lek 2004;61(6):636-9.

5. Dakak W, Oliver TI. Ventricular septal defect. https://www.ncbi.nlm.nih.gov/books/NBK470330/

6. Eidem BW, O'Leary PW, Cetta F: Echocardiography in Pediatric and Adult Congenital Heart Disease (2nd Edition). Philadelphia, Wolters Kuwer, 2015

7. Akhta F, Bikhari SRA. Down syndrome (trisomy 21). https://www.ncbi.nlm.nih.gov/books/NBK526016/

8. Fisher RG, Moodie DS, Sterba, Gill CC. Patent ductus arteriosus in adults-long-term follow-up: Nonsurgical versus surgical treatment. J Am Coll Cardiol 1986;8:280-284

9. Luu Q, Choudhary P, Jacson D, Canniffe C, McGuire M, Chard R, Clermajer DS. Ebstein's anomaly in those surviving to adult life – A single centre experience. Heart, Lung and Circulation 2015;24:996-1001.

10. Dabizzi RP, Teodori G, Barletta GA, Caprioli G, Baldrighi G, Baldrighi V. Associated coronary and cardiac anomalies in the tetralogy of Fallot. An angiographic study. Eur Heart J 1990;11(8):692-704.

11. Mizuno A, Niwa K, Matsuo K, Kawada M, Miyazaki A, Mori Y, Nakanishi N, Ohuchi H, Watanabe M, Yao A, Inai K. Survey of reoperation indications in tetralogy of fallot in Japan. Circ J. 2013;77(12):2942-7.

12. Faidutti B, Christenson JT, Beghetti M, Friedli B, Kalangos A. How to diminish reoperation rates after initial repair of tetralogy of Fallot? Ann Thorac Surg 2002;73(1):96-101.

13. Warnes CA. Transposition of the great arteries.

Echo Image Enhancing Agents
J Todd Belcik, BS, ACS, RDCS (AE) (PE), FASE

Definition

Ultrasound enhancing agents (UEA's) utilized in echocardiography have become a routine tool for Sonographers to better assess left ventricular endocardial border in technically difficult/suboptimal studies. The introduction of microbubbles via intravenous (IV) line has been documented to improve endocardial border delineation resulting in more accurate assessments of left ventricular wall motion (LVWM) and LV ejection fraction (LVEF%) as well as better visualization of structural abnormalities such as LV thrombus. UEA's also allow qualitative and quantitative assessment of myocardial perfusion and coronary blood flow in both resting and stress echocardiography.

Left Ventricular Ultrasound Enhancing Agents

Echocardiography Indication

For use in pediatric (Lumason® only) adult patients with suboptimal echocardiograms to opacify the left ventricular chamber and improve delineation of the left ventricular endocardial border.

Table 16.1: Commercially Available Ultrasound Enhancing Agents

Agent	Mean Diameter Range (um)	Percent less than 10μm	Gas	Shell composition
Optison® a,c	3.0 - 4.5	95%	Perfluoropropane	Human albumin
(perflutren protein type-A microspheres)	**Indication:** (1) for use in patients with suboptimal echocardiograms to opacify the left ventricle and to improve the delineation of the left ventricular endocardial borders			
Definity® a,d /	1.1 - 3.3	98%	Perfluoropropane	Phospholipid
Luminity b,d (perflutren lipid microspheres)	**Indication:** (1) for use in patients with suboptimal echocardiograms to opacify the left ventricular chamber and to improve the delineation of the left ventricular endocardial border			
Lumason a,e / SonoVue b, e	1.5 - 2.5	≥99%	Sulfur hexafluoride	Amphiphilic phospholipids
(sulfur hexafluoride lipid-type A microspheres)	**Indication:** (1) in echocardiography to opacify the left ventricular chamber and to improve the delineation of the left ventricular endocardial border in adult and pediatric patients with suboptimal echocardiograms; (2) in ultrasonography of the liver for characterization of focal liver lesions in adult and pediatric patients; (3) in ultrasonography of the urinary tract for the evaluation of suspected or known vesicoureteral reflux in pediatric patients			

a) Approved for use in USA by FDA; b) Approved for use in UK and Europe ; c) GE Healthcare (Princeton, NJ); d) Lantheus Medical Imaging (North Billerica, MA) e) Bracco Diagnostics (Milan, Italy)

Recommendations and Guidelines
American Society of Echocardiography [1,2]

- Very low-MI (VLMI) and low-MI imaging techniques should be utilized for optimal LVO
- Per 2014 ASE guidelines, it is recommended UEA's should be administered either by a bolus (≤0.5 mL) injection followed by slow (10 to 20 sec) saline flush or a continuous infusion per package insert using VLMI imaging to minimize apical microbubble destruction and basal segment attenuation [1]
- As per 2008 ASE guidelines, UEAs should be used when two or more LV segments cannot be visualized adequately for the assessment of global LV function and regional wall motion assessment (LVEF and RWM) and/or in settings in which the study indication requires accurate analysis of regional wall motion (RWM). [2]
- Use in all patients requiring quantitative assessment of LVEF for prognostic or management of the clinical condition, UEA's should be used.
- Use in all patients in whom LV thrombus cannot be ruled in or out with unenhanced (2D) imaging
- Use should be considered in patients in whom structural abnormalities of the left ventricle (non-compaction cardiomyopathy, apical hypertrophy pseudoaneurysms, aneurysms, and masses) cannot be adequately assessed with unenhanced (2D) imaging.
- Use for differential diagnosis in patients with cardiac masses to assess the vascularity of the cardiac mass
- Use should be considered during TEE for assessment of atrial appendage with significant spontaneous contrast or cannot be adequately visualized with unenhanced (2D) imaging
- Use in all technically difficult ICU and ED patients to more quickly and accurately diagnose potentially life-threatening conditions and to reduce the need for downstream diagnostic testing.
- In patients presenting to the ED with suspected myocardial ischemia (and non-diagnostic ECG), regional function and myocardial perfusion assessment with UEAs adds incremental diagnostic and prognostic value and may reduce health care costs. Myocardial perfusion imaging (MPI) should be considered at centers with sonographer and physician expertise in performance and interpretation of MPI.
- MCE with VLMI imaging may be used in post-STEMI patients to evaluate for LV systolic function, intracavitary thrombi, and microvascular flow within the infarct territory at institutions with sonographer and physician expertise in performance and interpretation of MPI.

European Association of Echocardiography

- All commercially available UEA's are suitable for assessment of LV function, structural LV abnormalities and myocardial perfusion (Class I, Level B).

- Ultrasound enhancing agent specific imaging modalities should be used (Class I, Level B).

- The low MI methods are particularly useful, as they provide simultaneous assessment of wall motion and myocardial perfusion and require less UEA compared with methods using higher MI (Class I, Level B).

- For the optimal assessment of LV structure, switching to intermediate MI imaging is preferable (Class IIa, Level B). UEA's are adequate for the assessment of LV function and diagnosis of structural LV abnormalities such as apical hypertrophy, aneurysms, cardiomyopathies and thrombi (Class I, Level A).

- Infusion of UEA's is optimum for the assessment of myocardial perfusion and for perfusion assessment of cardiac masses (Class I, Level A).

- For infusion of the UEA's, a special pump that agitates the UEA is preferable (Class IIa, Level B).

- Simultaneous infusion of UEA's with Dobutamine or adenosine can be performed through the same IV cannula (Class I, Level B).

- Should be considered when apical hypertrophy and diverticula, pseudeoaneurysms, myocardial rupture, non-compaction and LV thrombi are suspected but not clearly documented or excluded on unenhanced (2D) images (Class I, Level B).

- For perfusion may be used in patients with cardiac masses suspicious of a tumor to distinguish it from a thrombus when CMR is not available or inconclusive (Class IIa, Level C).

- May be considered when unenhanced (2D) images are inconclusive for the diagnosis of LAA thrombus

- May be used to assess the aortic pathology if unenhanced (2D) and Doppler images are suboptimal or ambiguous in patients with acute aortic syndromes and in patients undergoing thoracic endovascular aortic repair procedures. (Class IIa, Level C).

- Stress echocardiography (SE) for the assessment of RWMA for the detection of myocardial ischemia should be performed with UEA'S when two or more contiguous segments are not adequately visualized at rest (Class I, Level A) or during deep inspiration mimicking cardiac motion during stress (Class IIa, Level C).

  - In patients with less than 2 segments not well-visualized, an UEA should be given when myocardial perfusion is assessed in addition to LV wall motion using low MI contrast imaging.

  - Low MI ultrasound enhancing agent specific imaging modalities should be used for SE irrespective of whether only wall motion or both wall motion and perfusion are assessed (Class I, Level C). [1]

16

Echo Image Enhancing Agents / Recommendations and Guidelines

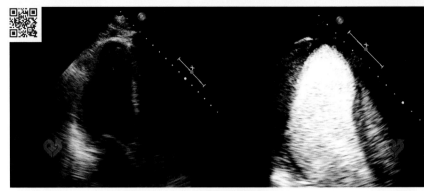

Figure 16.1: **Left ventricular wall motion 2D and LVO**

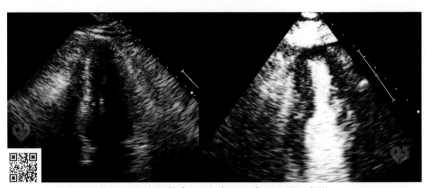

Figure 16.2: **Apical left ventricular opacification 2D and LVO**

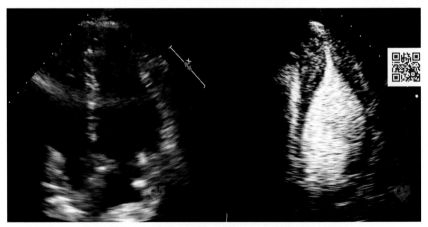

Figure 16.3: **Apical hypertrophic cardiomyopathy (HCM) 2D and LVO**

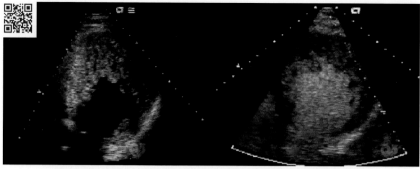

Figure 16.4: **Left ventricular non-compaction cardiomyopathy (LVNC) 2D and LVO**

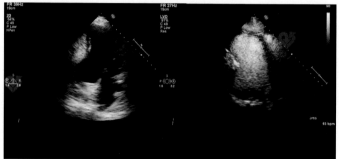

Figure 16.5: **Left ventricular true aneurysm 2D and LVO**

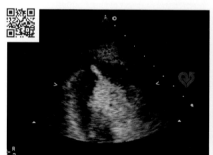

Figure 16.6: **Left ventricular diverticulum LVO**

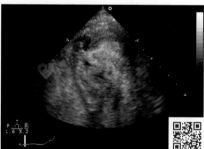

Figure 16.7: **Left ventricular rupture LVO**

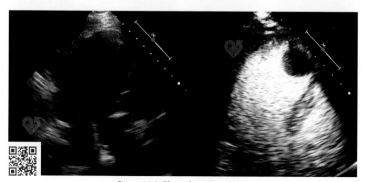

Figure 16.8: **Thrombus 2D and LVO**

16

Echo Image Enhancing Agents

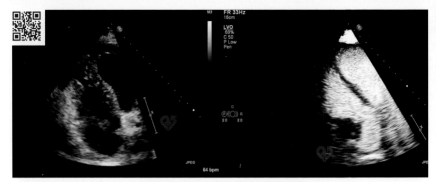

Figure 16.9: **Right atrium mass 2D and LVO**

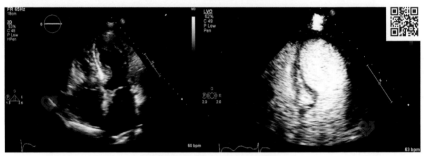

Figure 16.10: **Takotsubo 2D and LVO**

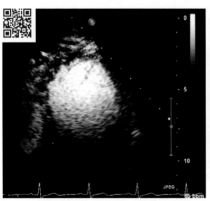

Figure 16.11: **Attenuation**

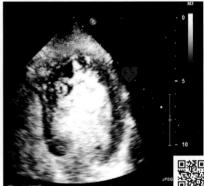

Figure 16.12: **Destruction**

Safety

Current FDA guidelines for all commercially available ultrasound enhancing agents (Optison™, Definity®, and Lumason®) state that these products are not to be administered to patients in whom the following conditions are known or suspected:

- Hypersensitivity to perflutren (Optison™ and Definity®)
- Hypersensitivity reactions to sulfur hexafluoride lipid microsphere components or to any of the inactive ingredients in Lumason®
- Hypersensitivity to blood product, or albumin (applies to Optison™ only)

As of 2019, **EVERY** UEA's approved for use in the United States by the US Food & Drug Administration carries the same Black Box Warning which states: *Serious cardiopulmonary reactions, including fatalities, have uncommonly occurred during or following (1) perflutren-containing microsphere administration, (2) sulfur hexafluoride lipid microspheres. Most serious reactions occur within 30 minutes of administration Assess all patients for the presence of any condition that precludes administration. Always have resuscitation equipment and trained personnel readily available.*

In special populations such as pregnancy, lactating women, or children, there are no safety data published in pregnant patients or children under age 5 for echocardiography, thus it is considered Class B drug. Sonographers should consult with physicians if UEA's is warranted in pregnant patient to determine risk-benefit.

Adverse Reactions

Rare adverse reactions occur in approximately 1 in 10,000 (1:10,000) after administration of UEA's, thus the ASE advises and the Intersocietal Accreditation Commission (IAC) mandates that a policy be in place for early identification and rapid response to these acute and severe reactions. All staff should be familiar with both early identification of an allergic reaction and the appropriate treatment. Allergy kits which include auto-injectable epinephrine should be available and easily accessible in all areas where UEA's are in use.

Guidelines for Equipment Setup and Contrast Agent Administration

Ultrasound machine settings

- Preferably, use the very low-MI (VLMI) modalities provided by vendor of machine
- VLMI ideally should be 0.10 to 0.20 to minimize microbubble destruction
- Optimize transmit focus location (usually far-field location at level of mitral annulus)
- Optimize TGCs and gain
- Minimize near-field gain

IV Setup and Ultrasound Enhancing Agent (UEA) preparation

- Store ultrasound enhancing agent as directed and check its expiration date before use
- Insert 22-gauge or larger IV catheter into a large antecubital vein, preferably in the arm opposite the sonographer's imaging position. If possible, avoid the arm that has blood pressure cuff
- For stress studies using UEA's, avoid the antecubital vein to minimize potential IV flow problems if arm is bent during administration at peak HR
- When a quantitative UEA protocol requires simultaneous administration

IV Administration, Bolus method

Resting study

- Rate of bolus injection is generally 0.5 to 1.0mL/s
- After bolus or diluted bolus injections, administer a slow saline flush per package insert (2-5mL over 3-5 seconds)
- When the UEA is seen in right ventricle, slow or stop saline flush
- Acquire views (Apical 4ch, 2ch, 3ch, and PSAX) with optimal LV endocardial border delineation *without* foreshortening views.
- Administer additional IV doses as required for optimal LV cavity opacification (up to maximum dose allowed per package insert)

Dobutamine stress study

- UEA can be administered simultaneously through the Dobutamine infusion line via side port of extension tubing or use of Y-connection extension set.
- Avoid 90° angle connections; avoid having IV line and blood pressure cuff on same arm
- Dobutamine infusion acts as flush, thus no saline flush may be necessary.
- Rest imaging: administration as above
- Acquire Apical 4ch, 2ch, 3ch, PSAX for Dobutamine stages per laboratory protocol (example: Baseline, Low-Dose, Peak Dose, and Recovery)
- If attenuation occurs as a result of rapid bolus, use "Flash" feature (is equipped) to send several frames of high MI to destroy microbubbles or use Color Flow Doppler for a 1-3 seconds to destroy microbubbles.
- If lack of effect is seen, determine if an administration issue such as impeded IV, low concentration as result of inadequate resuspension of microbubbles in solution, or, whether mechanical index is set too high (>0.30)

Treadmill stress study

- Rest imaging: administration as above
- While patient is on treadmill, inject UEA about 30 seconds before exercise termination
- Transfer patient to imaging bed
- Begin acquiring images of Apical 4-chamber, 2-chamber, 3-chamber, and PSAX making sure not to foreshorten images

- If additional UEA dose(s) needed for better LV endocardial border delineation, administer UEA dose followed by slow saline flush up to maximum dose allowed per package insert.

- If attenuation occurs as a result of rapid bolus, use "Flash" feature (is equipped) to send several frames of high MI to destroy microbubbles or use Color Flow Doppler for a 1-3 seconds to destroy microbubbles.

- **NOTE:** For Supine bicycle exercise, administer UEA at each stress stage (baseline, intermediate, peak, and recovery) similar to Dobutamine stress echo above

IV Administration, Infusion Method

- Dilute UEA in 9mL of saline in a 10mL syringe or a 50mL bag of saline (per package insert)

- Adjust/titrate the infusion rate in accordance with the appearance of UEA in the LV cavity, generally 150 to 200mL/h, if using the 50mL bag of saline, or if using the 10mL syringe, as a slow push of 0.5 to 1.0mL every few minutes

- An optional method for administration of UEA as continuous infusion can be performed an syringe infusion pump (ideal) or hand push (acceptable) in lieu of the hanging bag method of suspended UEA

When low-MI imaging presets are used for LVO, the appearance of the microbubbles within the myocardium may become so robust that clear endocardial border distinction between myocardium and the LV cavity may become obscured. This can be managed by utilization of "Flash" or "Burst" modes which sends several high-MI (>0.70) frames to destroy microbubbles within the myocardium. It is important to destroy microbubbles only within the myocardium and not the LV cavity which results in better delineation of LV endocardial border where LV myocardium opacification is darker than LV cavity opacification.

Table 16.2: Practical Guidelines and Ways to Avoid Common Pitfalls	
Using Contrast Agents for Image Acquisition	• Start at apical window and have the patient in a bed with a cutout
	• To improve image quality and decrease shadowing
	• Use respiratory movements
	• Move transducer to change its position within intercostal space either medially or laterally
If shadowing cannot be eliminated	• Attempt to direct shadow through center of left ventricle
If swirling of the UEA or "underfilling" of the LV apex appears	• Reduce mechanical index (MI)
	• Increase administration/titration rate/verify microbubbles are uniformLy re-suspended
	• Administer additional UEA dose(s) followed by rapid saline flush (dosing up to maximum per package insert)
	• Adjust transmit focus to LV apex
If attenuation occurs	• Wait a few seconds to see if resolves as UEA concentration decrease
	• Use "Flash"/"Burst" feature to send several frames of high MI to destroy microbubbles

Myocardial Perfusion Imaging

• Ultrasound enhancing agents have been for many years used in research for the assessment of myocardial perfusion. Microbubbles possess a linear relationship between concentration and detection intensity as microbubbles behavior similar to red blood cells with in the microcirculation, i.e. capillaries.

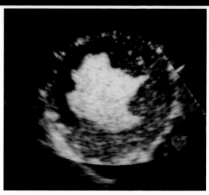

Figure 16.13: **Example of myocardial perfusion defect**

• Clinically, myocardial perfusion imaging allows quick assessment of known or suspected coronary artery disease (site of lesion and collateralization), acute myocardial infarction (risk area during occlusion and efficacy of post-PCI therapy), and evaluation of myocardial viability (post-MI no reflow and identification of hibernating myocardium in chronic CAD) and can be performed at bedside.

• According to the ASC Guidelines Myocardial perfusion imaging is should be performed by skilled trained sonographers and physicians. [1]

• To perform Myocardial Perfusion Imaging, a technique call "Burst-Replenishment" is required which utilizes any of the very low MI contrast-enhanced ultrasound modalities (Power Modulation, Pulse Inversion, and Contrast Pulse Sequencing (CPS)) during a steady state administration of microbubbles.

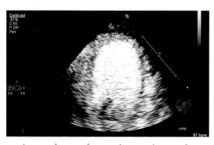

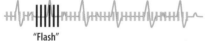

"Flash"

Figure 16.14: **Illustration of real-time burst replenishment perfusion imaging using very low MI (VLMI) technique for assessment of LV function and myocardial perfusion. During infusion of microbubbles, imaging is performed at very low MI (<0.18) followed by several high MI (0.74 to 1.0) to destroy microbubbles within the myocardium then reverting back to VLMI (yellow frames) to assess the replenishment kinetics of myocardial tissue. (Red = destruction frames, Yellow = imaging frames)**

The Burst-Replenishment sequence can be described into 3 phases:

1) **Pre-destruction** which is baseline steady state at very low MI (VLMI) imaging

2) **Destruction** ("Flash" or "Burst") by delivering several frames of high MI (<0.80) to destroy microbubbles within the myocardium

3) **Post-destruction** which ultrasound system reverts back to VLMI imaging to allow visualization of myocardium opacification or filling.

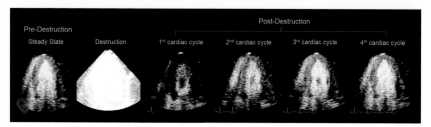

Figure 16.15: **Burst-replenishment sequence**

During myocardial perfusion imaging, there are 3 major determinants in assessing myocardial blood flow:

Signal intensity

The "brightness" or opacification of the myocardium when microbubbles are present which denotes myocardial blood volume (A)

• A perfusion defect at rest indicates either 1) myocardial ischemia/infarction, 2) artifact, or 3) technical issues. It is important to understand the pitfalls such as:

  - Failure to visualize signal due to attenuation (rib, lung, and microbubbles)
  - Destruction of microbubbles in the apical myocardium due to beam overlap of ultrasound scan lines in the near field
  - Inadequate dosing/concentration to visualize presence of microbubbles in myocardium
  - Improper overall gain and compression settings

Rate of filling

How fast the "brightness" or opacification reaches plateau which denotes myocardial blood velocity (β).

• **At rest:** microbubbles traverse the capillary beds at the same rate of red blood cells which is ~1mm/sec. With a ultrasound beam elevation of ~4 to 5mm, the elevational plane should be completely saturated/filled in ~5 seconds

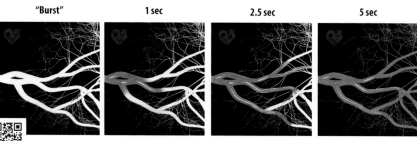

Figure 16.16: **Illustration of rate of filling**

- **At stress:** Myocardial blood velocity must increase to meet oxygen/nutrient demand of the myocardial tissue, thus the ultrasound beam elevation should be demonstrate homogeneous refill/plateau within ~1-2 seconds.

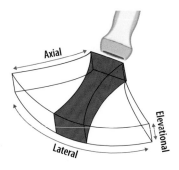

Myocardial perfusion defects observed during hyperemia not evident at rest are indicative of myocardial ischemia

Figure 16.17: **Ultrasound beam elevation**

Pattern of filling

Transmural differences in myocardial blood volume and velocity between epicardium and subendocardium.

- **Subendocardial to epicardial:** perfusion defects begin as a reduction in blood flow at the subendocardium (arterioles, capillaries) which may progress outwards towards the epicardium (arteries, arterioles), known as wave front ischemia/necrosis. A reduction in blood flow may not be seen during resting perfusion under normal resting conditions, but may be present during stress perfusion imaging (Dobutamine, Regadenoson, Dipyridamole, Adenosine) as coronary blood flow is limited due to coronary stenosis demand mismatch.

- **LV regional shape changes:** may be indicative of ischemia such as irregular contour of the apex, mid-inferior segments, C-shape of the basal inferior segment or global LV geometric changes.

- **Location:** basal LV segment perfusion defects with normal mid-to-distal perfusion of the same coronary artery distribution are most likely artifact. True basal LV perfusion defects will also result in perfusion defect downstream within the same LV wall/perfusion territory.

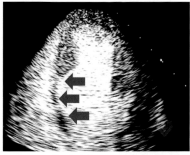

Figure 16.18: **Classic C-shaped configuration of the basal septum indicative of perfusion defect of involving RCA coronary artery**

Quantitative Analysis

Myocardial perfusion imaging allows for both qualitative and quantitative analysis of myocardial blood flow. Using the equation:

Myocardial Blood Flow (MBF) = Myocardial blood volume (A) x blood velocity (β)

A = Signal intensity (myocardial blood volume)

β = Rate of filling (myocardial blood velocity)

MBF (myocardial blood flow) = volume (A) x Velocity (β)

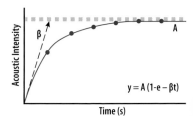

$$y = A(1-e-βt)$$

Figure 16.19: **Quantitative myocardial perfusion replenishment curve**

For myocardial perfusion, the primary determinant of myocardial blood flow is myocardial blood velocity (β). Quantitative analysis requires measuring the acoustic intensity and rate of filling of a specified region of interest (ROI). In Figure 16.21, the ROI's are drawn within the mid-to-distal septum (LAD) and displayed on as:

$$y = A (1\text{-}e - \beta t)$$

y is myocardial acoustic intensity (AI) at a pulsing interval (PI) of t

A is the plateau AI representing MBV

β is the rate constant representing the mean myocardial blood flow velocity from the slope of the time-intensity curve

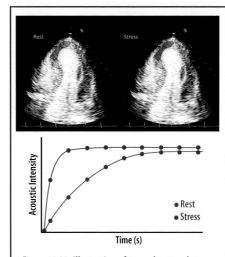

Figure 16.20: **Illustration of normal rest and stress burst replenishment curve**

The difference between rest and stress is known as coronary flow reserve which in the absence of CAD, should increase 4 to 6 fold during exercise/stress. However, in this example of rest (red) and stress (blue), the β-reserve (velocity difference between stress and rest) is significantly reduced to 1.33, indicative of a significant obstruction during demand ischemia of the mid to distal LAD perfusion territory.

The difference between the maximal blood flow and resting blood flow in the coronary arteries is known as Coronary Flow Reserve (CFR).

$$y = A (1\text{-}e - \beta t)$$

y = myocardial acoustic intensity (AI) at a pulsing interval (PI) of t

A = plateau AI representing MBV

β = rate constant representing the mean myocardial blood flow velocity from the slope of the time-intensity curve

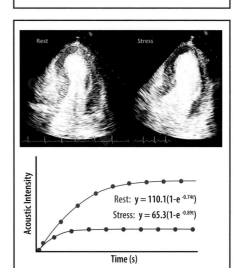

	A	β	A x β	β-reverse
Rest	108.1	0.74	79.99	**1.33**
Stress	61.3	0.98	60.07	

Figure 16.21: **Quantitative analysis of A, β, A x β at rest and stress in patient with perfusion defect of mid to distal LAD as well as mid to distal LCx territories.**

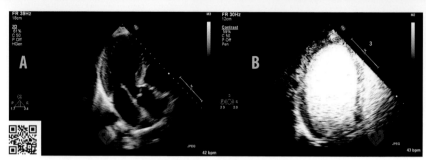

Figure 16.22: **Example of patient with known CAD S\P stent of LAD.**
(A) normal LV wall motion and EF. (B) MPI demonstrates subendocardial ischemia of distal LAD territory.

Future Applications

Contrast-enhanced ultrasound (CEUS) will include ultrasound-targeted drug and gene delivery, sonothrombolysis, molecular imaging, and utilization of ultrasound bioeffects to augment tissue blood flow.

References

1. Roxy Senior1, Harald Becher, Mark Monaghan, Luciano Agati, Jose Zamorano, Jean Louis Vanoverschelde, and Petros Nihoyannopoulos. Contrast echocardiography: evidence-based recommendations by European Association of Echocardiography European Journal of Echocardiography (2009) 10, 194–212

2. Thomas R. Porter, MD, FASE (Chair), Sahar Abdelmoneim, MD, J. Todd Belcik, BS, RCS, RDCS, FASE, Marti L. McCulloch, MBA, RDCS, FASE, Sharon L. Mulvagh, MD, FASE, Joan J. Olson, BS, RDCS, RVT, FASE, Charlene Porcelli, BS, RDCS, RDMS, FASE, Jeane M. Tsutsui, MD, and Kevin Wei, MD, FASE. Guidelines for the Cardiac Sonographer in the Performance of Contrast Echocardiography: A Focused Update from the American Society of Echocardiography. J Am Soc Echocardiogr 2014;27:797-810.

3. Optison Package Insert

4. Definity Package Insert

5. Lumason Package Insert

Michelle Bierig, PhD, ACS, RCS RDCS, RDMS, CPHQ, FSDMS, FASE

Exercise Echocardiography

Definition

A noninvasive diagnostic method which combines baseline echocardiographic imaging with a peak/post exercise in order to detect ischemia and assess known or suspected coronary artery disease (CAD).

Rationale

If a patient with significant coronary artery disease exercises, ischemia will be induced in the region subtended by a narrowed coronary artery. This will be demonstrated as an abnormality of contractility (thickening and/or motion) that can be visualized by echocardiographic imaging.

Indications

• Evaluation of patients with symptoms suggestive of CAD
• Evaluate patients with known CAD
• Risk stratify patients before non-cardiac surgery, after myocardial infarction, or interventional procedures and prior to starting an exercise/diet program
• Ambiguous stress ECG examination (e.g., women)

Objectives

• To evaluate left ventricular global and segmental systolic function
• To identify viable, hibernating or stunned myocardium
• To evaluate hemodynamics in valvular/pulmonary hypertension/ cardiomyopathic heart disease

Contraindications

Absolute
• Acute myocardial infarction (within two days)
• Unstable angina
• Uncontrolled cardiac arrhythmias
• Symptomatic valvular aortic stenosis (mean resting gradient >50mmHg)
• Uncontrolled symptomatic heart failure
• Acute pulmonary embolus/pulmonary infarction
• Acute myocarditis/pericarditis/infective endocarditis
• Acute aortic dissection

Table 17.1: Calculating Target Heart Rates	
Maximal Heart Rate	220 minus age (in years)
Pharmacologic Stress	85% of age predicted maximal heart rate for at least one minute
% Maximal Heart Rate Achieved	Maximal Heart Rate Achieved/Maximal Heart Rate
Double Product	Maximal Heart Hate achieved X Systolic Blood Pressure
Rate Pressure Product	Heart Rate (bpm) X Systolic Blood Pressure (mmHg)

Relative

• Left main coronary artery stenosis
• Moderate stenotic valvular heart disease
• Electrolyte abnormalities
• Severe arterial hypertension
• Tachyarrhythmias/bradyarrhythmias
• Hypertrophic cardiomyopathy and other forms of outflow tract obstruction
• Mental/physical impairment leading to the inability to exercise
• High degree of atrioventricular block

Physiologic Basis

The normal response to exercise is an increase in left ventricular contractility (thickening and excursion). In the presence of CAD, stress induced myocardial ischemia results in a decrease/cessation of contractility in the myocardial region supplied by the stenosed vessel. The ischemic wall(s) will appear hypokinetic, akinetic or dyskinetic. Termination of stress is at maximal effort (symptom limited) with a goal of at least 90% (85% for pharmacologic stress) of the age predicted maximum heart rate for at least one minute and a double product of >25,000.

Methods

Exercise	*Pharmacologic*	*Historical/other*
• Treadmill	• Dobutamine	• Atrial pacing: direct
• Supine bicycle	• Dobutamine-atropine	• Atrial pacing: esophageal
• Upright bicycle	• Dipyridamole	• Arbutamine
• Isometric	• Dipyridamole-dobutamine	• Cold pressor
	• Adenosine	• Mental
	• Regadenoson	• Hyperventilation

Table 17.2: Two-Phase Exercise Echo Protocol
1. Explain the test to the patient
2. Position electrodes to ensure that echo windows are unobstructed
3. Obtain resting echo images (digital capture)
4. Exercise patient
5. Prepare probe and system for immediate post-exercise study
6. Obtain and record (digital capture) post-exercise images rapidly
7. Select post exercise images, shuffle and review pre- and post-exercise images

Patient Preparation

- Patient should be NPO three hours before the examination
- Patient history
    - Risk factors for CAD
    - Previous history of CAD (e.g., PTCA, MI, CABG)
    - Previous test/procedures and/or medications
    - Goal of examination/ indication
- Patient informed of procedure and consent form signed
- 12 lead ECG placement (modified)
- Obtain a resting blood pressure
- Obtain a resting 12 lead ECG
- Patient is instructed on the importance of the time from when the exercise ends and the echo examination begins and encouraged to exercise to the best of their ability
- Inform patient for the need to control breathing during post exercise image acquisition. This cooperation will assist the sonographer in acquiring high quality images within the limited time requirements.

Exercise Protocol

1. Standard Bruce protocol (most common but may depend on institution)
2. Modified Bruce protocol (utilized in patients with lower exercise capacity)
3. Naughton protocol

Resting Images

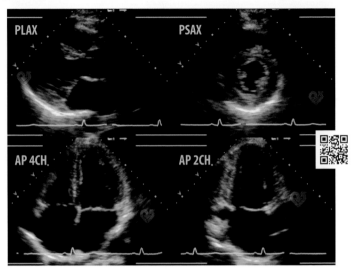

Figure 17.1: **Resting images for stress echo**

- Resting (baseline) images are captured for the following views at a scan depth that optimizes the LV and RV. When endocardial borders are not well visualized in all segments, ultrasound enhancing agents should be utilized.
  - Parasternal long-axis (substitute apical 3/long axis chamber when using contrast)
  - Parasternal short-axis at the level of the papillary muscle
  - Apical 4-chamber
  - Apical 2-chamber
  - Additional views:
    - Apical long-axis
    - Apical 4-chamber with posterior tilt
    - Parasternal/apical short-axis of the left ventricular apex
    - Subcostal 4-chamber and/or short axis
    - Evaluation of the presence and severity of mitral regurgitation
    - Evaluate mitral valve inflow pattern, E/e'
    - Evaluate SPAP using the tricuspid regurgitation peak velocity

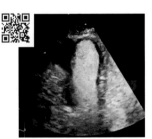

Figure 17.2: **Use of apical 3-chamber in place of parasternal long axis when contrast is used**

- During the resting examination, evaluate image quality, global and segmental left ventricular systolic function. If resting echo has not been performed, it may be helpful to evaluate diastolic ventricular function, coexisting valvular heart disease (e.g., valvular aortic stenosis, mitral regurgitation), cardiomyopathy, pericarditis.
- Note the patient's position relative to the bed

- Consider ultrasound enhancement agents (e.g., Lumason, Definity, Optison) (recommended when any wall segments are not well visualized)

Endpoints

- Symptom limited stress is the primary endpoint with patients unable to continue (e.g., fatigue, dyspnea, chest pain)
- Achievement of predicted heart rate (90% of maximum heart rate for one minute)
- Atrial/ventricular tachyarrhythmias (e.g., SVT, AF)
- Severe angina pectoris
- ≥2mm ST segment depression in comparison to baseline or ST elevation
- Systolic blood pressure >220/120mmHg or blood pressure drops >40mmHg during exercise to below baseline
- Equipment failure

Post Exercise

- The sonographer should begin the timer as soon as the treadmill stops and exercise ends

- The sonographer has approximately 60 seconds from the time the treadmill stops to obtain peak/post exercise images and continue to scan at least two minutes post exercise. If new segmental wall motion abnormalities occur, sonographer should continue to scan until wall motion returns to normal.

- Obtain the imaging windows obtained during the resting imaging session

- Choose the best post images keeping in mind endocardial definition, on axis views and tend to choose those images acquired earliest which have the highest heart rate (select multiple beats per window if possible)

- Shuffle images to display imaging by view (e.g. rest parasternal long axis next to stress parasternal long axis)

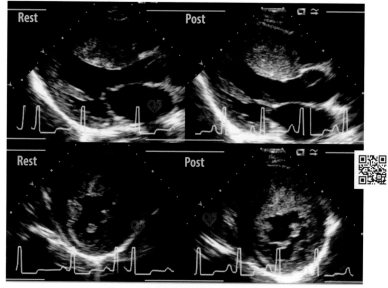

Figure 17.3: **PLAX and PSAX comparison**

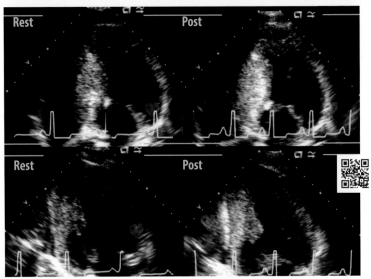

Figure 17.4: **Apical 4-chamber and Apical 2-chamber comparison**

Table 17.3: Wall Motion Score Index

Wall Motion	Score	Definition
Normal/hyperkinesis	1	Systolic wall thickening >40%
Hypokinetic	2	Systolic wall thickening <30%
Akinetic	3	Systolic wall thickening <10%
Dyskinetic	4	Systolic wall thinning with myocardial segment moving outward during systole
WMSI =	$\dfrac{\text{Sum of wall motion scores}}{\text{Number of segments visualized}}$	

Note: In normal subjects, the percent of systolic thickening of the interventricular septum is somewhat less than that of the free wall of the left ventricle.

A normal contracting left ventricle has a wall motion score index of 1.

Patients with a wall motion score index of >2.0 are abnormal.

Recovery

- Monitor vital signs
- Obtain 12 lead ECG at two minute intervals for 10 minutes or until blood pressure and heart rate returns to within 10 beats of baseline heart rate

Interpretation

- Note patient symptoms during exercise (e.g., workload performed, heart rate, blood pressure response)
- Evaluate exercise electrocardiography information (e.g., ECG changes, presence of arrhythmias)
- Evaluate global and segmental left ventricular systolic function pre- and post-exercise

- Assign a wall motion score to each wall segment well visualized and calculate a wall motion score index
- Utilizing a ultrasound enhancing agents (e.g. Lumason, Optison, Definity) improves the evaluation of global/segmental ventricular function by decreasing intra-observer interpretation variability and improves reader confidence

Table 17.4: Interpretation by Segmental Wall Motion Analysis

Rest	Stress	Interpretation
Normal wall motion	Hyperdynamic and contractility	Normal
Normal wall motion	New wall motion abnormality or lack of hyperdynamic wall motion	Ischemia
Wall motion abnormality (akinesis to dyskinesis)	Worsening (hypokinesis to akinesis)	Ischemia/Infarct
Wall motion abnormality	Unchanged	Infarct
Hypokinetic/Akinetic wall motion (biphasic response)	Improved to normal wall motion myocardium	Viable

Normal Response

- All walls become hyperdynamic with symmetric wall thickening and equal excursion in all segments *(Figure 17.4)*

- Ejection fraction measured at rest and peak imaging increases (minimum increase in ejection fraction of 5% is normal response)

- Left ventricular end-systolic dimension decreases

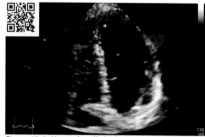

Figure 17.5: Normal wall thickening and contraction at peak exercise

- Note: Studies have demonstrated a benign prognosis following normal exercise echocardiography (annual event rate of cardiac death and nonfatal myocardial infarction of <1%).

Abnormal Response

- New segmental wall motion abnormalities (utilize wall motion score index) *(Figure 17.5) (Table 17.3)*

- Resting hypokinetic wall segment that worsens with exercise may represent hibernating myocardium

- Global systolic dysfunction (decreased ejection fraction)

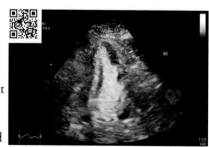

Figure 17.6: Apical wall motion abnormality visualized at peak exercise. Note decreased myocardial filling in segments with abnormal contraction.

- Increased left ventricular end-systolic and/or end-diastolic chamber dimension/volume
- Shape change of ventricle
- Increased right ventricular dimensions
- New/increased mitral regurgitation
- Significant increase in pulmonary artery pressures
- Reduced mitral annulus E/e' ratio as compared to rest E/e' ratio
- Decrease in global longitudinal strain

Interpretation Pitfalls

False-Negative

- Suboptimal study due to inadequate exercise capacity/beta-blocker therapy (primary cause)
- Poor image quality. Quick heart rate recovery resulting in peak imaging acquired at a lower heart rate that peak heart rate. Delayed image acquisition post-stress (greater than 60 seconds past treadmill stopping)
- Left ventricular hypertrophy (especially "small" left ventricular cavity)
- Hypertensive exercise response may cause wall motion abnormalities or cavity dilatation in the absence of CAD
- Single vessel disease
- Disease of the left circumflex (apical long axis view may be useful)

False-positive

- Non-ischemic causes of wall motion abnormalities (e.g., hypertensive response to exercise, left ventricular hypertrophy, syndrome X, coronary artery spasm, diabetes mellitus, dilated cardiomyopathy)
- Long-standing systemic hypertension
- Hypertrophic obstructive cardiomyopathy
- Reduction in motion of the basal inferior wall/basal interventricular septum due to tethering/mitral annular calcification/mitral valve replacement
- Abnormal interventricular septal motion (e.g., left bundle branch block, RV pacing, post-op septum)

Dobutamine Stress Echocardiography

Definition

Dobutamine stress echocardiography is a pharmacologic alternative to exercise echocardiography for those who are unable to exercise or have specific indications. The advantages of Dobutamine include:

- Useful in patients who cannot exercise
- Useful in patients who are able to exercise but a specific question is posed (e.g., myocardial viability)

- Allows echo/Doppler evaluation throughout the procedure
- Allows immediate detection of an abnormal response facilitating cessation of stress.

Pharmacology

- Dobutamine is a synthetic catecholamine that augments myocardial contractility and increases heart rate thus increasing the work of the heart and myocardial oxygen requirements. Normal heart muscle becomes hyperkinetic with the administration of Dobutamine. In the presence of significant coronary arterial stenosis, myocardial ischemia is produced, resulting in segmental wall motion abnormalities or resulting in the inability of the affected region(s) to augment their systolic thickening and excursion. Dobutamine is administered intravenously and has a half-life of two minutes.

Patient Preparation

- Patient should abstain from oral intake for three hours before the test
- The procedure, side effects of Dobutamine (e.g., palpitations, tingling, flushing, headache) and potential complications should be explained
- Patient consent form should be obtained
- Cardiovascular history should be obtained with patient's height and weight included

- Place ECG leads with modification if necessary to allow for echo imaging
- Obtain a resting baseline 12 lead ECG and blood pressure
- Place a 20 gauge needle or larger with stopcock in an arm vein
- A pre-mix solution consisting of 250mg of Dobutamine in 250mL of NaCl is prepared

Dobutamine Dosage Calculation

To determine the number of mL/hr which equals 1mcg/kg/min:

- Determine the patient's weight in kilograms (pounds/2.2) and utilize the following equation:

Weight (kg) x 60 min/100mg/mL

- The answer will provide the number of mL/hr, which equals 1mcg/kg/min. To determine the amount of Dobutamine to be administered, multiply the mL/hr by 5, 10, 20, 30 and 40 respectively

Procedure

1. Obtain a baseline echocardiogram to screen for image quality, ventricular function, valvular disease, cardiomyopathy and pericardial disease

2. Obtain the following baseline (beat systole preferred) views on digitization:
   - Parasternal long-axis
   - Parasternal short-axis of the left ventricle at the level of the papillary muscle
   - Apical 4-chamber
   - Apical 2-chamber
   - Apical long axis (may be a substitute or additional fifth view when using ultrasound enhancing agent)
   - Additional views:
     - Evaluation of the presence and severity of mitral regurgitation
     - Evaluate mitral valve inflow pattern, E/e'
     - Evaluate SPAP using the tricuspid regurgitation peak velocity

3. Infuse Dobutamine (starting rate 5mcg/kg/min or 10mcg/kg/min)

4. At 2 minutes 30 seconds, begin obtaining views, blood pressure and 12 lead ECG

5. Increase Dobutamine infusion to 10mcg/kg/min at 3 minutes

6. At 5 minutes 30 seconds, obtain a second set of views, blood pressure and 12 lead ECG

7. Increase Dobutamine infusion to 20mcg/kg/min at 6 minutes

8. At 8 minutes 30 seconds, obtain a third set of views, blood pressure and 12 lead ECG

9. Increase the Dobutamine infusion to 30mcg/kg/min at 9 minutes

10. At 11 minutes 30 seconds, obtain a fourth set of views, blood pressure and 12 lead ECG

11. Increase the Dobutamine infusion to 40mcg/kg/min at 12 minutes

12. At 14 minutes 30 seconds, obtain a fifth set of views, blood pressure and 12 lead ECG

13. At 15 minutes, obtain 12 lead ECG, note heart rate and increase Dobutamine infusion up to 50mcg/kg/min until peak heart rate is achieved.

If no endpoint is reached, Dobutamine infusion is continued (up to 50mcg/kg/min) with atropine sulfate (0.5 mg) administered to increase heart rate. Additional doses of 0.25 to 0.5 mg may be repeated at 1 minute intervals to a maximum of 2 mg may be administered.

It is recommended that baseline and peak images always be captured for digital comparison. Based on clinical necessity and laboratory preference, the remaining images may be a combination of low stress, intermediate stress, post atropine images or recovery images.

Table 17.5: Dobutamine Stress Echo Protocol

1. Explain the test to the patient

2. Hook up 12 lead ECG and BP monitoring

3. Begin IV

4. Obtain resting echo digital images

5. Begin Dobutamine infusion at 5 or 10mcg/kg/min

6. Monitor ECG, BP and echocardiogram throughout infusion

7. Obtain low-dose images

8. Increase Dobutamine infusion by 10mcg/kg/min every 3 minutes up to a maximum dose of 40mcg/kg/min or until achieving 85% of the age-predicted maximal heart rate (atropine may be required)

Endpoints

- Development of a new segmental wall motion abnormality or worsening of preexisting segmental wall motion abnormality
- >1mm of horizontal or downsloping ST segment depression at 80 msec after the J point with segmental wall motion abnormality
- Angina pectoris
- Achievement of greater than either 85% of maximum predicted heart rate determined by age
- Systolic blood pressure ≥210/120mmHg
- Symptomatic hypotension, fall in systolic blood pressure of >40mmHg (evaluate for ischemia or left ventricular outflow tract obstruction or give saline if hypovolemic)
- Atrial or ventricular tachyarrhythmias
- Significant increase in gradients across abnormal cardiac valves
- Maximum dose of 50mcg/kg/min
- Adverse effects from the Dobutamine (e.g., nausea, vomiting, headache)
- Patient requests ending test

Recovery

Evaluate vital signs, obtain 12 lead ECG at 2-minute intervals and record echo images when the heart rate reaches below 100 or within 10 of baseline heart rate. After 10 minutes, if patient is stable (e.g., patient is asymptomatic with heart rate, blood pressure and ECG returned to baseline) the examination is completed.

Recovery Images

Digitize recovery images when heart rate is at or within 10 beats of baseline heart rate

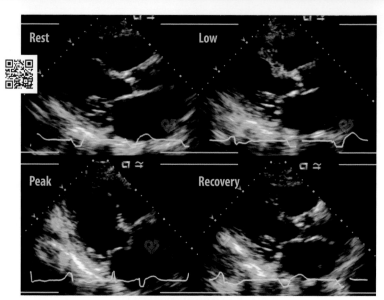

Figure 17.7: **Dobutamine PLAX comparisons**

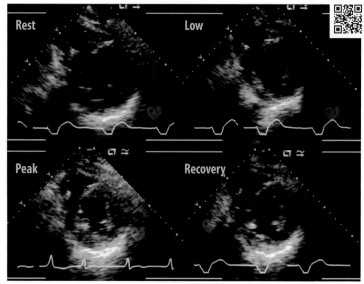

Figure 17.8: **Dobutamine PSAX comparison**

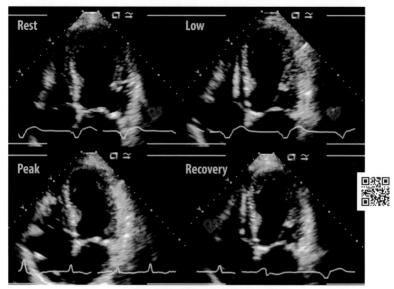

Figure 17.9: **Dobutamine apical 4-chamber comparison**

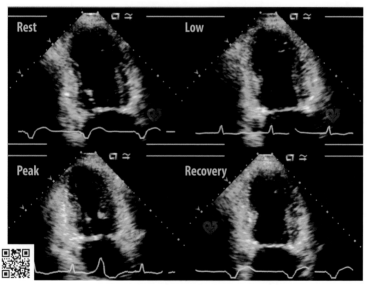

Figure 17.10: **Dobutamine apical 2-chamber comparison**

Interpretation

- Similar to exercise echocardiography
- The normal response to Dobutamine infusion is hyperdynamic wall motion and increased ejection fraction
- Abnormal response is hypokinesia, akinesia or dyskinesia or failure of a wall to increase systolic thickening and excursion or an increase in left ventricular volume

17

Stress Echocardiography / Dobutamine Stress Echocardiography

- Improvement of a hypokinetic, akinetic segment during administration of low dose Dobutamine (5 to 10mcg/kg/min) suggests the presence of viable myocardium
- Determine wall motion score index
- Determine E/e' ratio at rest and peak dose (especially useful in patients with shortness of breath indication)
- Utilizing an ultrasound enhancing agent (e.g., Lumason, Definity, Optison) is indicated when any segment is not visible

Myocardial Viability

- Performed in patients to evaluate if revascularization could improve myocardial contractility and left ventricular function.
- Evaluating myocardial response to a low dose and a high dose of Dobutamine in four different clinical scenarios, with resting akinetic/hypokinetic segment:
  - **Monophasic (sustained) response:** If the myocardium is viable with no stenosis of the coronary artery subtending the akinetic/hypokinetic myocardium, myocardial contractility increases continuously with a low dose and a high dose of Dobutamine.
  - **Biphasic response:** If the myocardium is viable but the coronary artery that supplies the myocardium is severely stenotic, myocardial contractility improves initially with a low dose of Dobutamine but worsens with high dose. This is a typical biphasic response for hibernating myocardium and suggests increased potential of recovery of function.
  - **Nonphasic response:** When myocardium is scarred, with no myocardial viability, there is no myocardial thickening at rest or with either a low dose or a high dose of Dobutamine.
  - **Ischemic response:** A worsening of function without contractile reserve suggests a stress-induced ischemic myocardium due to a flow-limiting stenosis (ischemia).

Important to Note

- Strain and strain rate echocardiography permit quantification of segmental wall motion abnormalities and provides additional information in a stress echocardiography protocol.
- Three-dimensional or triplane imaging allows rapid acquisition and with continued improvements in image quality may result in increased use of this modality.
- Myocardial contrast perfusion (imaging utilizing ultrasound enhancing agents with a mechanical index of less and 0.15) may improve the sensitivity of stress echocardiography and provides incremental assessment for improving diagnostic accuracy.

Stress Echocardiography in the Non-ischemic Evaluation

Diastolic Stress Echocardiography

- Utilized in patients with shortness of breath, fatigue, poor exercise capacity, and potential heart failure to detect diastolic filling impairment with exercise.
- Supine bike is the preferred stress modality around a heart rate of 100 to 110 bpm.
- The mitral valve E/A, E/e' ratio may be used to estimate filling pressures with exercise. Healthy individuals will show a similar increase in mitral valve peak E wave velocity and mitral annular e' peak velocity. Patient with increased filling pressures with exercise demonstrate an increased E/e'.
- At rest, mitral E, mitral A and annular e' velocities should be recorded, along with the peak velocity of the TR jet from multiple windows. The same parameters are recorded during exercise or 1 to 2 minutes after termination of exercise when E and A velocities are not merged, because increased filling pressures usually persists for a few minutes.
- The test is considered positive when all three conditions are met during exercise:
  - Exercise average E/e' >14 or E/e' (septal) >15
  - Exercise TR peak velocity >2.8 m/s
  - Rest Septal e' peak velocity <7cm/s or lateral e' <10cm/sec

Cardiomyopathy

- Hypertrophic Cardiomyopathy
  - Exercise stress echocardiography is utilized in symptomatic patients to induce a left ventricular outflow tract obstruction gradient of >50mmHg
  - Obstruction may be due to systolic anterior motion of the mitral valve or due to hemodynamic changes in ventricular loading conditions.
  - Evaluation of E/e', outflow tract obstruction, systolic pressure, blood pressure, mitral regurgitation in addition to the routine exercise parameters should be included.

Dilated Cardiomyopathy

- Exercise and dobutamine stress echocardiography can help differentiate ischemic from non-ischemic cardiomyopathies by utilizing traditional stress parameters as well as strain changes in mitral regurgitation
- Changes to cardiac synchronization and evaluation of cardiac resynchronization can be used in dobutamine stress echocardiography

Native Valve Disease

- Exercise stress echocardiography for mild or moderate asymptomatic Aortic Stenosis aims to elicit symptoms whereas dobutamine stress echocardiography is used to evaluate low flow, low gradient aortic stenosis. This technique evaluates changes in the aortic gradient with dobutamine.

- Exercise stress echocardiography evaluates hemodynamic quantitative and qualitative changes in Mitral Regurgitation

- Exercise stress echocardiography is used in patients with Aortic Regurgitation to elicit symptoms rather than evaluate changes in regurgitation

- Exercise or dobutamine stress echocardiography can be used to evaluate changes in Mitral Stenosis severity

- Stress echocardiography can also be used in the evaluation of post valve procedures, pulmonary hypertension, athlete's heart and congenital heart disease

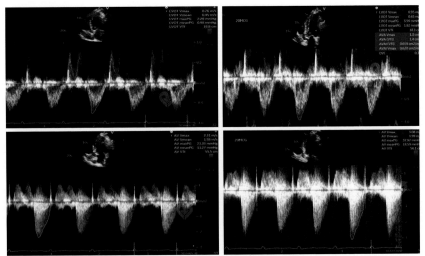

Figure 17.11: **Baseline and peak dobutamine infusion LVOT and Aortic valve waveforms seen in a patient with Aortic Stenosis.**

References

1. Gibbons RJ, Balady GJ, Bricker JT, Chaitman BR, Fletcher GF, et al. ACC/AHA 2002 guideline update for exercise testing: summary article. A report of the American College of Cardiology/American Heart Association Task Force on Practice Guidelines (Committee to Update the 1997 Exercise Testing Guidelines). J Am Coll Cardiol. 2002 Oct 16;40(8):1531-40.

2. Pellikka PA1, Nagueh SF, Elhendy AA, Kuehl CA, Sawada SG; American Society of Echocardiography recommendations for performance, interpretation, and application of stress echocardiography. J Am Soc Echocardiogr. 2007 Sep;20(9):1021-41.

3. Lancellotti P1,2, Pellikka PA3, Budts W4, Chaudhry FA5, Donal E6, et al. The clinical use of stress echocardiography in non-ischaemic heart disease: recommendations from the European Association of Cardiovascular Imaging and the American Society of Echocardiography. Eur Heart J Cardiovasc Imaging. 2016 Nov;17(11):1191-1229.

Transesophageal Echocardiography
Ken Horton, ACS, RCS, FASE

Definition

A specialized type of cardiac ultrasound which allows for real time imaging of the heart by means of a transducer mounted on a flexible gastroscope and positioned behind the heart via the esophagus.

Types

- Multiplane
- 3D

Indications

- Cardiac source of embolism (e.g., thrombus)
- Infective endocarditis
- Prosthetic heart valve dysfunction (regurgitation, perivalvular abscess, stenosis)
- Diseases of the aorta (e.g., dissection)
- Pre-cardioversion in patients with atrial fibrillation (screen for left atrial thrombus/left atrial appendage thrombus)
- Intracardiac masses (tumors)
- Congenital heart disease (e.g., atrial septal defect, ventricular septal defect)
- Evaluation of native valve disease (e.g., valvular regurgitation; valvular stenosis; flail mitral valve)
- Pericardial disease (e.g., loculated pericardial effusion; constrictive pericarditis)
- Complications of myocardial infarction (ventricular septal rupture, papillary muscle rupture)
- Intraoperative studies (adequacy of valvuloplasty procedures, congenital heart disease repair, assessment of left ventricular global and segmental function, myotomy/myectomy evaluation of intracardiac air)
- Evaluation of the critically ill/injured
- Technically difficult transthoracic exam
- High likelihood of non-diagnostic transthoracic imaging
- Re-evaluation of prior TEE findings for interval change
- Imaging support of surgical and transcatheter interventions (procedure planning, procedure guidance, post-procedure assessment)

Contraindications

- Uncooperative/unwilling patient
- Dysphagia
- Mediastinal radiation
- Active upper gastrointestinal bleeding
- Penetrating/blunt chest trauma
- Recent gastroesophageal surgery
- Known esophageal pathology (e.g., malignancy, diverticulum, varices, fistulas, stricture)
- Extreme oropharyngeal muscle weakness
- Severe, uncontrolled bleeding disorders, active upper gastrointestinal hemorrhage
- Unstable respiratory status
- Unstable cervical spine

Complications

- Anaphylaxis
- Arrhythmias
- Aspiration
- Asthma attack
- Blood tinged sputum
- Heart failure
- Death
- Esophageal perforation
- Hematemesis
- Hypertension
- Hypotension
- Hypoxemia
- Laryngospasm
- Minor pharyngeal bleeding
- Parotid swelling
- Sore throat
- Transient laryngeal nerve paralysis
- Vasovagal reaction

Equipment/Materials

- High quality ultrasound machine with TEE probe
- Sedation (conscious sedation, general anesthesia)
- Reversal agents (Romazicon IV, Narcan IV)
- Suction cannister with tubing and tip
- O2 nasal prongs with connection to O2
- Pulse oximeter
- Blood pressure monitoring
- Gloves (sterile/unsterile)
- Bite block
- Emesis basin
- Intravenous access
- Sterile normal saline with three-way stopcock for agitated saline study
- Tongue blades
- Pharyngeal anesthetic (Xylocaine spray, Xylocaine viscous/Xylocaine jelly)
- Water-soluble lubricant (e.g., KY jelly)
- Endotracheal intubation tray with various size endotracheal tubes
- ECG electrodes
- Patient gowns
- Goggles/mask when indicated
- "Crash cart"
- Signed consent form
- TEE report sheet

Pre-procedure

- Verify order and time
- Patient should fast for four to six hours prior to the examination
- Obtain a patient history emphasizing:
  - Allergies
  - H/O bleeding disorders
  - Difficulty in swallowing
  - Current medical problem
  - Thoracic radiation
  - Hematemesis
  - Explain the procedure to the patient and obtain a signed consent
- Remove patient dentures
- Check CPR equipment
- Insert IV line
- Administer prophylactic antibiotics
- Anesthetize the pharynx
- Administer the IV sedation (e.g., Phenergan, Demerol, Diazepam, Valium), Midazolam (Versed)
- Select appropriate TEE probe
- Place patient in left lateral decubitus position with neck flexed. Place a bite guard in the patient's mouth, apply gel to the tip of the slightly flexed probe and insert probe through the bite guard while asking the patient to swallow. The index finger may be used to guide the probe. Advance probe 30 to 35cm.
- In the operating room the patients are supine and under general anesthesia

Table 18.1: Multiplane TEE Examination			
Transgastric LV (35 to 40cm)		**Transgastric RV**	
0 to 30°	Short-axis of left ventricle	0°	Short-axis right ventricle
40 to 60°	Short-axis of left ventricle	30°	Short-axis tricuspid valve
90°	Left ventricle 2-chamber	90 to 100°	RVIT
120°	Left ventricle long-axis	110 to 130°	RVIT
Midesophageal (30 to 35cm)		**Upper esophagus (25 to 30cm)**	
0°	4-chamber	0 to 30°	Aortic valve
30 to 60°	4-chamber	40 to 60°	Short-axis aortic valve
90°	LV 2-chamber	60 to 75°	Short-axis aortic valve with pulmonic valve
130 to 150°	LV long-axis	90 to 100°	Short-axis aortic valve with pulmonic valve
Descending thoracic aorta		130 to 150°	Long-axis of aorta, aortic valve, mitral valve
0°	Short-axis of aorta, long-axis of aortic arch		
80 to 110°	Long-axis of aorta		

3D TEE

- Integral component of diagnostic examination
- Utilized for pre-procedure planning of surgical and transcatheter interventions
- Utilized for intra-procedural guidance of surgical and transcatheter interventions
- Utilized for post-procedure assessment on surgical and transcatheter interventions

Post-procedure

- Upon removal check probe for evidence of bleeding
- Check mouth/pharynx for injury
- Monitor vital signs for 20 to 30 minutes
- Patient should remain NPO until gag reflex returns (1 to 2 hours), be informed that performing tasks such as driving or operating moving equipment should not be done for 12 to 24 hours, report a sore throat if it persists for more than two days, contact a physician immediately if bleeding from the mouth occurs, IV site is painful or if fever develops.
- Post-procedure care of the probe
  - Point of care enzymatic cleaning (enzymatic sponge)
  - Transport probe for high level disinfection in a biohazard suitable container
  - High Level Disinfection
    - Soak probe in enzymatic cleaner
    - Rinse probe
    - Soak in high level disinfection solution (Metricide OPA)
- Check probe for visible signs of physical damage (bites/crimps along shaft of probe, cracks in transducer face)
- Perform electrical safety check

Table 18.2: Transesophageal Echocardiography Cross Sections

Window (depth from incisors)	Cross Section	Multiplane Angle Range	Structures Imaged
Upper esophageal (20 to 25cm)	Aortic arch long-axis	0°	Aortic arch, left brachio v
	Aortic arch short-axis	90°	Aortic arch, PA, PV, left brachio v
Mid esophageal (30 to 40cm)	Four-chamber	0 to 20°	LV, LA, RV, RA, MV, TV, IAS
	Mitral commissural	60 to 70°	MV, LV, LA
	Two-chamber	80 to 100°	LV, LA, LAA, MV, CS
	Long-axis	120 to 160°	LV, LA, AV, LVOT, MV, asc aorta
	RV inflow-outflow	60 to 90°	RV, RA, TV, RVOT, PV, PA
	AV short-axis	30 to 60°	AV, IAS, coronary ostia, LVOT, PV
	AV long-axis	120 to 160°	AV, LVOT, prox asc aorta, right PA
	Bicaval	80 to 110°	RA, SVC, IVC, IAS, LA
	Asc aortic short-axis	0 to 60°	Asc aorta, SVC, PA, right PA
	Asc aortic long-axis	100 to 150°	Asc aorta, right PA
	Desc aorta short-axis	0°	Desc thoracic aorta, left pleural space
	Desc aorta long-axis	90 to 110°	Desc thoracic aorta, left pleural space
Transgastric (40 to 45cm)	Basal short-axis	0 to 20°	LV, MV, RV, TV
	Mid short-axis	0 to 20°	LV, RV, papmm
	Two-chamber	80 to 100°	LV, MV, chordae, papmm, CS, LA
	Long-axis	90 to 120°	LVOT, AV, MV
	RV inflow	100 to 120°	RV, TV, RA, TV, chordae, papmm
Deep transgastric (45 to 50cm)	Long-axis	0 to 20° (anteflexion)	LVOT, AV, asc aorta, arch

Brachio v, Brachiocephalic vein; PA, pulmonary artery; PV, pulmonic valve; LV, left ventricle; LA, left atrium; RV, right ventricle; RA, right atrium; MV, mitral valve; TV, tricuspid valve; IAS, interatrial septum; LAA, left atrial appendage; CS, coronary sinus; AV, aortic valve; LVOT, left ventricular outflow tract; prox, proximal; RVOT, right ventricular outflow tract; SVC, superior vena cava; IVC, inferior vena cava; RPA, right pulmonary artery; asc, ascending; desc, descending; papmm, papillary muscles.

Mid-esophageal Views

Level: Mid-esophageal
Structures Visualized:
- Aortic valve
- LVOT
- Left atrium/Right atrium
- Left ventricle/Right ventricle/IVS
- Mitral valve ($A_2A_1 - P_1$)
- Tricuspid valve

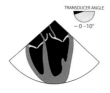
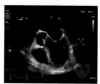

Figure 18.1: **ME 5-chamber**

18

Transesophageal Echocardiography / Mid-esophageal Views

Level: Mid-esophageal
Structures Visualized:
- Left atrium/Right atrium
- IAS
- Left ventricle/Right ventricle/ IVS
- Mitral valve (A_3A_2 - P_2P_1)
- Tricuspid valve

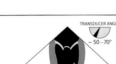
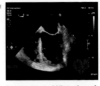

Figure 18.2: **ME 4-chamber**

Level: Mid-esophageal
Structures Visualized:
- Left atrium
- Coronary Sinus
- Left ventricle
- Mitral Valve (P_3 - $A_3A_2A_1$ - P_1)
- Papillary muscles
- Chordae tendinae

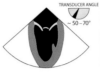
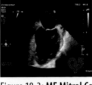

Figure 18.3: **ME Mitral Commissural**

Level: Mid-esophageal
Structures Visualized:
- Left atrium
- Coronary sinus
- Left atrial appendage
- Left ventricle
- Mitral valve (P_3 - $A_3A_2A_1$)

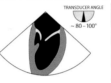
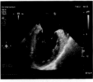

Figure 18.4: **ME 2-chamber**

Level: Mid-esophageal
Structures Visualized:
- Left atrium
- Left ventricle
- LVOT
- RVOT
- Mitral valve (P_2 - A_2)
- Aortic valve
- Proximal ascending aorta

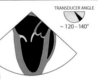
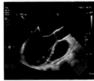

Figure 18.5: **ME long axis**

Level: Mid-esophageal
Structures Visualized:
- Left atrium
- LVOT
- RVOT
- Mitral valve (A_2 - P_2)
- Aortic valve
- Proximal ascending aorta

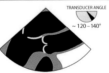
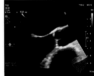

Figure 18.6: **ME AV LAX**

Level: Mid-esophageal
Structures Visualized:
- Aortic valve
- Right atrium
- Left atrium
- Superior IAS
- RVOT
- Pulmonary Valve

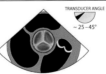
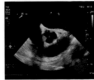

Figure 18.7: **ME AV SAX**

Level: Mid-esophageal
Structures Visualized:
- Aortic valve
- Right atrium
- Left atrium
- Superior IAS
- Tricuspid Valve
- RVOT
- Pulmonary Valve

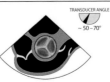
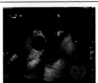

Figure 18.8: **ME RV inflow outflow**

Level: Mid-esophageal
Structures Visualized:
- Right atrium
- Left atrium
- Mid-IAS
- Tricuspid Valve
- Superior vena cava
- Inferior vena cava/coronary sinus

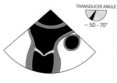 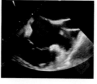

Figure 18.9: **ME modified bicaval**

Level: Mid-esophageal
Structures Visualized:
- Left atrium
- Right atrium/appendage
- IAS
- Superior vena cava
- Inferior vena cava

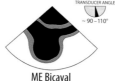 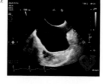

Figure 18.10: **ME bicaval**

Level: Mid-esophageal
Structures Visualized:
- Left atrial appendage
- Left upper pulmonary vein

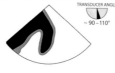 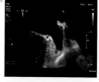

Figure 18.11: **ME left atrial appendage**

Level: Upper-esophageal
Structures Visualized:
- Mid-ascending aorta
- Right pulmonary artery

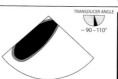 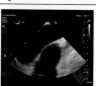

Figure 18.12: **UE ascending aorta LAX**

Level: Upper-esophageal
Structures Visualized:
- Mid-ascending aorta
- (SAX)
- Main/bifurcation
- pulmonary artery
- Superior vena cava

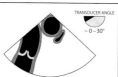 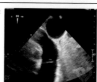

Figure 18.13: **UE ascending aorta SAX**

Level: Upper-esophageal
Structures Visualized:
- Mid-ascending aorta
- Superior vena cava
- Right pulmonary veins

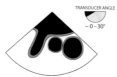 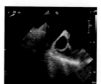

Figure 18.14: **ME right pulmonary vein**

Level: Upper-esophageal
Structures Visualized:
- Pulmonary vein (upper and lower)
- Pulmonary artery

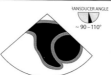 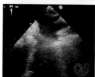

Figure 18.15: **UE R&L pulmonary veins**

18

Transesophageal Echocardiography / Mid-esophageal Views

Transgastric Views

Level: Transgastric
Structures Visualized:
- Left ventricle (base)
- Right ventricle (base)
- Mitral valve (SAX)
- Tricuspid valve (short-axis)

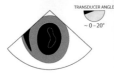 TRANSDUCER ANGLE ~0–20°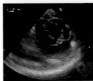

Figure 18.16: **TG basal SAX**

Level: Transgastric
Structures Visualized:
- Left ventricle (mid)
- Papillary muscles
- Right ventricle (mid)

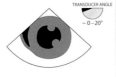 TRANSDUCER ANGLE ~0–20°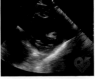

Figure 18.17: **TG mid papillary SAX**

Level: Transgastric
Structures Visualized:
- Left ventricle (apex)
- Right ventricle (apex)

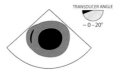 TRANSDUCER ANGLE ~0–20°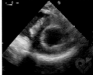

Figure 18.18: **TG apical SAX**

Level: Transgastric
Structures Visualized:
- Left ventricle (mid)
- Right ventricle (mid)
- Right ventricular outflow tract
- Tricuspid Valve (SAX)
- Pulmonary Valve

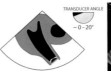 TRANSDUCER ANGLE ~0–20°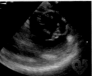

Figure 18.19: **TG RV basal view**

Level: Transgastric
Structures Visualized:
- Right atrium
- Right ventricle
- Right ventricular outflow tract
- Pulmonary valve
- Tricuspid Valve

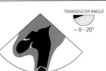 TRANSDUCER ANGLE ~0–20°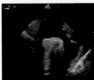

Figure 18.20: **TG RV inflow-outflow**

Level: Transgastric
Structures Visualized:
- Left ventricle
- Left ventricular outflow tract
- Right ventricle
- Aortic valve
- Aortic root
- Mitral Valve

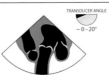 TRANSDUCER ANGLE ~0–20°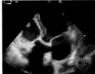

Figure 18.21: **Deep TG 5-chamber**

Level: Transgastric
Structures Visualized:
- Left ventricle
- Left atrium/appendage
- Mitral valve

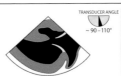 TRANSDUCER ANGLE ~90–110°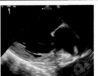

Figure 18.22: **TG 2-chamber**

Level: Transgastric
Structures Visualized:
- Right ventricle
- Right atrium
- Tricuspid valve

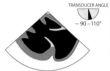 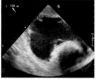

Figure 18.23: **TG RV inflow**

Level: Transgastric
Structures Visualized:
- Left ventricle
- Left ventricular outflow tract
- Right ventricle
- Aortic valve
- Aortic root
- Mitral valve

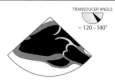 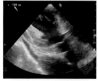

Figure 18.24: **TG LAX**

Aortic Views

Level: Transgastric to Mid-esophageal
Structures Visualized:
- Descending aorta
- Left thorax
- Hemiazygous and Azygous veins
- Intercostal arteries

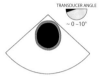 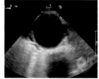

Figure 18.25: **Descending aorta SAX**

Level: Transgastric to Mid-esophageal
Structures Visualized:
- Descending aorta
- Left thorax

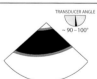 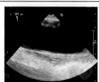

Figure 18.26: **Descending aorta LAX**

Level: Upper esophageal
Structures Visualized:
- Aortic arch
- Innominate vein
- Mediastinal tissue

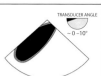 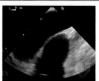

Figure 18.27: **UE aortic arch LAX**

Level: Upper esophageal
Structures Visualized:
- Aortic arch
- Innominate vein
- Pulmonary artery
- Pulmonary valve
- Mediastinal tissue

 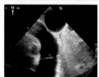

Figure 18.28: **UE aortic arch SAX**

18

Transesophageal Echocardiography / Aortic Views

Protocol for 3D TEE Echocardiography Image Acquisition

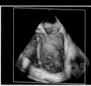

Figure 18.29: Left Ventricle

1. Obtain a view of the left ventricle from the 0°, 60°, or 120° mid-esophageal positions

2. Use the biplane mode to check that the left ventricle is centered in a second view 90° to the original.

3. Acquire using wide-angle, multi-beat mode

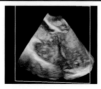

Figure 18.30: Right Ventricle

1. Obtain a view of the right ventricle from the 0° mid-esophageal position with the right ventricle tilted so that it is in the center of the image

2. Acquire using wide-angle, multi-beat mode

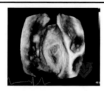

Figure 18.31: Interatrial Septum

1. 0° with the probe rotated to the interatrial septum

2. Acquire using narrow-angle, single-beat or wide-angle, multi-beat modes

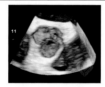

Figure 18.32: Aortic Valve

1. Obtain a view of the aortic valve from either the 60° mid-esophageal, long-axis view

2. Acquire using either the narrow-angle, single-beat or the wide-angle, multi-beat modes

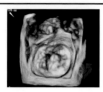

Figure 18.33: Mitral Valve

1. Obtain a view of the mitral valve from the 0°, 60°, 90°, or 120° mid-esophageal views

2. Use the biplane mode to check that the mitral valve annulus is centered with the acquisition plane in a second view 90° to the original.

3. Acquire using narrow-angle, single-beat mode

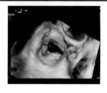

Figure 18.34: Tricuspid Valve

1. Obtain a view of the tricuspid valve from either the 0° to 30° mid-esophageal, 4-chamber view tilted so that the valve is centered in the imaging plane or the 40° transgastric view with anteflexion

2. Acquire using a narrow-angle, single-beat mode

3D Echocardiography
Rick Meece, ACS, RDCS, RCS, RCIS, FASE

Definition

3D echocardiography is used to improve a cardiac sonographer's ability to view, evaluate, measure, and manipulate visualization of the heart and inherent structures in 3D space from virtually any orientation for diagnostic enhancement in addition to the conventional 2D echocardiographic examination.

3D Matrix Array Transducer Architecture and Use

All 3D echocardiographic images are acquired in what is termed as "volumes" derived from thousands of voxels, which consist of a geometrically cubed area (cm³) compared to the flat 2D pixel in conventional echocardiography. 3D imaging is possible using both trans-thoracic (TTE) and trans-esophageal (TEE) matrix-array transducers, designed with orthogonally arranged multiple 2D scanning beams which enable such voxel-based reconstruction. Volumes or datasets may be acquired with limited region of interest (ROI), or "narrow angle" datasets, or a larger region inclusive of the majority of the heart, or "wide angle" datasets. Depth or Zoom capabilities are on most vendor cart options for image manipulation. Operating frequencies generally range between 2.5 to 5MHz, as high as 7MHz in transesophageal imaging modes. Temporal resolution for 3D images may be expressed as Volume or Voxel Rate or VR, synonymous with frame rate (MHz) in 2D echocardiography. Matrix-array 3D transducers are commonly used for simultaneous bi-planar (X-Plane) 2D imaging in two steerable orthogonal views, defaulted at primary 0 degrees, and orthogonal 90 degrees. When viewing and cropping 3DE images, the sonographer should remain aware they are viewing three-dimensional constructed objects on a two-dimensional screen or plane. On-cart image enhancing tools assist to overcome this reality with various rendering tools which affect perception of depth and tissue integrity, while highlighting variations or abnormalities. Advances in 3D visualization remains in evolution through simultaneous echo or CT images overlaid on fluoroscopy (Fusion).

Other emerging applications utilize software based virtual and augmented reality (AR) for future use in surgical and structural intervention in hybrid imaging procedural labs. Such tools and improvements have established transesophageal 3D echocardiography as essential, indeed in many procedures, a gold standard for primary imaging guidance during transcatheter device implantation as an adjunct to fluoroscopy.

Types or Modes of 3D Echocardiographic Imaging

Three primary 3D dataset acquisition modes are used and displayed on high definition 2D screens, each of which is chosen based on the region of interest (ROI) and the primary diagnostic purpose of the dataset being acquired:

Live 3D

Real-time or "Live" 3D imaging

- Used to widen and deepen structural visualization as compared to conventional 2DE.

- Using Live 3D imaging, a sonographer may easily narrow or widen the angle of viewing while adjusting both the depth and position of a dynamic voxel-based dataset.

- For more discrete regions, Live 3D may yield better overall spatial and temporal resolution than other Zoom approaches (described below) depending on the matrix beam depth and size of the ROI.

- As you widen the angle and depth of the voxels in live 3D mode to view a larger area, there will be deterioration of spatial and temporal image quality based on scan line density, requiring use of alternative higher resolution methods, depending on the primary goal of the 3D imaging.

3D Zoom

- 3D Zoom datasets

- Obtained as real-time or "live", but contain more specific and adjustable ROI using two 2D boxes as the pre-cropping guide (much like color flow) from two orthogonal views which are 90 degrees in variance.

- In Zoom imaging, voxels are literally magnified, with no change in density or "zoomed". When zoomed to fill the viewing screen, there is qualitative loss in detail as the viewing screen itself yields no change in resolution as the image is enlarged.

- The advantage is an increase in the overall flat screen area of visualization of the region for viewing structures and abnormalities more closely.

- 3D Zoom also has a capability of being acquired with multiple cardiac cycles which improves spatial and temporal resolution, particularly for TEE visualization for interventional planning.

- An alternative to using Live 3D Zoom imaging is to simply magnify the Live real-time 3D image, yielding similar visualization results, but inherently will not enlarge smaller regions as Zoom does, making them appear smaller on the viewing screen.

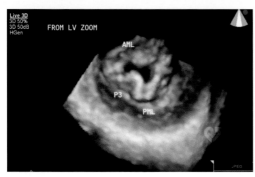

Figure 19.1: **Live 3D Zoom from a TTE examination of severe congenitally myxomatous mitral valve from left ventricular perspective. Labels of leaflet position were placed for assisting correct nomenclature in diagnostic viewing**

3D Full Volume

- A 3D "full volume" is collected using single or multiple cardiac cycles (with apnea), for the purpose of larger, if not complete, encapsulated regions of the heart containing some or all of the cardiac chambers, valves, and structures.

- Full volumes are most often used where Live 3D cannot obtain a large enough ROI without unacceptable loss in temporal and spatial resolution below a benchmark of diagnostic value.

- Full volumes are primarily used for accurate software-assisted 3D quantitation of chamber size and volume displacement (ejection fraction), yet to be investigated global strain, or with multi-plane reconstruction (MPR) to view multiple simultaneous 2D views or "cut-planes" (C-Planes).

- MPR skills are essential for appropriate alignment of the C-Planes to measure dimensions and areas of structures, similar to computed tomography (CT) or cardiac magnetic resonance imaging (CMRI).

- A specific 2D view or plane extracted from a full volume is often referred to as a "C-Plane" denoting a 2D cut plane from a 3D full volume.

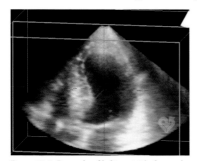

Figure 19.2: **Example of left ventricle focused 3D full volume obtained from 4-chamber view cropped at 50% of depth showing image gain balance and minimal attenuation, artifact, or fall-out.**

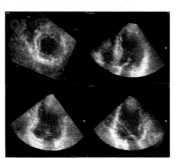

Figure 19.3: **Left ventricle 3D full volume MPR based 2D cut planes of Apical four, two, and 3-chamber views, with transverse SAX view at papillary level. This shows all regions of left ventricle are present within volume and all wall segments visualized. This demonstrates an optimal 3D volume for software-assisted quantitation of left ventricular volumes and functional derivatives.**

3D Echocardiography / Types or Modes of 3D Echocardiographic Imaging

Live 3D and Full Volume Color Doppler Datasets

• Until recent improvements in transducer beam former and processing speeds, useful 3D volumes containing Doppler color flow had limited diagnostic and prognostic value compared to 2D color Doppler due to very low temporal acquisition rates.

• New higher voxel rate (MHz or VR) capabilities using HVR (high volume rate) settings enable much higher VR dynamically during important flow cycles such as regurgitation. This enables identification and measurement of regurgitant jet origins in complex valvular disease, calculation and measurement of regurgitant vena contracta areas, and MPR based C-Plane visualization of color jets from the 3D dataset.

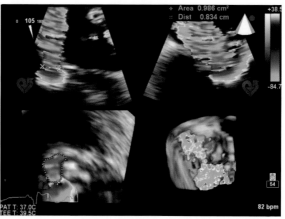

Figure 19.4: TEE 3D color flow volume of tricuspid regurgitation in MPR. Longitudinal planes of TR jet at upper left and right showing vena contracta dimension. The transverse C-plane across the TR vena contracta shows the measurement of VC area at lower left.

3D Echocardiography Scanning Protocols

The American Society of Echocardiography (ASE) has suggested appropriate 3D scanning approaches.

Focused or limited: The focused approach is a routine and productive protocol performed within a clinical TTE. Focused 3D exams may be generally appropriate with a primary purpose for specifically improved visualization of a valve (bicuspid aortic valve, mitral prolapse) or structure (masses, lesions) or software-assisted chamber quantitation involving the left ventricle, right ventricle, and left atrium.

Complete 3D evaluation: A complete 3D echo evaluation with images acquired from multiple windows is more commonly performed via TEE, and may involve multiple valves, the inter-atrial septum, and any of the cardiac chambers or vessels. In patients with established valve and/or functional pathology from a previous clinical TTE, the complete TEE based 3D examination provides more in-depth diagnostic value in conditions requiring consultation for potential of surgical or transcatheter intervention. Just as is the case with 2D TEE, 3D TEE images have high spatial clarity due to proximal internal access, enabling higher frequency imaging and less surrounding tissue attenuation and artifact.

2D Guided Acquisition of 3D Volumes

The architecture of 3D matrix-array transducers dictates some level of incremental sacrifice of scan line density compared to conventional 2D probes. However, these differences are largely addressed through modernized processing and re-design, which have generated increasingly small transducer footprint and improvement of scan line density. It remains true that a poor quality 2D image predicts likelihood of an even lower quality 3D image with little to no improvement in diagnostic value. Therefore the 2D examination is used as the sonographer's imaging benchmark in whether truly diagnostic 3D images may be obtained, and if they will add prognostic value to the examination.

Three useful steps have been suggested in the acquisition and use of 3D datasets, (1) optimization preceding collection, (2) acquisition according to technique (full volume, single vs. multi-cycle) and conditions (heart rhythm and respiration), and (3) rendering, cropping, or use of software assisted quantitation.

Successful acquisition of diagnostic 3D volumes should be achieved through observation and optimization of the initial 2D images using a systematic approach:

• Careful determination of a patient's highest quality acoustic windows based on what needs to be evaluated. Once discovered, images are improved with optimization tools in your 2D image balance (I-Scan, AutoScan, Tissue Equalization), finalizing the image balance with TGC and LGC regional adjustments.

• The patient's heart rhythm and heart rate will determine which acquisition approach will produce a useful 3D volume. If a rhythm is regular and 50-75 beats per minute, a higher resolution multi-cycle dataset should be acquired with good patient coaching and cooperation to maximize both spatial and temporal resolution. In the case of frequent atrial or ventricular extrasystoles or atrial fibrillation, most systems now have an option to acquire a single cycle dataset retrospectively at a setting enabling higher temporal rate combined with a slight decrease in spatial resolution. This same approach is also a likely consideration for patients who have a heart rate at ≥80 beats per minute where temporal rate is paramount.

• Effective use of breath hold apnea (rarely deep inspiration) with the patient is essential as a final step for the best quality image. Live 3D imaging, excessive respiration induces translational motion which distorts structures as they move within the fixed ultrasound beam. When obtaining a multi-cycle 3D volume for large chamber quantification, respiration will introduce stitching artifact between the 2-6 narrow angle volumes being obtained, rendering the dataset unusable for viewing or quantitation.

3D Echocardiography / 3D Echocardiography Scanning Protocols

Table 19.1: 3D Full Volume Acquisition Protocol

Step	Process	Pitfall	Solution
1	Observe electrocardiogram for regular rhythm	Ectopy, atrial fibrillation, low voltage	Reposition electrodes closer to heart; use single cycle high frame rate setting by vendor specification
2	Position patient, obtain best window for focused 3D image, practice breath arrest, attempt 4 cycle volume for chambers	Poor compliance, inadequate apnea	Consider use of lower or single cardiac cycle setting with higher temporal rate to decrease time of breath hold
3	Re-optimize your optimal acoustic window and use image balance tool per vendor specification	May require modified angulation (ie, lateral/apical) acoustic window to include entire ROI	Retain window which encompasses best 2D resolution
4	Adjust TGC/lateral gain compensation for final balance from near field to maximum depth	Apical or near field appears over gained or attenuated	Increase/Decrease TGC and LGC or move focal zone to ROI
5	Coach patient to remain motionless and maintain stable transducer scanning position – do not move scanning hand!	Moving hand or transducer position alters image balance and negates steps 3-5	Repeat steps 3-5
6	Go to full volume mode – use the initial 2D bi-plane views to validate complete region of interest will reside within 3D volume	Only part of ROI is in 90 degree orthogonal view	Incrementally adjust transducer position to put ROI within both windows. Re-optimization may be needed.
7	Set pre-acquisition full-volume to highest voxel rate obtainable based on rhythm and conditions	Use 1-4 cycle setting which yields >15 VR regardless of heart rate to ensure diagnostic value	IF VR >15MHz cannot be achieved based on chamber size and/or heart rate, diagnostic quality may be affected
8	Have patient perform appropriate breath arrest and acquire 3D image	Patient moves or breathes; stitching artifact noted in post cropping of volume dataset (if multi-cycle)	Rehearse acquisition and breath hold with patient, repeat attempt for 3D volume capture

ROI, Region of interest; TGC, time gain compensation; LGC, lateral gain compensation

Common Applications for Transthoracic 3D Echocardiography

Chamber Quantification

Left Ventricle

The left ventricle 3D full volume is the most commonly ordered or indicated focused imaging as an adjunct to the complete 2D echocardiogram. 3D echo based LV volumes have been validated against CMRI as a gold standard to have accuracy and significant prognostic value for patient evaluation, treatment, and serial study follow up. The purpose is for accurate measurement of left ventricular end-diastolic volume, end systolic volume, and ejection fraction. These are indicated by appropriateness criteria in patients with enlarged chambers, hypertrophic and idiopathic cardiomyopathies, valve regurgitation and stenosis, and decreased ejection fraction with ischemia induced regional wall motion abnormalities not well appreciated by conventional 2D Simpson's Bi-Plane calculation. A caveat of 3D images for software-assisted chamber quantification is that use of ultrasound contrast cannot be used in the majority of software programs due to infiltration of the agent into the myocardium, which interferes with the speckle-tracking mechanism of the software. Therefore, a 3D full volume of diagnostic value must be obtainable without the use of intra-venous LVO contrast enhancement.

Right Ventricle

Recently, the FDA has approved semi-automated and fully automated 3D echocardiography based right ventricular quantitation, and is available both on-cart and through PACS based offline software applications. Acquiring a 3D volume of the right ventricle is identical to any other chamber using the Table 19.1 approach, using a right ventricle focused imaging technique which centers the entire right ventricle within the sectors with no regard to other structures. The same attention in the use of MPR C-Planes to ensure all regions and walls are visualized should be followed.

Left Atrium

Measures of left atrial volumes may also be performed using 3D echocardiography. Acquisition techniques for 3D echo based left atrial size and volume displacement are identical to other chambers and these are commonly measured within the same dataset as a left ventricular capture with allowed depth to include the left atrium. Tissue enhancement of atrial walls and temporal resolution or VR remains important as incremental changes in left atrial size and compliance exist in a smaller chamber.

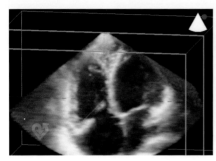 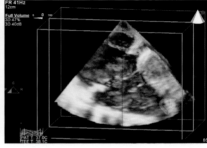

Figure 19.5: **Example of RV focused angulation for acquisition of TTE (left) and TEE (right) multi-cycle full volume datasets viewed with 50% depth cropping. Note the pre-acquisition image gain balance using TGC and LGC to enhance apical regions, bands and trebeculations where attenuation and fall-out are common.**

Cardiac Valves

Diagnostic and prognostic value of 3D TTE imaging of the cardiac valves as compared to the standard of care TEE in patients with significant pathology remains debatable and is largely associated with patients having very good acoustic windows. Because TTE imaging has more distance and variant angles from valves compared to TEE with most views from the ventricular side of valves, the common loss of spatial clarity on the pathology side of the valve structures often prevents diagnostic value beyond the 2D examination.

3D Imaging

If a concurrent 2D comprehensive valve examination reveals a significant disease, i.e., severe stenosis or regurgitation, this effectively demonstrated with the 2D and Doppler color flow images with enough information to indicate a complete 2D and 3D transesophageal examination at the referring or interpreting physician's discretion. Exceptions to this are patients who may be precluded from having a TEE anatomically, by personal choice, or other testing issues safely. Conversely, the 3D TTE imaging of the valve may be adequate to confirm a suspected sub-clinical pathology, such as less severe aortic valve stenosis with low gradients, bicuspid aortic valve pathology, masses, or mitral valve prolapse not requiring further investigation.

3D Color Flow

3D volume-based Doppler color flow datasets are becoming more commonly requested with an aim of capturing regurgitant jets in three dimensions for measurement of diameters, areas, and calculations. Usefulness of 3D color datasets are evaluated in a case by case basis regarding acoustic quality and adequate temporal resolution, ensuring the peak phase of color flow regurgitation is capable of being accurately evaluated.

Other Structures and Abnormalities

Any cardiac valve or structure may potentially be well seen or interrogated by 3D TTE imaging in patients exhibiting exceptional quality acoustic windows. If a particular valve, vessel, structure, mass, or defect appears well delineated in the 2D examination, even in the absence of other quality windows, using Live 3D imaging of the same structure may yield highly diagnostic images.

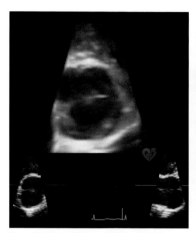

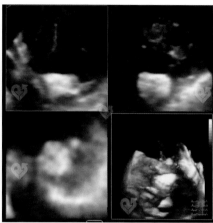

Figure 19.6: **Live 3D Zoom TTE viewing of a non-stenotic true two-leaflet bicuspid valve in a 27 year old patient not detected on outpatient 2D exam. Note only two commissures directly opposed from one another with two ovaloid sinuses of Valsalva.**

Figure 19.7: **calcific osseous mass imbedded within the mitral posterior annulus. This was suspected to be a myxoma until a 3D TTE full volume of the mass was viewed in MPR mode in dynamic motion.**

Common Applications for 3D Transesophageal Echocardiography

Complete 3D Examination

If significant pathology regarding a patient's welfare has been deemed a question large enough to warrant further echocardiographic evaluation, the sonographer may be assisting in a multitude of various 3D imaging approaches during TEE evaluation in order to view and perform measurements for surgical or interventional planning. The primary caveat in clinical TEE imaging is the inability to control or direct a moderately sedated patient's respirations. Any type of multi-cycle acquisition attempts will have to be observed and rehearsed to determine if they are obtainable in sedated conditions.

TEE 3D Imaging Modes

Depending on the level and number of combined pathologies, one or all of the imaging methods previously described may be used in different ways with specific purpose in the diagnostic flowchart, making for a more complete 3D examination. An example would be a patient with severe mitral valve prolapse, severe mitral regurgitation, left ventricular enlargement, reduced LVEF, left atrial enlargement, and combined question of the right ventricular size and function; all of which would be commonly present with longer term chronic mitral regurgitation from severe prolapse. In such a patient you might have an example algorithm:

Table 19.2: Use of Modalities and Diagnostic Applications	
TEE 3D zoom of mitral valve	Qualitative evaluation of valve and leaflets
TEE 3D zoom color flow	Location of MR jet(s)
TEE live 3D color flow	Size, depth, vena contracta of MR jet
TTE Full Volume of Left Ventricle	Measure size, volumes, EF%
TTE left atrium from full volume	Left atrial volume index
Live 3D of tricuspid valve with color flow	Measure TV annulus and TR vena contracta

Mitral Valve

The most common view for the mitral valve is the "surgeon's view" from 3D Zoom mode, from the same perspective seen during atriotomy from the left atrium with the commissures aligned horizontally and the aortic valve at 12 o'clock position above the anterior leaflet. While this can be acquired from any of the mid-esophageal angles, the 0 degree, or 4-chamber is used most in practice. Modern TEE transducers have fast processing, and a single cycle acquisition will suffice in most situations.

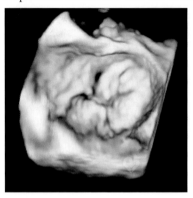

Figure 19.8: **Zoom of mitral valve oriented to the surgeon's view with significant prolapse of P-2 segment and associated A-3 and P-3 prolapse.**

Imaging protocol for TEE 3D Zoom Valve Acquisition

- Observe inherent rhythm and choose acquisition mode according to need or preference
- Have operator obtain 0 to 20 degree 4-chamber view with MV/TV centered in sector

- Optimize 2D image with balance between frequency and temporal rate
- Reduce supra-valvular speckles in atrium or over gain with TGC reduction
- Go to 3D Zoom mode and ensure entire valve apparatus is within the bi-plane views
- Select 3D Zoom Volume and ensure VR >14 (MHz)
- Adjust Gain and Compression to optimize image
- If Mitral, align and rotate to surgeon's view orientation
- Capture 3D Zoom volume dataset(s)

Uses of 3D imaging for the mitral valve will include MPR for mitral stenosis, leaflet pathology and length measurements, tenting heights and angles, and interventional guidance imaging.

Tricuspid Valve

The tricuspid valve is rapidly as high an interest as the mitral valve in a demand for comprehensive evaluation. This is partly due to the improved imaging and tools now available, and the overall morbidity correlation of right-sided failure as left heart failure and valvular disorder progresses. The location and tri-leaflet structure of the tricuspid valve demands the sonographer is familiar with bi-plane, 3D Zoom, and Live 3D imaging techniques, as any may apply best depending on cardiac orientation, rotation, and level of pathology.

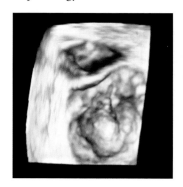 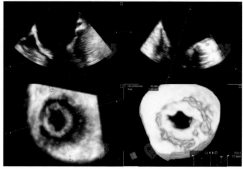

Figure 19.9: On left, a 3D Zoom of mitral valve with severe prolapse and flail chordae of a highly diseased P2 mitral leaflet segment. Oblique orientations as this often lend improved visualization. On right, a multi-planar reconstruction (MPR) of a 3D Zoom mitral valve and apparatus for measurement of the valve at leaflet tips for mitral valve area planimetry. The planes are placed at the mitral leaflet edges in the two upper planes level and then traced in the lower left SAX view where measures could be performed.

3D Echocardiography / Common Applications for 3D Transesophageal Echocardiography

Aortic Valve

TEE based 3D imaging of the aortic valve is a standard of care evaluation in patients with suspected or known severe aortic disease, and especially stenosis. While most information is obtained with the clinical TTE and Doppler information, 3D TEE images more clearly confirm the morphology of the valve leaflets, leaflet motion, improve visualization of regurgitant AR jet origins and direction. Many institutions use of MPR from a 3D Zoom volume to perform measurement of key structures and areas for sizing for transcatheter aortic valve replacement (TAVR) devices in some patients.

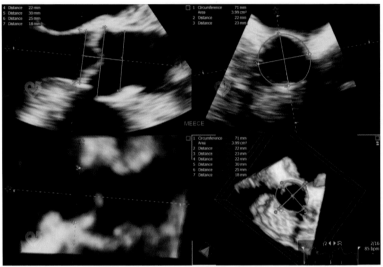

Figure 19.10: **View of a LAX orientation and acquisition of 3D Zoom of a stenotic aortic valve in MPR alignment. Note measures of LVOT diameter, sinus, sino-tubal junction (STJ), and area of LVOT annulus. This technique is used in some higher volume centers for patients who are not candidates for CT angiography with contrast due to renal failure for TAVR sizing.**

Pulmonic Valve

Pulmonic leaflets are quite thin, and often difficult to clearly image with either 2D or 3D imaging in the absence of pathology. As with any structure or mass, if present, there is always a potential for improvement in visualizing various pathologies using Live 3D imaging. Live 3D of the RVOT and infundibulum can be helpful in measurement of the RVOT diameter or area, as well as dynamic observation of infundibular hypertrophic disease combined with Doppler imaging.

The Left Atrial Appendage (LAA)

LAA is also commonly appreciated with 3D imaging due to transcatheter intervention using left atrial appendage occlusion devices. The LAA size and morphology is visualized, and MPR used to align planes along the very complex shape in order to measure for sizing of the device chosen for implantation.

Table 19.3: Applications for 3D Echocardiography				
	TTE	TEE	Common 3D Image Type	Emerging Use
Left Ventricle				
Volumes	X	X	Full	3D GLS
Shape or Deformation	X		Full	Torsion, Twist
Ejection Fraction	X	X	Full	
LV Mass	X	X	Full	Vendor Dependent
Right Ventricle				
Volume	X	X	Full	Strain
Shape or Deformation				n/a
Ejection Fraction	X	X	Full	
Left Atrium				
Volume	X		Full	
Mitral Valve Assessment				
Anatomy	X	X	Zoom	3D Models
Stenosis	***	X	Zoom	
Regurgitation	***	X	X	
Tricuspid Valve Assessment				
Anatomy	X	X	FV, Zoom	Intervention
Stenosis	X	X	FV, Zoom	
Regurgitation	***	X	All Modes	3D Color VC area
Pulmonic Valve Assessment				
Anatomy	***	X	Live, Zoom	Intervention
Stenosis				
Regurgitation				
Aortic Valve Assessment				
Anatomy	X	X		
Stenosis	X	X		TAVR
Regurgitation	***			X
Infective Endocarditis	X	X		X
Prosthetic Valves			Live, Zoom	TAVR ViV
Guidance of Transcatheter Procedures*		X	Live, Zoom	e.g., Mitraclip, LAA, TAVR

*** Limitations in spatial and temporal resolution for image and Doppler may affect diagnostic value

3D Echocardiography / Common Applications for 3D Transesophageal Echocardiography

Speckle Tracking Echocardiography Strain Imaging

Jeffrey C. Hill, BS, ACS, FASE

The American Society of Echocardiography and the European Association of Cardiovascular Imaging Industry Task Force established nomenclature and definitions in the effort to create a common standard for two dimensional (2D) strain imaging.[1] 2D global longitudinal strain (GLS) is now an integral part of the comprehensive echocardiogram, with its primary application in myopathic diseases and in patients undergoing chemotherapy.

Fundamentals of Strain and Myocardial Mechanics

Strain describes the deformation of an object. For instance, the linear strain can be defined as the ratio of the change in length (ΔL) to its original length (L_0), as shown in the equation below.

$$\text{Strain (\%)} = \frac{L - L_0}{L_0} = \frac{\Delta L}{L_0}$$

Lo = original length; L = current length; ΔL = change in length

Strain is a dimensionless quantity with no unit, and often expressed as a percentage by multiplying the value by 100%. The sign of strain reflects the state of the deformation, in a linear case, tension, or compression. For example, as shown in the equation below, a negative strain value (-20%) indicates a decrease in length from 10 to 8 and the compression of an object from either the circumferential (short) or the meridional (long) axis.

$$\text{Strain (\%)} = \frac{8 - 10}{10} = \frac{-2}{10} = -0.2 \times 100 = -20\%$$

Strain, the deformation of an object, can be related to stress, which is the internal force experienced by the object. The relationship between strain and stress is compliance.[2] Given a certain level of tissue compliance, as wall stress increases, the strain increases accordingly.[3,4]

Speckle Tracking Echocardiography

Speckle tracking echocardiography (STE) is a method in which the ultrasound speckles (i.e., motion of the kernel) are tracked over time. Speckles are contained within the gray scale image and are created by the interference patterns that are generated by the reflected ultrasound.[1] Speckles are relatively stable allowing for tracking of myocardial motion, and the randomness of the speckle pattern allows for differentiation of the regional displacement. The region of speckles being tracked in a single frame is called the kernel.[2] The kernel represents the signature pattern of the reflected ultrasound and can be tracked frame by frame throughout the cardiac cycle *(Figure 20.1)*.

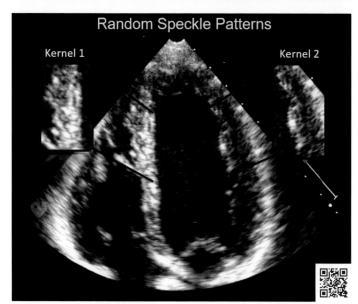

Figure 20.1: **Example of two kernels demonstrating the differences and randomness of the speckle patterns. Note the speckle patterns are completely different from one another allowing for regional tracking frame by frame throughout the cardiac cycle.** [2]

Fiber Architecture Shortening and Thickening

Due to the complex tethering and coordination, majority of the contribution of myocardial shortening is generated from the mid-myocardial and sub-endocardium with less contribution at the sub-epicardial level. Because of the angle of insonation between the ultrasound beam and the myocardium, the speckle pattern of the circumferential fibers at the mid-wall in the apical 4-chamber view and the true apex in the parasternal short axis view can be seen *(Figure 20.2)*. [4] During ventricular systole, the cardiac muscle undergoes cross-fiber shortening of the sub-epicardial wall (oblique), mid wall (circumferential) and sub-endocardium (longitudinal) to create overall "thickening" and contraction *(Figure 20.3)*. [4]

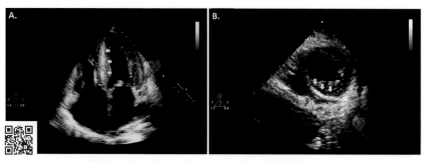

Figure 20.2: **Bright reflectors of the mid-wall circumferential fibers visualized along the inferoseptal wall (3 arrows) in the apical 4-chamber view (A). These reflectors can also be seen at the true apex (3 arrows) in the parasternal short axis view (B). This is due to the increased amplitude of the circumferential fibers that is created when rough surfaces are relatively orthogonal to the ultrasound beam.** [4]

| Sub-epicardial
Oblique Fibers | Mid-wall
Circumferential Fibers | Sub-endocardial
Longitudinal Fibers |

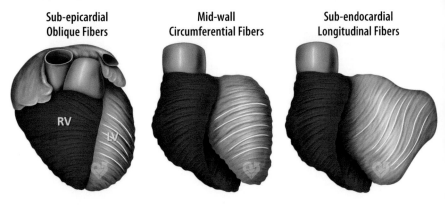

Figure 20.3: **Normal myocardial fiber architecture of the LV. Note the dramatic change in the direction of the fiber pattern between the three levels of the myocardium (white striations).**

STE Strain Imaging

There are three directional strains that can be measured by 2D STE. *(Figure 20.4)*:

- **Longitudinal strain** is measured from the apical views. The overall shortening at the endocardium can be measured *(Figure 20.5)*. The combined apical 4, 3, 2 chamber strains are averaged to calculate the global longitudinal strain (GLS) *(Figure 20.6)*. Normal GLS values ranges from -17 to -26%. [6] *(Table 20.1)*

- **Circumferential strain** is measured from the parasternal short axis. The overall shortening at the mid-wall can be measured *(Figure 20.8)*.

- **Radial strain** is also measured from the parasternal short axis. Combined shortening of the epicardial, longitudinal, and circumferential fibers creates overall thickening that can be measured *(Figure 20.9)*. Temporal relationship between contraction, strain and relaxation of the LV is described in Figure 20.10.

Longitudinal Strain (ε_l)

Shortening $\updownarrow$

Circumferential Strain (ε_c)

Shortening $\searrow \nearrow$

Radial Strain (ε_r)

Thickening $\longleftrightarrow$

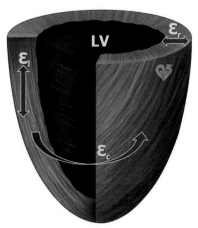

Figure 20.4: **Three directional strains (longitudinal, circumferential, radial) of the LV.**

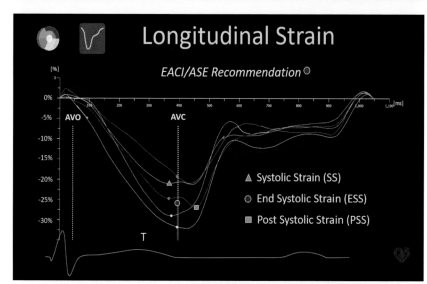

Figure 20.5: **Example of normal longitudinal strains obtained from the apical 4-chamber view. There are generally three peak strains that can be measured; systolic strain (SS) occurring when the heart is contracting during aortic valve opening (AVO) to aortic valve closure (AVC); end systolic strain (ESS) at AVC and; post systolic strain (PSS) occurring after AVC into early diastole. For consistency, the EACI/ASE recommends measuring ESS (red circle).** [1]

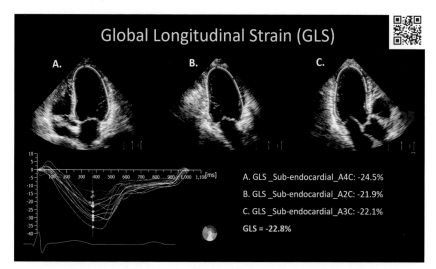

Figure 20.6: **Sub-endocardial peak systolic longitudinal strain for the calculation of global longitudinal strain (GLS) obtained from the apical 4-chamber (A), apical 2-chamber (B) and apical 3-chamber (C) views. An average of the peak strains (colored dots on the waveforms) from the three views allow for calculation of GLS. The GLS in this patient was -22.8%. In addition, the 18 segment bullseye can be constructed from the corresponding peak strains.** *(Figure 20.7)*

20

Speckle Tracking Echocardiography Strain Imaging

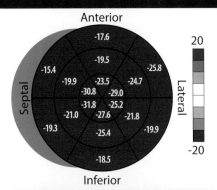

Figure 20.7: **GLS bullseye (18 segments)** representing peak systolic longitudinal strain values from the base, mid and apex from the apical 2, 3, and 4 chamber views. Deep red color in any given segment typically demonstrates normal strain values.

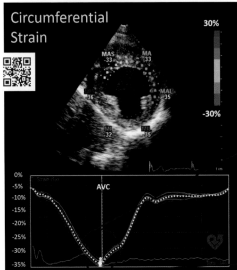

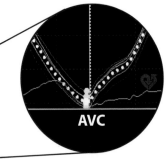

Figure 20.8: **Circumferential strain obtained from the parasternal short axis view at the level of the papillary muscles in a normal subject. Like the normal longitudinal strain example in Figure 20.5, observe how well synchronized the LV is, as the peak waveforms occur at aortic valve closure (AVC). Peak ave. circumferential is -34%.**

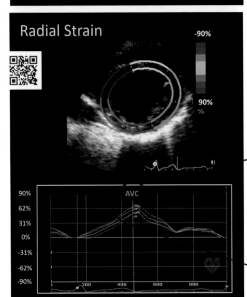

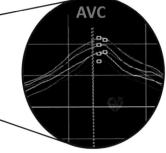

Figure 20.9: **Radial strain obtained from the parasternal short axis view at the level of the papillary muscles in a normal subject. Like the normal example in Figure 20.8 observe how well synchronized the thickening is, as the peaks strains (squares) are aligned. Importantly, timing of peak strains occur just after AVC. Peak ave. radial strain is 53%.**

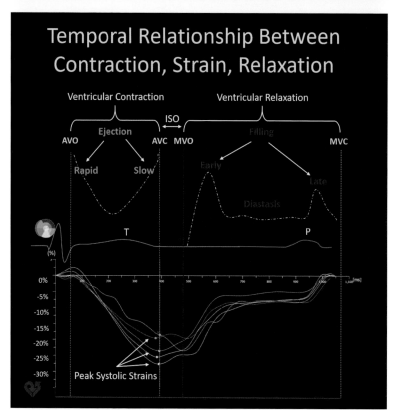

Temporal Relationship Between Contraction, Strain, Relaxation

Figure 20.10: **Relationship between contraction, strain and relaxation.** At the beginning of ventricular contraction the aortic valve opens (AVO), early rapid ejection occurs, followed by myocardial contraction. Note the strain waveforms begin to increase. Peak ejection occurs on or about the T wave on the ECG and begins to slow thereafter. At this point regional contraction is translated to peak strain. Peak systolic strain occurs before and at (white arrows below) aortic valve closure (AVC). Once the aortic valve closes, the myocardium begins to lengthen during the isovolumic relaxation (ISO) period prior to mitral valve opening (MVO). At the point of MVO the myocardium has completed most of its relaxation (i.e., untwisting). Note the strain waveforms begin to rapidly decrease and plateau at the point of diastasis. The strain waveforms return back to the zero baseline as filling is completed at the end of the P wave on the ECG with subsequent mitral valve closure (MVC). See Figure 20.5 for further description of peak strain and event timing.

Table 20.1: Normal GLS Ranges by Gender and Race				
	White	**Black**	**Asian**	**Other**
Male				
GLS %	-17 to -24	-17 to -25	-17 to -25	-18 to -24
Female				
GLS %	-18 to -26	-18 to -26	-18 to -26	-18 to -25

Table 20.1: Normal global longitudinal strain (GLS) in different gender and race representing the 95 percentile of the overall population. GLS values vary significantly and are highest in females. Information adapted and modified from: Asch et al., *J Am Soc Echocardiogr.* 2019. [6]

Clinical Application of STE Strain Imaging

Clinical application of GLS may include:

- Global assessment of systolic function
- Subclinical disease (e.g., chemotherapy, amyloidosis, Friedreich ataxia, hypertrophic cardiomyopathy, left ventricular hypertrophy, ventricular noncompaction, arrhythmogenic RV cardiomyopathy)
- Ventricular function pre- and post- congenital heart disease repair (e.g., tetralogy of Fallot)
- Ventricular function pre- and post- valve repair/replacement
- Coronary artery disease (e.g., acute ischemic myocardium, stunned myocardium, viable myocardium)

Technical Tips

Sonographer's systematic approach to the acquisition of STE strain imaging:

- Review the prior study including the strain bullseye and GLS values
- Same cardiac sonographer performing strain throughout patient treatment
- Same ultrasound system and importantly strain software
- Optimize the 2D frame rate of at least 40 fps
- Minimize foreshortening of the 2D images
- Optimize the 2D depth required for the strain software
- Obtain blood pressure at the time of 2D image acquisition
- Acquire 2D images during shallow breathing or apnea
- Carefully inspect the strain waveforms and tracking
- Acquire at least 2 cardiac cycles and average the GLS

References

1. Voigt J.-U., Pedrizzetti G., Lysyansky P., Marwick T.H., Houle H., Baumann R, et al. Definitions for a common standard for 2D speckle tracking echocardiography: Consensus document of the EACVI/ASE/industry task force to standardize deformation imaging. J Am Soc Echocardiogr 2015;28:183-93.

2. Basic concepts. Motion and deformation. Stoylen. [n.d.]. Retrieved from http://folk.ntnu.no/stoylen/strainrate/Basic_concepts.htmL

3. Murai D, Yamada S, Hayashi T, et al. Relationships of left ventricular strain and strain rate to wall stress and their afterload dependency. Heart and Vessels. 2017;32(5):574–583. doi:10.1007/s00380-016-0900-4.

4. Mor-Avi V, Lang RM, Badano LP, et al. Current and evolving echocardiographic techniques for the quantitative evaluation of cardiac mechanics: ASE/EAE consensus statement on methodology and indications endorsed by the Japanese Society of Echocardiography. Eur J Echocardiogr. 2011;12(3):167–205. doi:10.1093/ejechocard/jer021

5. Ho SY, Nihoyannopoulos P. Anatomy, echocardiography, and normal right ventricular dimensions. Heart. 2006;92 Suppl 1(Suppl 1):i2–i13. doi:10.1136/hrt.2005.077875

6. Asch FM, Miyoshi T, Addetia K, et al. Similarities and Differences in Left Ventricular Size and Function among Races and Nationalities: Results of the World Alliance Societies of Echocardiography Normal Values Study. J Am Soc Echocardiogr. 2019;32(11):1396-1406.e2. doi:10.1016/j.echo.2019.08.012

Cardiac Transplantation
Sue Phillip, RCS, FASE

Indications

The ACC/AHA guidelines include the following indications:

- Refractory cardiogenic shock requiring intra-aortic balloon pump counter-pulsation or left ventricular assist device (LVAD)
- Cardiogenic shock requiring continuous intravenous inotropic therapy
- Peak VO2 (VO2max) less than 10mL/Kg per min
- NYHA class of II or IV despite maximized medical and resynchronization therapy
- Recurrent life-threatening left ventricular arrhythmias despite an implantable cardiac defibrillator, antiarrhythmic therapy, or cather-based ablation
- End-stage congenital heart disease with no evidence of pulmonary hypertension
- Refractory angina without potential medical or surgical therapeutic options.

Absolute Contraindications

- Systemic illness with limited life expectancy
- Irreversible pulmonary hypertension
- Clinically severe symptomatic cerebrovascular disease
- Active substance abuse (drug, tobacco, or alcohol)
- Inadequate social support or cognitive-behavioral disability
- Multisystem disease with severe extracardiac dysfunction

Surgical Technique

- **Orthotopic (biatrial or bicaval)** — The recipient's heart is excised and the donor heart is placed in the correct anatomical position (most common)
- **Heterotopic ("piggyback")** — The donor heart is placed in the right chest alongside the recipient organ and anastomosed in a way to allow blood to pass through either or both hearts

Complications

- Acute cellular rejection (ACR) rejection (endomyocardial biopsy for monitoring, performed under fluoroscopic or echocardiography)
- Cardiac allograft vasculopathy (CAV)
- Side effects of immunosuppression therapy
- Right ventricular (RV) failure immediate post-transplant period
- Silent myocardial infarction (due to denervation)

Electrocardiogram

- Sinus rate >80 bpm in the denervated heart
- Conduction disturbances
- Supraventricular arrhythmias

2D

- 1 month post-op, increase in left ventricular mass and wall thickness, resolves after 3 months
- LVEF normalizes soon after transplant
- Decreased LVEF within the first year is a predictor for rejection or CAV
- May see paradoxical septal motion, post-op
- Biatrial enlargement with biatrial technique, may see suture lines
- Bicaval technique-may have a smaller right atrial size initially, large left atrium
- Right Ventricular systolic dysfunction
- Right atrial and right ventricular enlargement are common findings
- Post-biopsy, assess
- Tricuspid valve function, and assess for pericardial effusion
- Abnormal diastolic filling patterns, may also be due to other factors
- Doppler indices of mitral inflow are limited for detecting ACR

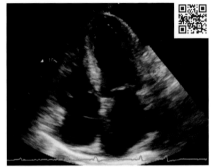

Figure 21.1: **Endomyocardial biopsy under echo guidance**

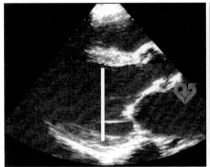

Figure 21.2: **Reduced global left ventricular systolic function pre-cardiac transplant**

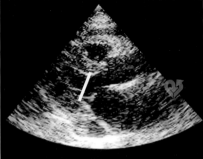

Figure 21.3: **Improved global left ventricular systolic function post-cardiac transplant**

Color Flow Doppler

- Tricuspid Regurgitation following endomyocardial biopsy

Tissue Doppler

- Early after transplant, LV e' and s' velocities are low and recover gradually.
- A systolic wall motion velocity of <10cm/s indicates a high likelihood of CAV
- Isovolumetric relaxation time <90ms, peak velocity may indicate ACR

Strain

- Lower LV Global Longitudinal Strain (GLS) and RV free wall strain
- Reduction of LV torsion of >25% from baseline may predict ACR

Stress Echo

- Exercise stress, low sensitivity due to the denervated transplanted heart to reach target heart rates
- Dobutamine Stress Echocardiography, moderate sensitivity for detecting angiographically significant CAV

Endomyocardial Biopsy with Echo Guidance

- Identify bioptome at the tip as it enters the right atrium and right ventricle *(Figure 21.1)*
- Clear view of the RV and the septum
- Complications: RV perforation, pericardial effusion, damage to the tricuspid valve chordae or valve. Right bundle branch block.

21

Cardiac Transplantation

Miscellaneous
David Adams, ACS, RCS, RDCS, FASE
Brigid Culey, BS, RDCS, FASE

22 Acquired Immune Deficiency Syndrome (AIDS)

Definition

The occurrence of immune deficiency in previously healthy individuals. Human immunodeficiency virus (HIV) is believed to be the etiology of acquired immune deficiency syndrome (AIDS). It destroys the essential conductor of the immune system—the CD4+ T cells.

Echo/Doppler

• Pericardial effusion is most common. Evaluate for cardiac tamponade/ constrictive pericarditis (up to 82%)

• Myocarditis (up to 52%)

• Dilated cardiomyopathy ("HIV heart muscle disease")

• Isolated right ventricular global systolic dysfunction

• Pulmonary hypertension

• Malignant infiltration (Karposi's sarcoma) (39%)

• Infective (marantic/NBTE) endocarditis (10%) (may suggest intravenous drug abuse)

• Valvular regurgitation (e.g., mitral, tricuspid)

The Aging Heart

Definition

Normal changes in cardiac structure due to aging.

Echo/Doppler

The expected cardiac changes include:

• Mitral annular calcification (hallmark finding)

• Fibrocalcific papillary muscle(s) changes (anterolateral papillary muscle greater than posteromedial papillary muscle)

• Thickened mitral valve leaflets

• Smaller mitral valve annulus dimension

• Aortic valve calcification/stenosis

• Sigmoid interventricular septum

• Left ventricular hypertrophy (normal IVSd and LVPWd: men 0.6 to 1.0cm; women 0.6cm to 0.9cm)

• Increased left ventricular mass index (normal LV Mass Index: men 49 to 115g/m^2; women 43 to 95g/m^2)

- Increased left atrial dimension
- Increased subepicardial fat
- Focal amyloid deposition in the myocardium/epicardium (>80 years of age)
- Decreased stroke volume
- Decreased cardiac output/cardiac index
- Preserved/slightly increased left ventricular ejection fraction
- Decrease (20%) in longitudinal shortening of the left ventricle (descent of the base) with an increase in systolic minor axis dimension (18%)
- Decreased aortic peak flow velocity, aortic average acceleration time, aortic velocity time interval (due to increased aortic root diameter)
- Atrioventricular valve regurgitation (e.g., mitral)
- Increased pulmonary artery systolic pressure
- Hypertensive hypertrophic cardiomyopathy (may be genetically determined)
- Progressive increase in mitral valve A velocity with a decrease in the mitral valve E/A ratio with increased isovolumic relaxation time
- Progressive decrease in the mitral annular TDI e' peak velocity, an increase in TDI a' velocity, a decrease in the e'/a' ratio and an increase in the TDI E/e' velocity ratio

Ankylosing Spondylitis

Definition

An autoimmune disease characterized by inflammation of the vertebral and sacroiliac joints.

Echo/Doppler

- Aortitis of the ascending aorta (dilatation of aortic annulus, sinus of Valsalva), aortic valve thickening, aortic valve prolapse, increased echogenicity of posterior aortic wall
- Subaortic bump at the base of the aortic valve non-coronary cusp (localized thickening of the anterior mitral valve base)
- Mitral valve prolapse
- Aortic or mitral regurgitation
- Left ventricular global systolic dysfunction
- Left ventricular diastolic dysfunction

Anomalous Origin of the Left Coronary Artery from the Pulmonary Artery

Echo/Doppler

- Left ventricular dilatation with global and segmental left ventricular systolic dysfunction

- Dilated right coronary artery best seen in the parasternal short-axis view of the aortic valve
- Left to right shunt entering the pulmonary artery distal to the pulmonary valve
- Mitral regurgitation

Aortic Atherosclerotic Plaques

Definition

- Atheroma located in the thoracic aorta which may represent a source of embolism.

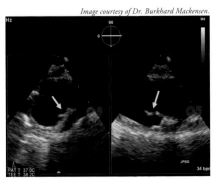

Image courtesy of Dr. Burkhard Mackensen.

Echo/Doppler

- Best observed with transesophageal echocardiography
- May be visualized in suprasternal, apical, subcostal views
- May present as atherosclerotic changes such as aortic wall calcification, thickening, ulceration, mural thrombi or atheromatous debris

Figure 22.1: TEE Biplane image of the transverse aortic arch showing atheroma (arrows)

- A plaque with a thickness of ≥4mm in ascending aorta/aortic arch; ≥5mm in descending thoracic aorta may indicate a risk group for an embolic event
- Pedunculated, (protruding, mobile debris) may represent an increased risk for embolism

Grading System for Severity of Aortic Atherosclerosis

- **Grade 1:** Intima thickness <2mm
- **Grade 2:** Mild – (focal or diffuse) intimal thickening 2 to 3mm
- **Grade 3:** Moderate – Atheroma >3 to 5mm (no mobile or ulcerated components)
- **Grade 4:** Severe – Atheroma >5mm (no mobile/ulcerated components)
- **Grade 5:** Complex – Grade 2, 3, 4 atheroma plus mobile or ulcerated components
- Careful evaluation of the aorta is important especially ascending aorta prior to cross clamping and cannulation of the aorta in cardiopulmonary bypass

Aortic Valve Prolapse (AVP)

Definition

AVP is defined as the downward displacement of one or more aortic valve leaflets below a line joining the points of attachment of the aortic valve leaflets

Echo/Doppler

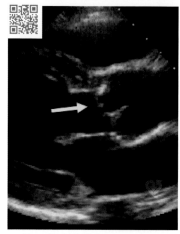

- AVP is best evaluated in the parasternal long-axis view
- The leaflets have a thick, redundant look with preserved systolic excursion
- Aortic regurgitation is the expected cardiac Doppler finding for aortic valve prolapse and may be significant

Figure 22.2: **PLAX showing prolapse (arrow) of the right coronary cusp (RCC) into the LVOT**

- AVP is most commonly associated with bicuspid aortic valve
- AVP has been associated with aortic root dilatation, infective endocarditis, mitral valve prolapse, tricuspid valve prolapse, perimembranous ventricular septal defect, severe mitral regurgitation

Aortic Valve Sclerosis

Definition

- Aortic valve sclerosis represents a degenerative process which occurs primarily in the elderly (up to 29% greater than 65 years of age). The etiologies include valvular stress, a primary degenerative process, or generalized atherosclerosis.

- May be a marker for increased risk of myocardial infarction, angina pectoris, heart failure, stroke and death.

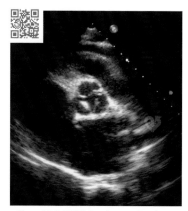

- May progress to significant aortic valve stenosis especially in the following: smokers, hypercholestermia, elevated serum creatinine and increased calcium levels.

Figure 22.3: **PSAX showing aortic valve thickening**

Echo/Doppler

- Thickened aortic valve leaflets with preserved systolic excursion
- Valve thickening may be localized, nodular or diffuse
- Can be categorized as:
  - Mild: valve thickness <4mm

22

Miscellaneous / Aortic Valve Prolapse (AVP)

- Moderate: 4 to 6mm
- Severe: >6mm
- Velocity across aortic valve is ≤2.5 m/s

22 Arrhythmogenic Right Ventricular Cardiomyopathy (ARVC)

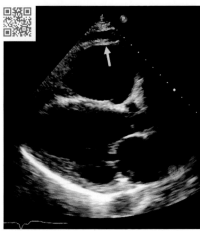

Figure 22.4: **PLAX showing a dilated RV & thin RV free wall (arrow) in a patient with ARVC**

Definition

- A right ventricular cardiomyopathy characterized by the fibrofatty sporadic/familial replacement of myocardium of the right ventricle.
- Affects young males (less than 50 years of age) associated with LBBB, ventricular tachycardia, syncope, thromboembolic events, heart failure, sudden death.
- May be referred to as arrhythmogenic RV dysplasia (ARVD)

Echo/Doppler

- Right ventricular dilatation, aneurysm, focal wall thinning, trabecular derangement/prominence, hyperreflective moderator band
- Right ventricular outflow tract dilatation (>30mm) (most common)
- Right ventricular segmental wall motion abnormalities in the absence of coronary artery disease
- Increased echogenicity of the affected area
- Left ventricular involvement (rare)
- Tricuspid regurgitation peak velocity <2.0 m/s (due to reduced ventricular systolic function)
- Contrast agents may be useful (e.g., Optison, Definity, Lumason)

Athlete's Heart

Definition

The differentiation of physiologic and pathologic changes in the athlete's heart is difficult to assess and may be confused with hypertrophic cardiomyopathy (HCM). These changes vary depending on the sport, level of training intensity and sex of the athlete.

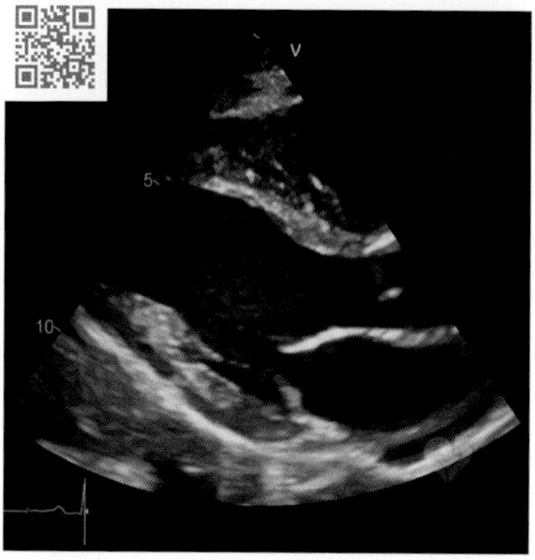

Figure 22.5: **PLAX of a typical athlete's heart showing mild LVH**

Echo/Doppler

- Dynamic exercise (e.g., running, skiing, soccer) generally will have large LV diastolic cavity dimension and increased wall thickness (eccentric hypertrophy), increased RV dimensions, increased IVC dimension

- Isometric (static) sports (e.g., weight lifting, wrestling, gymnasts) have higher values for wall thickness relative to cavity dimension (concentric LVH)

- Track sprinting, diving, field weight training events are at the lower end of the spectrum for cardiac adaptations to athletic training

- Female athletes have a smaller LV diastolic cavity dimension and wall thickness than male athletes training in the same sport

- It is believed that LV wall thickness seldom exceeds the normal limits of >1.3cm no matter the sport

- A posterior wall thickness of >16mm may indicate HCM

- Evaluate for hypertrophic cardiomyopathy, dilated cardiomyopathy, RV dysplasia (e.g., Uhl's anomaly, ARVC), coronary artery abnormalities, anabolic steroids (significant hypertrophy), premature coronary artery disease

- Cessation of exercise (for 6 to 8 weeks) causes a 2 to 5mm regression in wall thickness in athletic LVH but not in hypertrophic cardiomyopathy (reliable finding)

- Diastolic function may be enhanced in athletes in order to maintain stroke volume with increased heart rate.

- Typically bradycardic at rest (40-60 bpm)

Table 22.1: Normal Cardiac Dimensions in Athletic Individuals			
	Endurance-Trained Athletes	Combined Endurance and Strength-Trained Athletes	Strength-Trained Athletes
LVIDd (mm)	53.7	56.2	52.1
LVPWd (mm)	10.3	11.0	11.0
RWT	0.389	0.398	0.442
LVM (g)	249	288	267

From Pluim BM, Zwinderman AH, van der Laarse A, et al. Correlation of heart rate variability with cardiac functional and metabolic variables in cyclists with training induced left ventricular hypertrophy. Heart 1999;81:612-617

Table 22.2: Proposed Abnormal Findings in Athlete's Heart
• Left ventricular end-diastolic dimension >6.0cm
• Left ventricular end-diastolic wall thickness >1.3cm (rarely >1.7cm)
• IVSd to LVPWd ratio >1.5
• Concentric/eccentric remodeling (measured as LVPWd x 2/LVIDd ≥0.45 represents concentric remodeling; <0.30 represents eccentric remodeling)
• Left atrial dilatation
• Abnormal transmitral flow velocity (abnormal diastolic function)
• Mitral septal annular TDI e' <7cm/s
• Global longitudinal peak systolic strain is usually closer to normal than a true HCM.

Atrial Fibrillation

Definition

Atrial fibrillation is caused by multiple atrial ectopic foci. There is no well defined P wave, the QRS complex is normal although the ventricular rate is usually irregular.

Echo/Doppler

• Evaluate for etiology (e.g., mitral valve disease, cardiomyopathy, congenital heart disease)

• Determine:

• Presence of tachycardia induced dilated cardiomyopathy

- Left atrial dimension, area and volume

- Presence of atrial thrombus in the left atrium and left atrial appendage utilizing harmonics and multiple views (e.g., parasternal short-axis of the aortic valve, apical 2-chamber view) (TEE is preferred examination)

- Mitral valve E wave peak velocity, mitral valve deceleration time (the deceleration time should only be measured if the E velocity ends by the onset of the QRS complex) and TDI of the mitral valve annulus for evaluation of diastolic function

- E/e' septal ≥11 suggests increased filling pressures

- TV TDI S' <9cm/s and/or TV TDI septal e' <7 may predict increase risk for cardiac events in patients with HF and atrial fibrillation
- Left atrial appendage velocity (normal 46 ± 18cm/s) reduced (26.5 ± 19.6cm/s) in atrial fibrillation (TEE preferred examination)

• Pulmonary venous flow will demonstrate absent pulmonary vein A wave and blunted S wave

• Heart failure, systemic hypertension, previous thromboembolism, left ventricular systolic dysfunction, increased left atrial size, reduced left atrial appendage peak velocity (<20cm/s), dense left atrial spontaneous contrast ("smoke"), complex aortic atherosclerotic plaque are associated with increased risk of thromboembolism.

• TEE useful in ablation including evaluation of the pulmonary veins, left atrial appendage flow velocities, atrial septal puncture guidance, ensuring firm electrode-endocardial contact, detection of complications, monitoring effective atrial contraction

Chagas Disease (Trypanosoma Cruzi)

Definition

The initial infection with Trypanosoma occurs when young adults are bit, usually around the eye, by a reduviid bug. Approximately 1% develop acute myocarditis and pericarditis. The major cardiac manifestations of Chagas disease occur approximately 20 years after the initial infection and is present in 30% of the infected subjects. Cardiomegaly, heart failure, arrhythmias, thromboembolism, right bundle branch block and sudden death may occur.

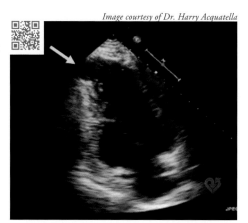

Image courtesy of Dr. Harry Acquatella

Figure 22.6: **Apical 2-chamber view of a focal aneurysm (arrow) in a patient with Chagas disease**

Echo/Doppler

Acute Phase

• Left ventricular dilatation, segmental wall motion abnormalities and/or decreased global left ventricular systolic function

• May demonstrate segmental myocardial hypokinesis (especially mainly involving the posteroapical region of the left ventricle)

Chronic Phase

• Several years after initial infection, 30% will develop "Chagas cardiomyopathy"

- Apical hypokinesia/akinesia, thin walled, thrombus filled left ventricular apical aneurysm (most common characteristic)
- Increased left/right ventricular dimensions with decreased left/right ventricular global systolic function (dilated cardiomyopathy)
- May have preserved interventricular septal motion with hypokinetic/akinetic left ventricular posterior wall motion
- Pericardial effusion
- Mitral regurgitation/tricuspid regurgitation

Chiari Network

Definition

- Mobile, web-like remnants of valves of sinus venosus usually seen in the right atrium near the opening of the inferior vena cava (IVC) and coronary sinus. It is usually of no clinical significance.

Echo/Doppler

- It may cause diagnostic confusion with right atrial pathologies such as thromboembolism by causing flow obstruction

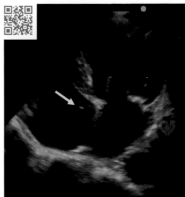

Figure 22.7: **Apical 4-chamber showing a chiari network in the RA (arrow)**

- Evaluate to ensure no thrombus is enmeshed in the network
- It may be associated with infective endocarditis, arrhythmias, and migraine
- It may act as a physical barrier during invasive procedures, such as catheterization
- Tricuspid regurgitation may be visualized by Doppler

Cocaine

Definition

Cocaine is the second most popular illegal recreational drug in the United States behind marijuana.

Echo/Doppler

- Acute myocardial infarction caused by coronary spasm (most common clinical presentation)
- Acute/chronic left ventricular dilatation/dysfunction
- Myocarditis leading to dilated cardiomyopathy
- Endocarditis
- Acute aortic dissection/rupture
- Marked elevation of blood pressure (left ventricular hypertrophy)
- Cardiac arrhythmias

Congenital Absence of the Pericardium

Definition

An uncommon entity that usually involves the left side of the pericardium. Complete bilateral and isolated right sided absence is rare. Congenital absence of the pericardium is more common in men than women (3:1), may have associated cardiac defects (e.g., atrial septal defect, ventricular septal defect) and may present on chest x-ray as a prominent pulmonary trunk, levoposition of the heart, lung interposition between the diaphragm and the base of the heart and/or a flattened, elongated left ventricular contour ("snoopy sign"). The electrocardiogram is often abnormal and may demonstrate right axis deviation, incomplete right bundle branch block or leftward displacement of the QRS transition zone.

Echo/Doppler

- Right ventricular dilatation
- Paradoxical interventricular septal motion
- Simulates right ventricular volume overload
- Vigorous left ventricular posterior wall motion
- Anterior displacement of the left ventricle during ventricular systole
- Cardiac hypermobility (cardioptosis)
- Abnormal swinging motion of the heart
- Unusual echocardiographic windows because heart often shifts resulting in marked lateral displacement of the parasternal long-axis and apical windows
- Localized (left) partial absence of the pericardium may present as left atrial appendage, left atrium, right atrium or right/left ventricular dilatation

Cor Pulmonale

Definition

Right heart failure due to intrinsic pulmonary disease. Echo/Doppler findings are similar to pulmonary hypertension.

Echo/Doppler

- Right ventricular hypertrophy/ dilatation
- Right ventricular systolic dysfunction
- D-shaped left ventricle during ventricular systole and diastole
- Right atrial dilatation (e.g., elevated right atrial pressure, tricuspid regurgitation)

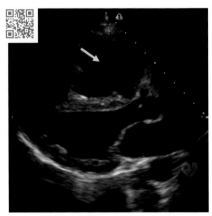

Figure 22.8: **PLAX showing a dilated RV (arrow) in a patient with Cor Pulmonale**

- Dilated inferior vena cava/hepatic veins
- Tricuspid regurgitation, Pulmonary regurgitation
- Decreased right ventricular outflow tract acceleration time
- May alter left ventricular/right ventricular diastolic filling pattern
- Determine the SPAP/MPAP/PAEDP/PVR at rest and exercise

Cor Triatriatum

Definition

A membrane which divides the body of the left atrium.

Echo/Doppler

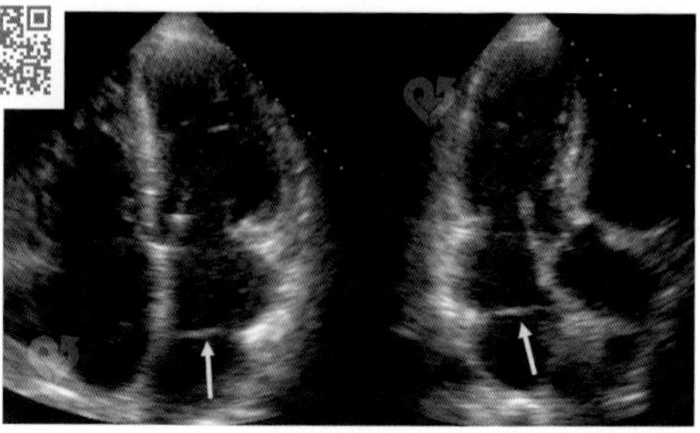

- Best views include parasternal/ apical long-axis, apical 4-chamber and subcostal 4-chamber

Figure 22.9: **Apical 4-chamber (L) and apical LAX (R) showing a membrane in the LA (arrows)**

- Membrane may be seen in the left atrium moving towards the mitral valve in diastole and away during ventricular systole
- Upper left atrial chamber receives the pulmonary veins and the lower left atrial chamber contains the left atrial appendage and the foramen ovale
- Associated defects include atrial septal defect (70 to 80%), persistent left superior vena cava, atrioventricular septal defect, aortic coarctation and anomalous pulmonary venous return
- Doppler may demonstrate turbulent flow, increased velocities and pressure gradient across the membrane
- Color flow Doppler is helpful in differentiating mitral supravalvular ring from cor triatriatum with the mosaic jet originating in the body of the left atrium while in supravalvular ring the mosaic jet forms downstream close to the left ventricle

Cushing's Disease

Definition

A syndrome resulting from hyper-secretion of the adrenal cortex in which there is excessive production of glucocorticoids.

Echo/Doppler

- Left ventricular hypertrophy
- Asymmetric septal hypertrophy

Diabetes

Definition

A disorder of carbohydrate metabolism which is characterized by hyperglycemia and glycosuria and resulting in inadequate production or utilization of insulin.

Echo/Doppler

- Premature coronary artery disease (stress echocardiography may be useful)
- Left ventricular global systolic dysfunction (diabetic cardiomyopathy with left ventricular dilatation)
- Left ventricular hypertrophy
- Left ventricular diastolic dysfunction (usually impaired relaxation)
- Abnormal strain/strain rate

Discrete Subaortic Stenosis (DSS)

Definition

Consists of a thin membrane attached from the left side of the interventricular septum to the anterior mitral valve leaflet. May progress to a thick fibromuscular collar or form a tunnel (tunnel subaortic stenosis).

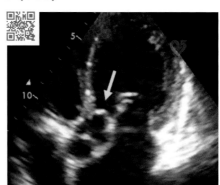

Figure 22.10: **Apical 5-chamber view of a subaortic membrane (arrow)**

Echo/Doppler

- Early systolic closure of the aortic valve (M-mode)
- Coarse systolic aortic valve flutter (M-mode)
- Thin membrane best seen in the parasternal long-axis, apical 5-chamber and apical long-axis views
- Aortic valve may appear thickened
- Associated defects include ventricular septal defect, aortic coarctation, bicuspid aortic valve, supravalvular mitral stenosis, persistent left superior vena cava, component of Shone's syndrome
- PW Doppler may locate high velocity below the aortic valve

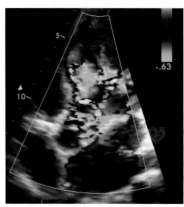

Figure 22.11: **Apical 5-chamber view of a subaortic membrane with color**

22

Miscellaneous / Diabetes

- CW Doppler (parabolic shape) may be used to determine peak velocity/peak pressure gradient/mean pressure gradient across membrane
- Color flow Doppler will demonstrate mosaic, high-velocity systolic jet below the aortic valve
- Aortic regurgitation is common

Diverticulosis of the Left Ventricle

Definition

A rare congenital cardiac malformation which may be confused with aneurysm.

Echo/Doppler

- A small circular echo free space arising from the left ventricle with all three layers of the heart intact
- Doppler may demonstrate low velocity, systolic-diastolic flow

Double Orifice Mitral Valve

Definition

A condition in which an accessory mitral valve orifice is present. Double orifice mitral valve may be created by the MitraClip in the cath lab or surgically by the Alfieri operation.

Echo/Doppler

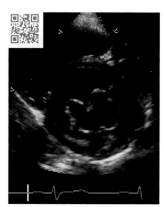

Figure 22.12: **PSAX view of a congenital double orifice MV**

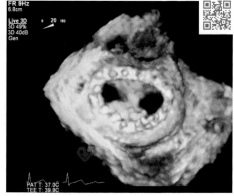

Figure 22.13: **3D TEE image of the MV from the surgeons view (LA). Note the double MV orifice created by an Alfieri stitch. An annuloplasty ring was also implanted.**

- Parasternal/subcostal short-axis of the mitral valve are the best views to identify the two mitral valve orifices

- Parasternal short-axis of the left ventricle at the level of the papillary muscles allows the visualization of abnormalities (e.g., abnormal papillary muscle rotation, single papillary muscle)
- Associated defects include AV septal defect, ventricular septal defect, Ebstein's anomaly, tetralogy of Fallot and aortic coarctation
- Doppler may demonstrate flow, stenosis and/or regurgitation, through both orifices

Ectopic Chordae/False Tendon/ Chordal Web/Aberrant Bands

Definition

Fibrous/muscular chords joining papillary muscle to papillary muscle, papillary muscle to ventricular free wall or ventricular septum to free wall. They can be single or multiple and located in the left and/or right ventricle. Important to report out since it may be a source of murmur, confused as a thrombus and a potential cause of catheter entrapment during an invasive procedure.

Echo/Doppler

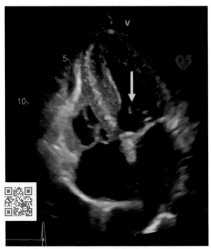

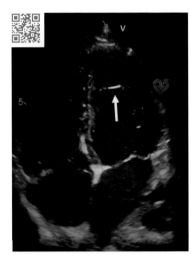

Figure 22.14: Apical 4-chamber in a patient with ectopic chordea (arrow)

Figure 22.15: Apical 4-chamber in a patient with a false tendon in the LV (arrow)

- String like structure(s) with free cavity course unrelated to the atrioventricular valves
- Color flow Doppler may be utilized to distinguish an ectopic chordae from thrombus. If there is an ectopic chordae, color flow Doppler (decrease velocity scale and wall filter) will be displayed on either side of the chord while if a thrombus, there will be a filling defect
- Contrast agents may be useful (e.g., Optison, Definity, Lumason)

Ehlers-Danlos Syndrome (EDS)

Definition

A heterogeneous group of connective tissue disorders with simple mendelian inheritance. The cardinal manifestations of EDS are hyperextensible ("stretchy") skin, hypermobile joints and easy bruising.

Echo/Doppler

- Aortic root dilatation (annuloaortic ectasia)
- Sinus of Valsalva aneurysm
- Aortic aneurysm (unruptured, ruptured)/dissection

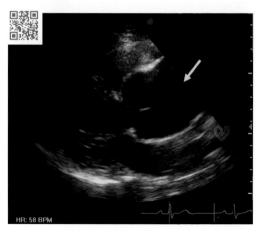

Figure 22.16: **PLAX in a patient with Ehlers-Danlos showing a dilated aortic root (arrow)**

- Dilatation of the proximal innominate artery
- Valvular prolapse (e.g., mitral valve, aortic valve)
- Valvular regurgitation (e.g., mitral regurgitation, aortic regurgitation)
- Evaluate for additional congenital defects (e.g., ASD, VSD, Tetralogy of Fallot, bicuspid aortic valve)

Fabry's Disease

Definition

An X-linked recessive inborn error of glycosphingolipid metabolism.

Echo/Doppler

- Classic mitral valve prolapse due to glycosphingolipid deposition
- Increased left ventricular wall thickness/mass which most likely represents progressive glycosphingolipid deposition in the myocardium
- Myocardial infarction (may mimic the findings of hypertrophic cardiomyopathy)
- Aortic root dilatation
- Mitral regurgitation (usually mild)
- Diastolic dysfunction

Flail Mitral Valve

Definition

Ruptured chordae/papillary muscle will result in the abnormal coaptation of the mitral valve. Can be caused by myocardial infarction or trauma.

Echo/Doppler

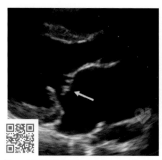
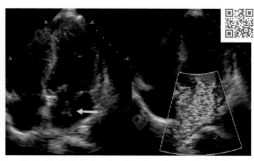

Figure 22.17: **PLAX in a patient with a flail anterior leaflet (arrow)**

Figure 22.18: **Apical 4-chamber views in a patient with a ruptured pap muscle (arrow) resulting in severe MR**

- Systolic flutter of the closure line (M-mode)
- Abnormal systolic motion of the effected mitral leaflet (M-mode)
- Systolic left atrial echoes (M-mode)
- Systolic inversion of the effected mitral leaflet and/or papillary muscle into the left atrium (2D)
- Doppler findings include mitral regurgitation, left atrial systolic antegrade flow, vertical striations superimposed on the typical regurgitant flow pattern
- Color flow Doppler may underestimate the severity of the mitral regurgitation due to the coanda effect (jet hugging wall or valve)

Friedreich's Ataxia

Definition

Cardiac abnormalities are a characteristic feature of the autosomal recessively inherited spinocerebellar degeneration known as Friedreich's ataxia (FA), which is the most common hereditary ataxia.

Echo/Doppler

- Concentric increase in left ventricular wall thickness (most common 68%) (may resemble hypertrophic cardiomyopathy)
- Globally decreased left ventricular systolic function, ejection fraction, fractional shortening (7%)
- Increased left atrial dimension
- Increased right ventricular mass (uncommon)
- Asymmetrical septal thickening (uncommon)
- Dilated cardiomyopathy (uncommon)

Glycogen Storage Disease (GSD)

Definition

A group of inheritable disorders or glycogen metabolism, resulting from specific enzymatic defects.

Pompe's Disease

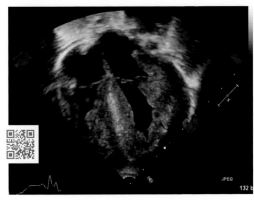

Figure 22.19: **Apical 4-chamber (inverted) in a child with Pompe's disease showing severe LVH**

• GSD type IIa, or Pompe's disease, is the classic form of infantile GSD and is autosomal recessive

• Basic defect is a-1,4 glucosidase deficiency, characterized by a progressive deposition of glycogen in all tissues, especially the myocardium, skeletal muscle and liver

Echo/Doppler

• Severe thickening of the interventricular septum, free wall and posterior left ventricle wall with a tumor-like appearance of the papillary muscles with small left ventricular cavity

• Poor global left ventricular systolic function

Heart Failure

Definition

The inability of the heart to meet the metabolic demands of the body. May be categorized as HFrEF (heart failure with reduced ejection fraction) and HFpEF (heart failure with preserved ejection fraction).

Etiology

• Myocardial damage (ventricular systolic dysfunction) (e.g., coronary artery disease, dilated cardiomyopathy)

• Pressure overload (e.g., systemic hypertension, valvular aortic stenosis)

• Volume overload (e.g., mitral regurgitation, aortic regurgitation)

• Diastolic dysfunction (20 to 40%) (e.g., left ventricular hypertrophy, restrictive cardiomyopathy)

History

- Dyspnea
- Orthopnea
- Paroxysmal nocturnal dyspnea
- Fatigue
- Cough
- Weight gain

Physical Examination

- Jugular venous distention
- Pulmonary rales
- Hepatomegaly
- Ascites
- Peripheral edema
- Pulsus alternans

Electrocardiogram

- Sinus tachycardia
- Left ventricular hypertrophy
- Left atrial dilatation/Right atrial dilatation/Biatrial dilatation
- Evidence for myocardial ischemia/infarction (e.g., pathologic Q waves)
- Low voltage (e.g., cardiac amyloidosis)

Chest X-ray/CMR/CT

- Cardiomegaly
- Pulmonary edema
- Pleural effusion

Cardiac Catheterization

- Confirms status of left ventricular function
- Determines the presence and severity of coronary artery disease
- Determines the presence and severity of valvular disease (e.g., stenosis, regurgitation)

22

Miscellaneous / Heart Failure

Echo/Doppler

Determine:

- Etiology (e.g., coronary artery disease)
- Global left ventricular systolic function (e.g., chamber dimensions, volumes, geometry, ejection fraction, index of myocardial performance)
- Diastolic function grade
- Presence and severity of valvular regurgitation (e.g., mitral, tricuspid)
- SPAP/MPAP/PAEDP/PVR
- Right ventricular systolic/diastolic function

Important to Note

- The causes for systolic heart failure (ejection fraction less than 40%) (HFrEF) include coronary artery disease with left ventricular damage, dilated cardiomyopathy, systemic hypertension, valvular heart disease.
- The causes of diastolic heart failure (normal or supranormal ejection fraction) (HFpEF) include coronary artery disease, left ventricular hypertrophy, small vessel disease (e.g., diabetes), restrictive cardiomyopathy (e.g., cardiac amyloidosis, sarcoidosis, hemochromatosis, scleroderma).

Holt-Oram (Heart-Hand) Syndrome

Definition

An autosomal dominant syndrome characterized by skeletal abnormalities and congenital cardiac defects.

Echo/Doppler

- Atrial septal defect (ostium secundum)
- Dilatation of right ventricle, right atrium, paradoxical motion of the ventricular septum consistent with right ventricular volume overload
- Ventricular septal defect (trabecular type)
- Complex congenital heart disease/vascular malformations
- Nonobstructive cardiomyopathy
- Mitral valve prolapse (10 to 20% of patients)

Hyperlipidemia

Definition

Concentration of triglycerides or cholesterol is increased in fasting plasma. As a working rule, hyperlipoproteinemia is considered to be present whenever the plasma cholesterol level exceeds 5.2mmol/L (200 mg/dL).

Echo/Doppler

- Echocardiographic features of coronary artery atherosclerosis
- Narrowing of the outflow tracts, characteristically at the sinotubular junction in the ascending aorta
- Immobility of valve leaflets and cusps
- Accelerated valve degeneration including sclerosis and calcification of the leaflets
- Infiltration of the myocardium
- Large depositions of lipid within the heart (uncommon)

Hyperlipomatous Interatrial Septum

Definition

Fatty infiltration of the interatrial septum seen mostly in older patients or those on long term steroid treatment.

Echo/Doppler

- Thickening of the proximal and distal interatrial septum (IAS) (dumbbell shape)
- The foramen ovale in the center of the IAS is usually spared since it does not contain fat cells

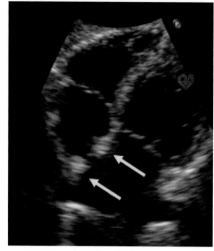

Figure 22.20: **Subcostal 4-chamber view showing a hyperlipomatous interatrial septum (arrows)**

Hyperthyroidism

Definition

A condition caused by excessive secretion of the thyroid glands which increases the metabolic rate causing an increased demand for food to support the metabolic activity.

Echo/Doppler

- Enhanced global left ventricular systolic function
- Hyperthyroid cardiomyopathy ("high-output" failure)
- Myocardial ischemia
- Pulmonary hypertension (>75mmHg possible)
- Increased left ventricular relaxation (decreased isovolumic relaxation time, mitral valve deceleration time)
- Global left ventricular systolic dysfunction (long term)

Hypothyroidism

Definition

A thyroid secretion deficiency resulting in a lowered basal metabolism.

Echo/Doppler

- Pericardial effusion/cardiac tamponade/constrictive pericarditis
- Decreased left ventricular global systolic function
- Left ventricular hypertrophy with abnormal myocardial texture
- Asymmetrical septal hypertrophy (ASH)
- Mitral valve prolapse
- Left ventricular diastolic dysfunction (usually impaired left ventricular relaxation)

Kawasaki Disease

Definition

Febrile illness of unknown etiology resulting in vasculitis. More commonly seen in children.

Also referred to as mucocutaneous lymph node syndrome.

Echo/Doppler

- Coronary artery aneurysm (usually proximal) (may be filled with thrombus)
- Left ventricular global and segmental systolic dysfunction
- Myocardial infarction
- Pericardial effusion (30%)
- Mitral regurgitation (30%)
- Aortic regurgitation (uncommon)
- Transesophageal echocardiography may be useful

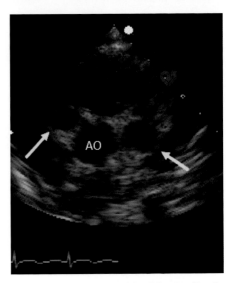

Figure 22.21: **PSAX at the AV level showing dilated proximal right and left coronaries (arrows)**

Left Bundle Branch Block (LBBB)

Definition

Delay or blockage of conduction in the main left bundle branch causing the left ventricle to contract after the right ventricle.

Echo/Doppler

- LBBB is best seen on M-mode as paradoxical septal motion due to the delay in LV contraction

Electrocardiogram

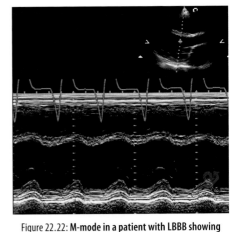

Figure 22.22: **M-mode in a patient with LBBB showing paradoxical septal motion**

Within 0.04 seconds of the onset of the QRS, there is a rapid downward motion of the interventricular septum ("beaking" of the interventricular septum). This downward motion lasts approximately another 0.04 seconds or until ventricular ejection when there is a rapid anterior motion lasting throughout ventricular ejection.

Loeys-Dietz Syndrome (Aortic Aneurysm Syndrome)

Definition

Autosomal dominant aortic aneurysm syndrome characterized by the triad of arterial tortuosity and aneurysms, hypertolerism and cleft palate caused by heterozygous mutations in the genes encoding transforming growth factor beta receptors.

Echo/Dopper Findings

- Aggressive arterial aneurysms (mean age of death 26 years of age)
- Vascular disease may be widespread
- Increased pregnancy related complications

Lung Transplantation

Definition

The grafting of lung tissue from donor to recipient.

Echo/Doppler

- Reduction in right ventricular dimension and right ventricular hypertrophy
- Improvement in right ventricular global systolic function
- Decrease in tricuspid regurgitation
- Decrease in pulmonary artery pressures

Lyme Disease

Definition

Caused by the tick-borne spirochete, Borrelia burgdorferi. Initial infection marked by rash, followed by weeks to months by involvement of other organ systems, including the heart, neurologic system and joints.

Echo/Doppler

- Severe atrioventricular node block associated with syncope
- Dilated cardiomyopathy

Marfan Syndrome

Definition

A hereditary condition of connective tissue, bones, muscles, ligaments and skeletal structures.

Echo/Doppler

- Proximal aortic dilatation (aortic annulus, sinuses of Valsalva, ascending aorta)
- Aortic dissection (most common cause of death)
- Multivalvular prolapse (especially mitral valve prolapse)

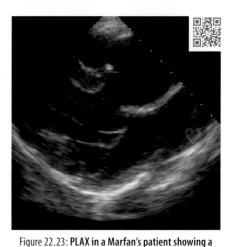

Figure 22.23: **PLAX in a Marfan's patient showing a dilated aortic root and mitral valve prolapse**

- Dilated mitral annulus
- Mitral annular calcification
- Left atrial compression
- Left ventricular volume overload pattern (left ventricular dilatation with hyperkinesis)
- Aortic and/or mitral regurgitation
- Coronary artery dissection
- Prophylactic repair of ascending aortic aneurysm in Marfan's has been recommended when the aortic diameter reaches 5.0cm or increase in diameter ≥0.5mm

Mitral Annular Calcification (MAC)

Definition

Idiopathic calcification of the mitral valve annulus is a common finding in the elderly. Calcification of the mitral valve annulus may be accelerated by systemic hypertension, aortic valve stenosis, hypertrophic cardiomyopathy, diabetes, mitral valve prolapse, obesity, disorders of calcium/ phosphorous metabolism, Marfan syndrome, Hurler's syndrome and chronic renal failure. It may be associated with coronary artery disease. Also referred to as submitral calcification and/or fibrosis

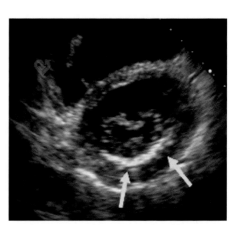

Figure 22.24: **PSAX MV level showing calcification/ fibrous of the mitral annulus (arrows)**

Echo/Doppler

- Echodense structure anterior to the left ventricular posterior wall at the atrioventricular junction best seen in the parasternal long-axis and apical views
- Appears as a semicircular linear band beneath the base of the posterior mitral valve leaflet in the parasternal short-axis view of the mitral valve
- Usually involves the posterior mitral valve annulus but may extend to the entire mitral valve annulus, ventricular wall, mitral valve posterior leaflet, left atrium and aortic root
- May become infected (e.g., abscess)
- May be a source of embolism (cerebral, retinal)
- Can be confused with mitral valve stenosis (mitral valve leaflets are usually thin and pliable in mitral annular calcification)
- May mimic cardiac tumor
- Mitral regurgitation (usually mild)
- Functional mitral stenosis is possible (especially if there is anterior mitral annular calcification) (determine mitral valve peak velocity, peak pressure gradient, mean pressure gradient, pressure half-time, mitral valve area)
- Determine the severity: (measure thickness of the calcification in the parasternal short-axis view of the mitral valve)
- Mild MAC: 1.5 to 5mm
- Moderate MAC: 6 to 10mm
- Severe MAC: >10mm

Mitral Valve Supravalvular Stenosing Ring

Definition

A membrane located at the level of the mitral valve annulus.

Echo/Doppler

- A thin band of echoes located just above the mitral valve or within the funnel of the mitral valve leaflets
- Mitral valve leaflets may appear thick and myxomatous
- Motion of the ring may be detected with the ring moving towards the mitral valve orifice in diastole and away from the leaflets during ventricular systole
- Associated with atrial septal defect, persistent left superior vena cava to the coronary sinus, aortic coarctation, ventricular septal defect and Shone's syndrome
- Doppler may demonstrate turbulent flow, increased velocities and pressure gradient similar to that which is seen in mitral valve stenosis

Non-communicating Intramural Hematoma (IMH)

Definition

May represent rupture of the vasa vasorum into the media and subadventitial regions (spontaneous intramural hemorrhage without intimal tear) (10 to 15% of aortic dissection). Associated with systemic hypertension, trauma. May be a precursor to aortic dissection (a dissection without an intimal tear).

Echo/Doppler

- Best visualized by transesophageal echocardiography (several planes of view may be required to identify IMH)
- Hemorrhage with crescentic/circular thickening of the aortic wall (>0.5cm)
- Central displacement of intimal calcification
- Layered appearance
- Length from 1 to 20cm
- Preserved aortic lumen with absence of intimal flap
- Contrast agents may be useful (e.g., Optison, Definity, Lumason)

Non-compaction of Ventricular Myocardium (Hypertrabeculation)

Definition

Noncompaction of the myocardium without an associated cardiac anomaly is a rare congenital disorder.

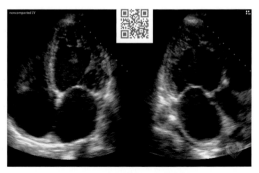

Figure 22.25: Apical 4-chamber and LAX in a patient with LV non-compaction. Note the spongy appearance of the apical myocardium.

Echo/Doppler

- Multiple prominent ventricular trabeculations and deep intratrabecular recesses (especially mid-lateral, mid-inferior, apical) ("spongy" appearance of myocardium)
- Dilated ventricle(s)
- Depressed global systolic ventricular function
- Diastolic dysfunction
- Multiple deep intratrabecular recesses communicating with the ventricular cavity as visualized on color flow Doppler (decrease color velocity scale, wall filter) (multiple views may be required including PSAX LV, PSAX cardiac apex, apical 4-chamber, apical long axis)
- Proposed echocardiographic criteria: Thickness of the noncompacted layer (NC) to compacted layer (C) are best measured in the short axis views at the mid and apical levels at end-systole with a ratio of >2:1 diagnostic (NC/C)
- Contrast agents may be useful (e.g., Optison, Definity, Lumason)

Noonan Syndrome

Definition

Noonan syndrome is inherited in an autosomal dominant manner and is characterized by congenital heart disease, short stature, abnormal facies and the somatic features of Turner's syndrome but a normal karyotype. Congenital heart defects are common in this genetic condition.

Echo/Doppler

- Valvular pulmonic stenosis (40%) with thickened, dysplastic pulmonary valve cusps
- Secundum atrial septal defect (33%)
- Ventricular septal defect (10%)
- Patent ductus arteriosus (10%)
- Localized anterior septal hypertrophy
- Diffuse right ventricular hypertrophy
- Left ventricular hypertrophy
- Partial atrioventricular canal with left ventricular outflow obstruction
- Constrictive pericarditis
- Dilatation of the ascending aorta

Obesity

Definition

Abnormal amount of body fat with an increased risk for diabetes, heart disease, and hypertension.

Table 22.3: Echo/Doppler		
Cardiac Hypertrophy	**Chamber Enlargement**	**Reduced left ventricular global systolic function**
• Increased interventricular septal thickness • Increased left ventricular posterior wall thickness • Decreased systolic amplitude of interventricular septum/left ventricular posterior wall • Increased right ventricular wall thickness • Increased left ventricular mass	• Increased left ventricular diastolic/systolic internal dimensions and volumes • Increased right ventricular dimensions • Increased left atrial dimension • Increased aortic root dimension	• Decreased stroke volume • Left ventricular diastolic dysfunction (impaired relaxation) • Strain/Strain rate may demonstrate subtle systolic and/or diastolic dysfunction

Parachute Mitral Valve

Definition

A congenital abnormality in which there is only one papillary muscle in the left ventricle and the chordae of the two mitral valve leaflets insert into this single papillary muscle.

Echo/Doppler

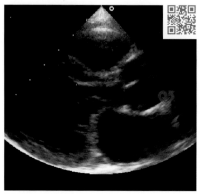

Figure 22.26: **PLAX in a patient with a parachute MV. Note the tethering of the MV leaflets in diastole.**

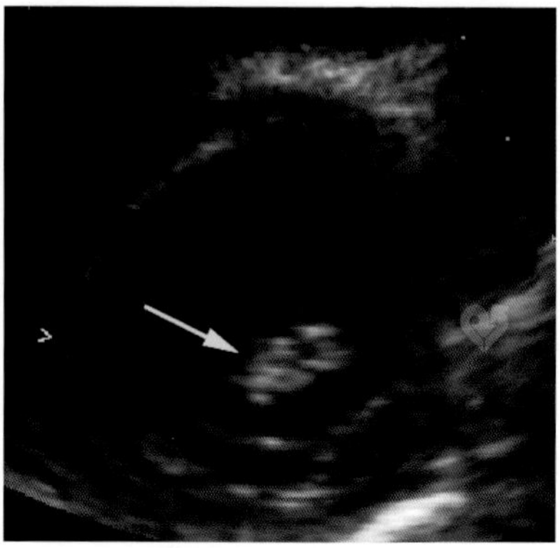

Figure 22.27: **PSAX level of the papillary muscles. Note the single pap muscle (arrow).**

- Single LV papillary muscle (usually posteromedial papillary muscle) best seen in the parasternal short-axis view of the left ventricle at the level of the papillary muscles
- Additional papillary muscle (usually small), may be present but receive no chordae tendineae
- Mitral valve leaflets and chordae are normal
- Doppler findings will be similar to mitral stenosis

Patent Foramen Ovale (PFO)

Definition

- PFO is failure of the primum and secundum atrial septa to fuse. This lack of fusion allows intermittent bidirectional blood flow between the atria.
- PFO is common (up to 30% of the adult population)
- Associated complications include cryptogenic stroke, paradoxical emboli, hypoxia with significant right to left shunt in COPD, complication in pulmonary embolism, decompression illness in divers, migraines

Echo/Doppler

- Intact atrial septum with shunting (may require TEE with agitated saline contrast exam)

- Valsalva maneuver/cough may enhance detection during saline contrast exam

- PFO is suggested if one microbubble appears in the left atrium within four cardiac cycles (if saline contrast appears after five cardiac cycles, pulmonary arteriovenous fistula may be present)

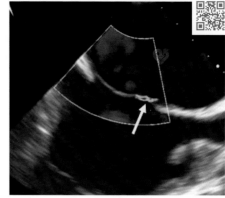

Figure 22.28: **TEE image of the IAS showing turbulent flow across a PFO (arrow)**

- Three or more saline contrast injections may be required (rest, Valsalva, cough)

- Recent study recommended 5 saline contrast injections: rest, Valsalva (2), cough, bed tilt with early Valsalva (10º feet down to decrease preload)

- Causes of false negative saline contrast exams include failure of the Valsalva maneuver or cough to transiently increase right atrial pressure, increased left atrial pressure, use of antecubital venous contrast injection when a prominent Eustachian valve is present

- Causes of false positive saline contrast exams include sinus venosus atrial septal defect, pseudocontrast caused by the Valsalva maneuver, pulmonary arteriovenous malformation mistaken as patent foramen ovale

Penetrating Aortic Ulcer (PAU)

Definition

A type of aortic dissection where a penetrating ulcer burrows deeply through the intima into the aortic media, precipitating a localized intramedial dissection and hematoma. PAU occur throughout the aorta but are more common in the thoracic and abdominal aorta.

Echo/Doppler

- Transesophageal echocardiography demonstrates a plaque that is crater-like ("dished out") ulcer with jagged edges, usually in the presence of extensive aortic atheroma. There is an absence of an intimal flap and false lumen

- Contrast agents may be useful (e.g., Optison, Definity, Lumason)

Persistent Left Superior Vena Cava (PLSVC)

Definition

The left horn of the sinus venosus persists and may drain to the coronary sinus, left atrium or left pulmonary vein.

22

Miscellaneous / Penetrating Aortic Ulcer (PAU)

Echo/Doppler

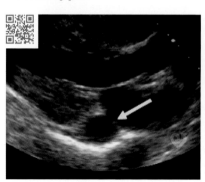

Figure 22.29: **DPLAX in a patient with a PLSVC and a dilated coronary sinus (arrow)**

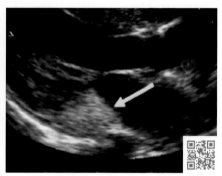

Figure 22.30: **PLAX in a patient with a PLSVC showing saline contrast in the dilated coronary sinus (arrow)**

- The PLSVC may be imaged from the suprasternal long-axis view with a leftward tilt
- Pulsed wave/color flow Doppler will demonstrate a low velocity, biphasic flow pattern away from the transducer in the persistent left superior vena cava
- Dilated coronary sinus best seen in the parasternal long-axis view and apical 4-chamber view with a posterior tilt
- Agitated contrast saline injected into a left arm vein demonstrates contrast in the coronary sinus before arriving into the right atrium

Fen-Phen

Definition

The appetite suppressants phentermine, fenfluramine and dexfenfluramine, alone or in combination, have been implicated as causing valvular heart disease. (3 to 15%). Complications uncommon with less than 6 months of use.

Echo/Doppler

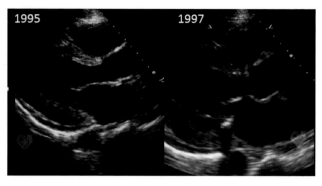

Figure 22.31: **PLAX images two years apart showing the MV changes from taking the Fen-Phen diet drug**

- Thickened mitral valve/chordae tendineae (similar to carcinoid)

- Thickened aortic valve
- Mild or greater aortic regurgitation (most common)
- Moderate or greater mitral regurgitation
- Pulmonary hypertension
- Severity of valvular regurgitation may regress over time

Pheochromocytoma
Definition

A tumor of chromaffin cells that secrete catecholamines and cause systemic hypertension. In approximately 80% of cases, pheochromocytomas are found in the adrenal medulla, but may also be found in other tissues derived from neural crest cells. They appear equally in both sexes, are bilateral in 10% of cases and are usually benign (95%).

Echo/Doppler

- Concentric left ventricular hypertrophy (20%)
- HCM with/without LVOT obstruction
- Myocarditis (acute) with catecholamine crisis
- Dilated cardiomyopathy
- Reversible dilatation
- Segmental wall motion abnormality(s)
- Tumor located in atrioventricular groove

Pregnancy
Definition

There are normal anatomic changes with pregnancy. These are mainly seen in the third trimester due to an increase in overall blood volume.

Echo/Doppler

- Increased heart rate, cardiac arrhythmias (e.g., PVC, PAC)
- Increased stroke volume, cardiac output
- Slight increase in all cardiac chambers and great vessles due to increased blood volume
- Small pericardial effusion (up to 20%)
- Increased left ventricular outflow tract/aortic valve peak velocity/right ventricular outflow tract
- Anatomic/hemodynamic parameters return to baseline (6 to 12 weeks)
- Peripartum (acute) cardiomyopathy (abnormal finding especially beyond six months postpartum) (1 in 10,000 pregnancies)

Important to Note

Examination should be performed with patient in left lateral position due to compression of the inferior vena cava in the supine position

Table 22.4: Normal Echocardiographic Parameters During Pregnancy at Term or Third Trimester			
Parameter	**Mean ± SD**	**Parameter**	**Mean ± SD**
LVIDd (mm)	47 ± 4	LA (mm)	38 ± 4
LV wall thickness (mm)	10 ± 1	RV (mm)	20 ± 1
LV mass (gm)	186 ± 39	Mitral annulus (mm)	24 ± 5
FS (%)	40 ± 7	Tricuspid annulus (mm)	27 ± 3
EF (%)	60 ± 4	Aortic root (mm)	30 ± 12

Pulmonary Embolism

Definition

Embolus (e.g., blood, tissue, air bubbles) in the pulmonary artery or one of its branches.

Echo/Doppler

- Actual visualization of the thrombus within right heart/pulmonary artery
- McConnell's sign (akinesia of the mid-free wall of the right ventricle with normal/hyperdynamic motion of the cardiac apex)
- 60/60 sign (SPAP <60mmHg and RVOT acceleration time <60 msec)
- Right ventricular and pulmonary artery dilatation
- Right ventricular global and segmental systolic dysfunction

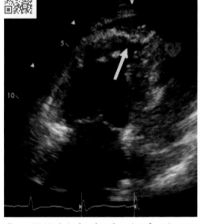

Figure 22.32: **Apical 4-chamber view focusing on the RV. The arrow points to the RV apex which demonstrated hyperdynamic motion (McConnell's sign).**

- Right atrial dilatation (normal RA volume: men 25 ± 7mL/m^2; women 21 ± 6mL/m^2)
- D-shaped left ventricle
- Abnormal interventricular septal motion
- Pericardial effusion
- Dilatation of the inferior vena cava
- Respiratory variation of mitral and tricuspid inflow (similar to cardiac tamponade)
- Tricuspid and/or pulmonary regurgitation
- Evidence of pulmonary hypertension
- Determine SPAP/MPAP/PAEDP/PVR

Important to Note

With a small pulmonary embolus, the right heart may appear normal.

Pulmonary Vein Stenosis

Definition

- Discrete narrowing of one or more of the pulmonary veins at or near the junction of the left atrium.
- Usually congenital but may be acquired due to catheter treatment of atrial fibrillation.

Echo/Doppler

- Difficult to identify with two-dimensional echocardiography
- Right ventricular hypertrophy
- Right ventricular dilatation
- Right atrial dilatation
- Color flow Doppler may demonstrate mosaic (turbulent) flow pattern
- PW Doppler may demonstrate increased peak systolic pulmonary vein velocity (>1.5 m/s) with a continuous flow pattern and phasic variation

Renal Failure

Definition

Failure of the kidneys to perform their essential functions.

Echo/Doppler

- Mitral annular calcification
- Mitral stenosis (functional)
- Aortic valve sclerosis/stenosis
- Pericardial effusion/cardiac tamponade/constrictive pericarditis
- Left ventricular systolic dysfunction (myocarditis, coronary artery vasculitis)
- Left ventricular hypertrophy
- Ground glass appearance of the myocardium
- Left ventricular dilatation with global systolic dysfunction (dilated cardiomyopathy)
- Mitral/aortic regurgitation
- Diastolic dysfunction
- Improvement of ventricular function post-renal transplantation

Rheumatoid Arthritis

Definition

A chronic autoimmune disease characterized by systemic arthritis.

Echo/Doppler

- Pericardial effusion/cardiac tamponade/constrictive pericarditis
- Leaflet fibrosis/nodules
- Left ventricular global systolic dysfunction (e.g., myocarditis, coronary artery disease)
- Myocardial nodules
- Valvular regurgitation
- Secondary amyloidosis
- Aortic aneurysm, wall thickening secondary to aortitis (rare)
- Secondary pulmonary hypertension (rare)
- Left ventricular diastolic dysfunction (impaired relaxation)

Scimitar Syndrome

Definition

Partial or total anomalous pulmonary venous connection of the right lung into the inferior vena cava (rare). "Scimitar" refers to the appearance of the anomalous right pulmonary vein on chest radiography. It produces a silhouette likened to an Arabic or Turkish sword (the scimitar) along the right border of the heart.

Echo/Doppler

- Partial or total anomalous pulmonary venous connection of the right lung into the inferior vena cava
- Sinus venosus atrial septal defect
- Dextrocardia

Scleroderma

Definition

Excessive connective tissue accumulation in the blood vessels, skin, joints, skeletal muscle and multiple organs.

Echo/Doppler

- Left ventricular systolic/diastolic dysfunction (up to 75%)
- Segmental wall motion abnormality(s)
- Left ventricular hypertrophy
- Valvular sclerosis
- Evidence of pulmonary hypertension
- Pericardial effusion/cardiac tamponade/constrictive pericarditis
- Mitral valve prolapse

Shone's Syndrome

Definition

A congenital heart condition characterized by multiple left heart defects.

Echo/Doppler

- Supravalvular mitral valve ring, parachute mitral valve
- Subaortic stenosis
- Bicuspid aortic valve
- Aortic coarctation

Syncope

Definition

A transient loss of consciousness due to inadequate blood flow to the brain.

Echo/Doppler

- Hypertrophic obstructive cardiomyopathy
- Aortic and/or mitral stenosis
- Hypovolemia (small left ventricle with hypercontractile function)
- Myxomatous mitral valve prolapse
- Left ventricular global systolic dysfunction
- Pulmonary hypertension
- Pulmonary embolism
- Myocardial infarction
- Intracardiac mass
- Pericardial effusion/cardiac tamponade
- Aortic dissection

Systemic Lupus Erythematosus

Definition

Chronic inflammatory disease which affects the musculoskeletal and mucocutaneous systems causing fatigue, myalgias, arthralgias, arthritis, photosensitivity and serositis.

Echo/Doppler

- Libman Sacks vegetations (noninfected valve mass) usually involving the mitral valve or aortic valve with the vegetation small in size (<1cm^2), irregular borders and no independent motion
- Pericardial effusion (10 to 15%)/Cardiac tamponade (<1%)/Constrictive pericarditis
- Mitral valve prolapse (5 to 10%)

- Left ventricular global/segmental systolic dysfunction (accelerated atherosclerosis, myocarditis, coronary artery embolism)
- Left ventricular diastolic dysfunction
- Pulmonary hypertension (up to 5%)
- Valvular regurgitation
- Valve stenosis (rare)
- Aortitis (rare)
- Coronary artery aneurysm (rare)
- Vascular thrombosis

Takayasu's Disease

Definition

An aortic arteritis with marked intimal proliferation and fibrosis and fibrous scarring and degeneration of the elastic fibers of the media which leads to localized aneurysm, post-stenotic dilatation and calcification of the aorta and its major branches.

Echo/Doppler

- Dilatation of the aortic root/aorta
- Increased echogenicity of the aortic root/aorta (similar to atherosclerosis)
- Left ventricular systolic dysfunction (myocarditis, coronary artery vasculitis)
- Aortic regurgitation
- Stenosis/occlusion of large vessels

Takotsubo Cardiomyopathy

Definition

Acute heart failure precipitated by sudden, intense emotional or physical stress. (e.g., death of a spouse, surgery, severe pain) Also referred to as stress cardiomyopathy, transient apical ballooning syndrome, "broken heart" syndrome.

Typical findings include chest pain in a woman (mean age 58 to 77), after an acute stressor, ST segment elevation/T wave inversion, small elevation of troponin/CK-MB levels, angiogram will demonstrate normal coronary arteries

Echo/Doppler

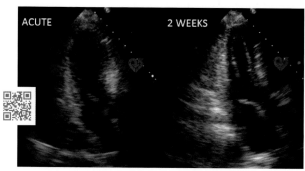

Figure 22.33: **Apical LAX views in a patient with Takotsubo CM with normal function returning two weeks later**

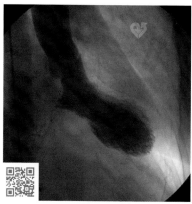

Figure 22.34: **Cath angiogram in the same patient with Takotsubo CM. The LV apex is aneurysmal.**

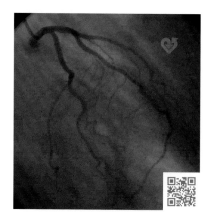

Figure 22.35: **Cath with normal coronaries in the same patient with Takotsubo CM**

- Reduced ejection fraction
- Classic finding includes apical regional wall motion abnormality with preserved basilar function (apical ballooning)
- Wall motion abnormalities may include mid-ventricular region, basal left ventricle, right ventricle
- Apical thrombus may be present
- Return of normal ventricular function occurs in the majority of patients within days to weeks
- Diagnosis is based on clinical criteria and may be difficult to distinguish from myocardial infarction without coronary angiography

Traumatic Heart Disease

Definition

Penetrating and nonpenetrating chest trauma can damage the myocardium, pericardium, cardiac valves and great vessels.

Echo/Doppler

Evaluate for the following:

- Pericardial effusion/cardiac tamponade
- Myocardial contusion seen as thick, bright signal with segmental wall motion abnormalities
- Thinning of the ventricular wall, true aneurysm, pseudoaneurysm, intramural thrombi (especially right ventricle)
- Laceration/tear of the myocardium, great vessels, ventricular/atrial septal defect
- Papillary muscle rupture
- Flail tricuspid/mitral valve leaflet
- Aortic valve trauma
- Aortic hematoma, aneurysm, dissection (especially in area of aortic isthmus) pseudoaneurysm
- Fistulas (e.g., aorta to right atrium)
- Comet tail artifact may indicate bullet
- Valvular regurgitation

Uhl's Anomaly (Parchment Heart)

Definition

Rarely seen dysplasia of the right ventricular myocardium.

Echo/Doppler

- Thin, hypokinetic right ventricular myocardium (may be biventricular)
- Right ventricular dilatation with poor global systolic function
- Right ventricular trabeculation may be absent
- Tricuspid regurgitation
- Tricuspid valve located in the correct position (versus Ebstein's anomaly)

Valsalva Maneuver

Definition

The Valsalva maneuver is performed by attempting to forcibly exhale while keeping the mouth and nose closed. May be useful in the echocardiography laboratory to evaluate patent foramen ovale, atrial septal defect, hypertrophic cardiomyopathy, diastolic function.

Four Phases of the Valsalva Maneuver

- **Phase 1** — Onset of straining with increased intrathoracic pressure. The heart rate does not change, blood pressure increases.

- **Phase 2** — Marked by a significant decrease in venous return with a reduction in stroke volume and pulse pressure as straining continues. The heart rate increases, blood pressure decreases, increased intrathoracic pressure is maintained. (useful in the evaluation of hypertrophic cardiomyopathy, diastolic function)

- **Phase 3** — Release of straining which results in a sudden decrease in intrathoracic pressure with increase in RV preload (useful in the evaluation of PFO, ASD)

- **Phase 4** — Sudden increase in cardiac output, aortic pressure (blood pressure overshoot) with return of heart rate to baseline

Proper Technique for Evaluation of Patent Foramen Ovale During Saline Contrast Exam

- While imaging, practice with patient straining for 5 to 10 seconds (blowing on their thumb) and releasing; adjust image if necessary

- Valsalva should be started 3 to 5 seconds before injection of saline contrast and should be held for at least 8 to 10 seconds

- Once contrast is seen in the right atrium, Valsalva may be released

- If the interatrial septum does not shift towards the left atrium, then the Valsalva is not being performed properly or the left atrial pressure is increased.

Valvular Strands

Definition

Thin, mobile, filamentous projections attached to the valvular leaflets (Lambl's excrescences) or prosthetic valves and may be multiple. May represent small, endothelial covered, fibrinous protuberances resulting from mechanical trauma.

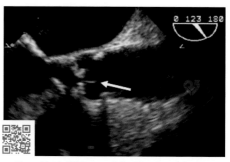

Figure 22.36: **TEE image of the AV and root showing Lambl's excrescences**

Echo/Doppler

- Best visualized by transesophageal echocardiography

- May be considered an embolic source when visualized with a prosthetic heart valve

Ventricular Assist Device (VAD)

Definition

A bridge to transplant and a blood pump that can augment or replace the function of a failing ventricle. Placed in the left or right ventricle to support patients with end-stage heart failure.

Echo/Doppler

- Evaluate the surgical results of the VAD implantation
- Evaluate overall structure, size, and function of the chambers
- Determine mitral regurgitation; with normal VAD, mitral regurgitation should decrease
- Determine the frequency of aortic valve opening and presence and severity of aortic regurgitation
- Evaluate apical inflow cannula position and the inflow with color and PW Doppler; cannula should be aligned with LVOT; PW Doppler assessment of the inflow cannula should be done in apical 4 and 2-chamber views (should be laminar flow); high velocity and turbulent flow suggest obstruction of the inflow cannula secondary to thrombus or intermittent ventricular wall obstruction
- Evaluate outflow cannula with color and PW Doppler; use high left parasternal long axis view to show end-to-side anastomosis to the midascending aorta
- Position of the interventricular septum with shift suggesting underfilled left ventricle; rightward shift suggesting poor left ventricular unloading
- Evaluate right ventricular dimension and function

Weight Reduction

Definition

Weight loss

Echo/Doppler

- Improved left ventricular fractional shortening/global systolic function
- Reduced left ventricular mass

Prediction of Intracardiac Pressures
Laura J Phillips, BS, RDCS, RVT

Definition

2D echocardiography combined with cardiac Doppler may be utilized to predict intracardiac pressures.

Right Atrial Pressure (RAP)

- Normal: 2 to 5mmHg
- To approximate the RAP, examine the IVC by 2D and substitute one of the following values for the actual RAP:

Table 23.1: **Right Atrial Pressure**			
Variable	**Normal** (0 to 5 [3]mmHg)	**Intermediate** (5 to 10 [8]mmHg)	**High** (15mmHg)
IVC diameter	≤2.1cm	>2.1cm	>2.1cm
Collapse with sniff	>50%	>50%	<50%
Secondary indices of elevated RAP			• Restrictive filling • Tricuspid E/e' >6 • Diastolic flow predominance in hepatic veins (systolic filling fraction <55%)

Ranges are provided for low and intermediate categories, but for simplicity, midrange values of 3mmHg for normal and 8mmHg for intermediate are suggested. Intermediate (8mmHg) RA pressures may be downgraded to normal (3mmHg) if no secondary indices of elevated RA pressure are present, upgraded to high if minimal collapse with sniff (<35%) and secondary indices of elevated RA pressures are present, or left at 8mmHg if uncertain.

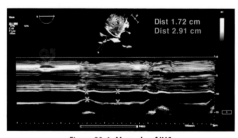

Dist 1.72 cm
Dist 2.91 cm

Figure 23.1: **M-mode of IVC**

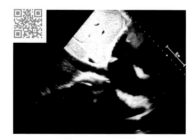

Figure 23.2: **2D IVC**

- Dilated hepatic veins with a dilated inferior vena cava suggests increased RAP
- A dilated coronary sinus (normal 4 to 8mm as measured in the apical 4-chamber with a posterior tilt) suggests increased RAP (May be dilated also with persistent left superior vena cava, coronary artery AV fistula, anomalous hepatic venous drainage to the coronary sinus, total anomalous pulmonary venous return or tricuspid regurgitation)

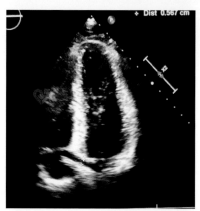

Figure 23.3: **Apical 4-chamber view with coronary sinus**

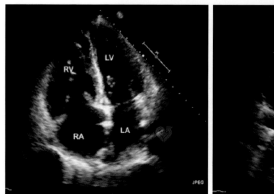

Figure 23.4: **Apical 4-chamber**

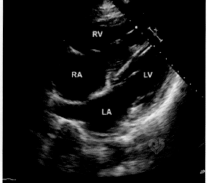

Figure 23.5: **Subcostal 4-chamber**

- In the absence of significant tricuspid regurgitation, a right atrium that is increased in dimension (especially when compared to the left atrium) suggests increased RAP

- A right atrial maximal volume measured at end-systole of >25 ± 7mL/m^2 for men and 21 ± 6mL/m^2 for women may suggest elevated RAP.

- Interatrial septal deviation towards the left atrium may indicate increased RAP

- A hepatic vein systolic fraction of <55% suggests a mean RAP of >8mmHg

- A dagger shaped CW tricuspid regurgitation velocity spectral display suggests increased RAP

- A decreased right ventricular isovolumic relaxation time (normal 54 ± 3.55 msec) suggests increased RAP

- A patient with left-sided heart disease and pulmonary hypertension may eventually develop elevated right heart pressures

Right Atrial Pressure Estimate Heptic Vein Flow in PAH Patients

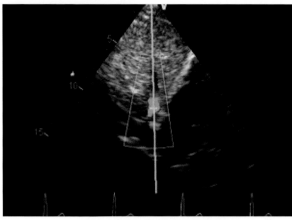

Figure 23.6: **Systolic filling fraction.**
Vs / (Vs +Vd) <55% sensitive and specific for increase

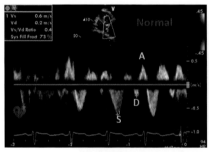

Figure 23.7: **Normal systolic predominace in hepatic vein flow**

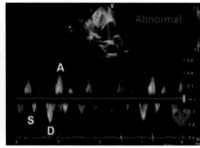

Figure 23.8: **Abnormal: Vs/Vd <1 (High RAP)**

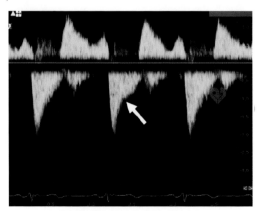

Figure 23.9: **CW Demonstrating the TR jet early equalization secondary to an increase in RAP**

Right Ventricular Diastolic Pressure (RVDP)

- Normal: mean 2 to 8mmHg
- In the absence of right ventricular inflow tract obstruction, the mean right atrial pressure reflects the RVDP
- An increase in the peak velocity of the atrial reversal (AR) wave of the hepatic vein may indicate increased right ventricular end-diastolic pressure
- An increase in the hepatic vein AR duration as compared to the tricuspid A wave duration may indicate increased RVEDP
- An increased D wave of the PW Doppler hepatic vein tracing may indicate increased RVDP
- A decrease in right ventricular ejection fraction suggests increased RVDP

Right Ventricular Systolic Pressure (RVSP)

- Normal: 15 to 30mmHg
- Importance: equals the systolic pulmonary artery pressure (SPAP) in the absence of right ventricular outflow tract (RVOT) obstruction
- Evidence of increased RVSP includes: right ventricular hypertrophy, right ventricular dilatation, flattened ("pancaked") interventricular septum throughout the cardiac cycle

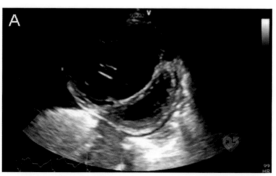

Figure 23.10: **2D PSAX of the LV demonstrating IVS flattening**

- The RVSP may be determined by the following formula (assuming the absence of RVOT obstruction):

$$\text{RVSP mmHg} = 4 \times (\text{TR peak jet velocity}^2) + \text{RAP}$$

- In the presence of a ventricular septal defect, the RVSP may be calculated by the formula (assuming the absence of RVOT obstruction):

$$\text{RVSP mmHg} = \text{Systolic BP} - 4 \times (\text{VSD peak systolic jet velocity}^2)$$

- In the presence of a patent ductus arteriosus (PDA) and assuming the absence of RVOT obstruction, the RVSP may be predicted by the formula:

SPAP/RVSP mmHg = Systolic BP − 4 x (PDA peak systolic velocity^2)

Systolic Pulmonary Artery Pressure (SPAP)

- Normal: 15 to 30mmHg
- In the absence of RVOT obstruction, SPAP equals RVSP
- In the presence of RVOT obstruction (e.g., valvular pulmonic stenosis), the SPAP may be predicted by the formula:

SPAP mmHg = RVSP (utilizing the tricuspid regurgitation method (see above) −

Pulmonic valve transvalvular peak pressure gradient

- In patients with a PDA, aortopulmonary window or Blalock-Taussig shunt, the SPAP may be determined by the formula:

SPAP mmHg = Systolic BP − 4 x (shunt peak velocity^2)

Mean Pulmonary Artery Pressure (MPAP)

- Normal: 9 to 18mmHg
- 2/3 of SPAP equals MPAP
- A shortened RVOT PW Doppler acceleration time (normal ≥120 msec) may indicate increased MPAP
- The actual MPAP may be calculated by the following formula:

MPAP mmHg = 4 x (pulmonary regurgitation peak velocity$^)$)+RAP
MPAP mmHg = 79 − 0.45 x RVOT acceleration time

- If the acceleration time is 120msec or less use the formula :

MPAP mmHg = 90 − 0.62 x RVOT acceleration time

Pulmonary Artery End-diastolic Pressure (PAEDP)

- Normal: 4 to 12mmHg
- The PAEDP may be predicted by the formula:

PAEDP mmHg = 4 x (pulmonary regurgitation end-diastolic velocity^2) + RAP

- In the presence of an arterial to pulmonary shunt patient ductus arteriosus (PDA), Blalock-Taussig shunt, the PAEDP may be predicted by the formula:

PAEDP mmHg = Diastolic BP − 4 x (end-diastolic velocity^2 of the shunt)

Pulmonary Vascular Resistance (PVR)

- Normal: 20 to 130 dyne-sec-cm^{-5}

PVR (WU) = Tricuspid regurgitation peak velocity (TRV) / RVOT $_{VTI}$ (VTI$_{RVOT}$) x 10 + 0.16

A TRV/VTI$_{RVOT}$ ratio of greater than 0.2 may indicate a PVR >2 Wood units (WU)

Left Atrial Pressure (LAP)

- Normal: mean 2 to 12mmHg
- A left atrium that is larger in dimension than the right atrium in the absence of significant mitral regurgitation infers increased LAP. This may best evaluated in the apical 4-chamber view.
- An increased left atrial maximum volume (>34mL/m^2) may indicate a LAP of >12mmHg
- LAP may be predicted in the presence of mitral regurgitation in the absence of left ventricular outflow tract (LOVT) obstruction by the formula:

LAP mmHg = Systolic BP − 4 x (mitral regurgitation peak velocity^2)

- The LAP may be predicted in the presence of a patent foramen ovale or atrial septal defect by the formula:

LAP mmHg = 4 x (peak PFO/ASD velocity^2) + RAP

- Mitral annular E/e' ratio >14 (average) >15 (lateral annulus), >13 (septal annulus) may indicate increased LAP
- Elevated pulmonary artery pressures due to left-sided heart disease implies elevated left atrial pressures
- Evidence of left ventricular systolic dysfunction implies elevated LAP

Left Ventricular Diastolic Pressure (LVDP)

- Normal: mean 3 to 12mmHg
- In the absence of left ventricular inflow tract (LVIT) obstruction, the estimated LAP represents LVDP
- The presence of poor left ventricular systolic function implies elevated LVDP
- In the presence of aortic regurgitation (AR), the left ventricular end-diastolic pressure (LVEDP) may be calculated by the formula:

LVEDP mmHg = Diastolic blood pressure − 4 x (AR end-diastolic velocity^2)

- A pulmonary vein AR wave peak velocity of >30cm/s indicates an increase in LVEDP
- A pulmonary vein AR flow duration of >30 msec compared to the mitral valve A wave duration indicates increased LVEDP of >15mmHg

- A shortened isovolumic relaxation time (IVRT) of <60 msec may indicate an increased LAP and LVEDP
- Mitral annular valve average E/e' ratio >14 may indicate increased LVEDP

Left Ventricular Systolic Pressure (LVSP)

- Normal: 100 to 140mmHg
- In the absence of LVOT obstruction, the systolic blood pressure equals the LVSP
- In patients with valvular aortic stenosis, the LVSP may be calculated by the formula:

LVSP mmHg = Systolic BP + peak aortic transvalvular pressure gradient

- In the presence of mitral regurgitation (MR), the LVSP may be predicted by the formula:

LVSP mmHg = 4 x (MR peak velocity^2) + LAP

- The LVOT obstruction (such as in HOCM), can be predicted by the formula:

LVOT obstruction mmHg = 4 x (MR peak velocity^2) + LAP – systolic blood pressure

Echo/Doppler Measurements and Calculations

Michael Rampoldi, ACS, RDCS, RVT, FASE

24 | M-mode Measurements

Table 24.1: M-mode of the Aortic Valve and Aortic Root

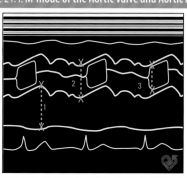

1	**Left Atrial End-Systolic Dimension (LA)**	Measure the greatest vertical distance between the leading edge of the posterior aortic wall and the anterior side of the posterior left atrial wall at end ventricular systole when the aorta is in its maximal anterior position (normal range: men 3.0 to 4.0cm; women 2.7 to 3.8cm) (Note: Left atrial volume measurement preferred (normal: $\leq$34mL/m^2)
2	**Aortic Root End-Diastolic Diameter (AoR)**	Measure the vertical distance from the outer-edge of the anterior aortic root to the inner-edge (leading-edge to leading-edge) of the posterior aortic wall at end-diastole (normal range 2.0 to 3.7cm)
3	**Aortic Valve Systolic Separation (ACS)**	Measure the maximal opening of the aortic valve cusps during the initial part of ventricular systole, using the internal borders of the aortic cusp echoes. The distance between the cusps may decrease slightly during ventricular systole (normal range 1.5 to 2.6cm)

Table 24.2: M-mode of the Mitral Valve

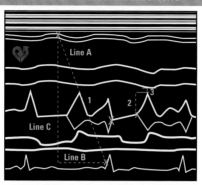

1	**E-F Slope (MV E-F)**	• Draw a diagonal line (Line A) through the steepest initial part of the E-F portion of the anterior mitral valve leaflet • Draw a horizontal line (Line B) near the bottom of the tracing rightward beginning at a point where Line A intersects one of the time lines on the tracing • Construct a vertical line perpendicular to Line B at a point along Line B that is exactly 1 sec from the intersection of Lines A and B. The length of this Line C, measured inmm, from where it intersects Lines A and B is the E-F slope of the anterior mitral valve leaflet inmm/s (normal range 70 to 150mm/s).
2	**D-E Excursion (Amplitude) (MV EXC)**	Measure the vertical distance from the point where the anterior and posterior mitral valve leaflets separate at the end of ventricular systole (D point) and an imaginary horizontal line that marks the maximal anterior motion of the anterior mitral leaflet in the beginning of ventricular diastole (E point) (normal range 18 to 28mm)
3	**E Point Septal Separation (EPSS)**	Measure the vertical distance from the mitral valve E point to the lowest point of the interventricular septum (normal range 2 to 7mm). An increased EPSS suggests a reduced ejection fraction.

Table 24.3: M-mode Measurements of the Left Ventricle [1]

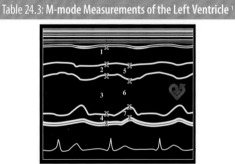

		Measurement	Normal Ranges
1	**Right Ventricular Dimension (RVIDd)**	**Vertical distance** Internal side of the anterior right ventricular wall to the right ventricular side of the septum in end-diastole	1.9 to 2.6cm Apical 4-chamber preferred for RV measurements
2	**IVS Diastolic Thickness (IVSd)***	**Vertical distance:** Right ventricular side of the IVS to the left ventricular side of the IVS at end-diastole	Men 0.6 to 1.0cm Women 0.6 to 0.9cm
3	**LVID End-Diastole (LVIDd)***	**Vertical distance** Endocardium of the IVS to the endocardium of the LVPW in end-diastole	Men 4.2 To 5.8cm Women 3.8 to 5.2cm
4	**LV Posterior Wall Diastolic Thickness (LVPWd)***	**Vertical distance** Endocardium of the LVPW to the epicardium in end-diastole	Men 0.6 to 1.0cm Women 0.6 to 0.9cm
5	**IVS Systolic Thickness (IVSs)***	**Systolic thickness of the IVS** the maximal vertical distance that occurs between the right ventricular and left ventricular sides of the IVS at end-ventricular systole	
6	**LVID End-Systole (LVIDs)***	**Vertical distance** Endocardium of the IVS at the lowest point of the septal motion to the endocardium of the LVPW	Men 2.5 to 4.0cm Women 2.2 to 3.5cm
7	**LVPW Systolic Thickness (LVPWs)***	**Systolic thickness of the LVPW** The maximal vertical distance between the endocardium and epicardium at end-ventricular systole	

*American Society of Recommendations [1]

- 2D targeted M-mode linear measurements of the interventricular septum, posterior wall and LV internal dimensions should be recorded from the parasternal long-axis view at the level of the LV minor axis, approximately at the mitral valve leaflet tips. These linear measurements can also be made directly from 2D images.

- Chamber dimensions and wall thicknesses can be acquired from the parasternal short-axis view of the LV using direct 2D measurements or targeted M-mode echocardiography provided that the M-mode cursor can be positioned perpendicular to the septum and LV posterior wall.

- A 2D method, useful in assessing patients with coronary disease, has been proposed. When using this method, it is recommended that the LV internal dimensions and wall thicknesses be measured at the mitral chordal level.

- End-diastole can be defined as the onset of the QRS complex, the first frame after mitral valve closure or the frame in the cardiac cycle in which the cardiac chamber dimension is largest. [2]

- End-systole is defined as the frame after aortic valve closure or the time in the cardiac cycle in which the cardiac chamber dimension is smallest. (For atrium end-systole is when chamber is largest in dimension)

Standard 2D Views and Wall Segments

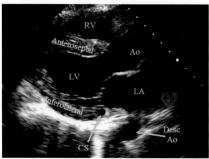

Figure 24.1: **Parasternal long-axis**

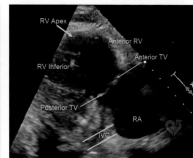

Figure 24.2: **Right ventricular inflow view**

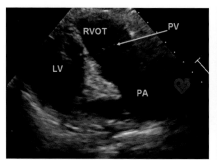

Figure 24.3: **Parasternal long-axis of the right ventricular outflow tract**

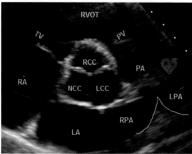

Figure 24.4: **Parasternal short-axis level of aortic valve**

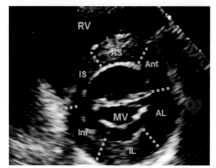

Figure 24.5: **Parasternal short-axis MV level**

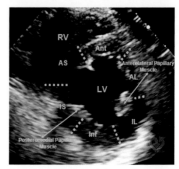

Figure 24.6: **Parasternal short-axis papillary**

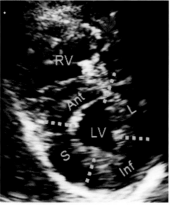

Figure 24.7: **Parasternal short-axis level of the apex**

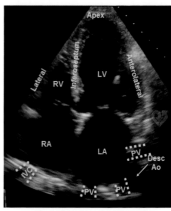

Figure 24.8: **Apical 4-chamber**

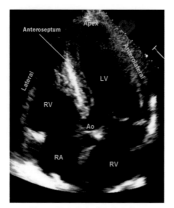

Figure 24.9: **Apical 5-chamber**

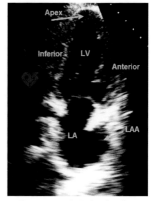

Figure 24.10: **Apical 2-chamber**

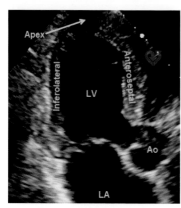

Figure 24.11: **Apical long-axis**

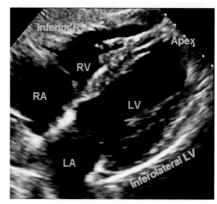

Figure 24.12: **Subcoastal 4-chamber**

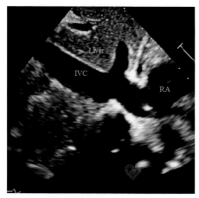

Figure 24.13: **Subcostal long-axis of inferior vena cava**

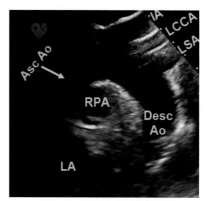

Figure 24.14: **Suprasternal notch**

24

Echo/Doppler Measurements and Calculations / Standard 2D Views and Wall Segments

2D Measurements

Table 24.4: Parasternal Long-Axis [1]

		Measurement	Normal Ranges
1	**Right Ventricular Minor Axis (RVIDd)***	**Inner-edge to inner-edge:** Anterior RV wall to the IVS-aortic junction	2.0 to 3.0cm Apical 4-chamber view preferred for RV measurements
2	**IVS Diastolic Thickness (IVSd)***	**Vertical distance:** Right ventricular side of the IVS to the left ventricular side of the IVS at end-diastole	Men 0.6 to 1.0cm Women 0.6 to 0.9cm
3	**LV Minor Axis End-Diastole (LVIDd)***	**Vertical distance:** Endocardium of the IVS to the endocardium of the LVPW at end-diastole	Men 4.2 to 5.8cm Women 3.8 to 5.2cm)
4	**LV Minor Axis End-Systole (LVIDs)***	**Vertical distance:** Endocardium of the IVS to the endocardium of the LVPW at end-systole	Men 2.5 to 4.0cm Women 2.2 to 3.5cm
5	**LV Posterior Wall Diastolic Thickness (LVPWd)***	**Vertical distance:** Endocardium of the LVPW to the epicardium at end-diastole	Men 0.6 to 1.0cm Women 0.6 to 0.9cm
6	**Aorta (AoRd)***	**Leading edge to leading edge:** At end-diastole at the valve plane perpendicular to the walls of the aortic root	
7	**Left Atrium End-Systole (LAs)***	**Leading edge to leading edge:** At the aortic valve plane, also perpendicular to the aortic root.	Men 3.0 to 4.0cm Women 2.7 to 3.8cm Volume measurement preferred

*American Society of Recommendations include:

• 2D targeted M-mode linear measurements of the interventricular septum, posterior wall and LV internal dimensions should be recorded from the parasternal long-axis view at the level of the LV minor axis, approximately at the mitral valve leaflet tips. These linear measurements can also be made directly from 2D images.

- Chamber dimensions and wall thicknesses can be acquired from the parasternal short-axis view of the LV using direct 2D measurements or targeted M-mode echocardiography provided that the M-mode cursor can be positioned perpendicular to the septum and LV posterior wall.

- A 2D method, useful in assessing patients with coronary disease, has been proposed. When using this method, it is recommended that the LV internal dimensions and wall thicknesses be measured at the mitral chordal level.

- End-diastole can be defined as the onset of the QRS complex, the first frame after mitral valve closure or the frame in the cardiac cycle in which the cardiac chamber dimension is largest.

- End-systole is defined as the frame after aortic valve closure or the time in the cardiac cycle in which the cardiac chamber dimension is smallest. (For atrium end-systole is when chamber is largest in dimension)

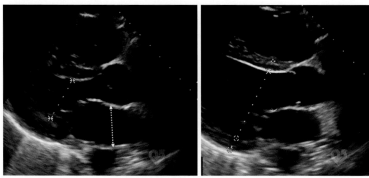

Figure 24.15: **Parasternal long axis**

Aortic Root and Ascending Aorta Measurements

Table 24.5: Aortic Root Dimensions in Normal Adults *(ASE Recommendations)*[1]				
	Absolute Values (cm)		**Indexed Values (cm/m)**	
Aortic Root	**Men**	**Women**	**Men**	**Women**
Annulus	2.6 ± 0.3	2.3 ± 0.2	1.3 ± 0.1	1.3 ± 0.1
Sinus of Valsalva	3.4 ± 0.3	3.0 ± .0.3	1.7 ± 0.2	1.8 ± 0.2
Sinotubular Junction	2.9 ± 0.3	2.6 ± 0.3	1.5 ± 0.2	1.5 ± 0.2
Proximal Ascending Aorta	3.0 ± 0.4	2.7 ± 0.4	1.5 ± 0.2	1.6 ± 0.3

Adapted from Roman et al. and Hiratzka et al.

Important to Note

- Measure the aortic root and ascending aorta at four levels (1 through 4) when clinically indicated.*

- Views used for measurements should be those that show the largest diameter of the aortic root (e.g., parasternal long-axis, right parasternal).*

- Measurement of the aortic diameter should be made perpendicular to the long-axis of the vessel using the inner-edge to inner-edge technique (aortic annulus measured inner edge to inner edge at end-systole) or leading-edge to leading-edge technique (for sinuses of valsalva, sinotubular junction and ascending aorta leading edge to leading edge at end diastole).*

- It is important to measure 1 through 3 for homograft placement, Ross procedure, stentless valve procedure, TAVI.

*American Society of Echocardiography Recommendations

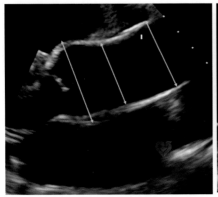

Figure 24.16: **SoV/Sinotubular junction/ascending aorta**   Figure 24.17: **Aortic annulus**

Biplane Simpson's Method of Discs (LA Volumes)

Steps in Acquiring Left Atrial Volumes

1. Acquire an apical 4-chamber view, zoom the left atrium, trace the left atrial cavity excluding the left atrial appendage and the pulmonary veins at ventricular end-systole (ventricular end-systole is defined as one frame immediately preceding mitral valve opening or when the left atrium is at its largest). Measure the left atrial end-systolic length from the mid mitral annulus to the superior portion of the left atrium. These steps will yield the left atrial end-systolic volume. The same steps are repeated at end-diastole for the left atrial end-diastolic volume.

2. The apical 2-chamber view is then acquired and the same end-systolic and end-diastolic measurements are performed (not shown)

3. The calculation of end-systolic volume, end-diastolic volume and ejection fraction will be calculated from the summation of areas from the diameters of 20 cylinders or discs of equal height.

4. The difference in left atrial lengths between the apical 4-chamber view and the apical 2-chamber view should be less than 5mm.

Right Atrial Volume

The recommended parameter to assess right atrial size is right atrial volume calculated using the single plane Simpson's method of discs or area-length method. (normal range: men $25 \pm 7mL/m^2$; women $21 \pm 6mL/m^2$)

Biplane Area-length Method (LA Volumes)

Steps in Acquiring Left Atrial Volumes

1. Acquire an apical 4-chamber view, zoom the left atrium, trace the left atrial cavity excluding the left atrial appendage and the pulmonary veins at ventricular end-systole (ventricular end-systole is defined as one frame immediately preceding mitral valve opening or when the left atrium is at its largest) Measure the length of the left atrium from the mid-annulus plane to the superior aspect of the left atrium.

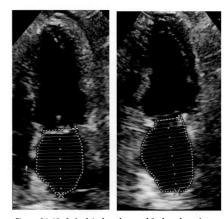

Figure 24.18: **Apical 4-chamber and 2-chamber views**

2. Acquire the apical 2-chamber view and the same end-systolic measurements are performed. In the area-length formula the length is measured in both the four and 2-chamber views and the shortest of these two length measurements is used in the formula:

Left atrial volume (mL) = 8/3pi x [(A1) x (A2) / (L)]

3. The difference in left atrial lengths between the apical 4-chamber view and the apical 2-chamber view should be less than 5mm.

4. Right atrial volume can be determined using the single plane area-length method in the apical 4-chamber view.

Biplane Simpson's Method of Discs (LV Volumes)

Steps in Acquiring Left Ventricular Volumes

1. Acquire an apical 4-chamber view, trace the left ventricular cavity at ventricular end-diastole (end-diastole can be defined as the onset of the QRS complex, the frame after mitral valve closure or the frame in the cardiac cycle in which the cardiac chamber dimension is largest). Measure the left ventricular end-diastolic length from the mid mitral annulus to the cardiac apex. This will yield the left ventricular end-diastolic volume. The same steps are repeated at end-systole (end-systole is defined as the frame after aortic valve closure or the time in the cardiac cycle in which the cardiac chamber dimension is smallest) to determine the ventricular end-systolic volume.

2. The apical 2-chamber view is then acquired and the same end-diastolic and end-systolic measurements are performed

3. The calculation of end-diastolic volume, end-systolic volume, stroke volume, cardiac output, cardiac index and ejection fraction will be calculated from the summation of areas from the diameters of 20 cylinders or discs of equal height

4. The percentage difference in length between the apical 4-chamber view and apical 2-chamber view should be less than 10%

5. The right ventricular end-diastolic, end-systolic volumes and ejection fraction may be determined in the apical 4-chamber view by using the single plane Simpson's method of discs

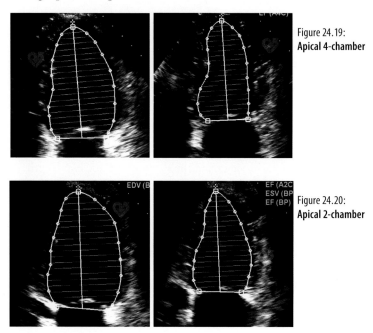

Figure 24.19:
Apical 4-chamber

Figure 24.20:
Apical 2-chamber

Left Ventricular Mass

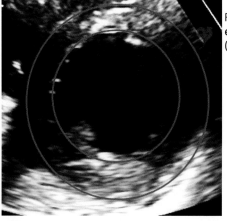

Figure 24.21: **Endocardial and epicardial trace of the left ventricle (end-diastole)**

Steps in Acquiring Left Ventricular Mass

1. Trace the epicardial border of the left ventricle at the level of the papillary muscles at end-diastole (end-diastole can be defined as the onset of the QRS complex, the frame after mitral valve closure or the frame in the cardiac cycle in which the cardiac chamber dimension is largest)
2. Trace the endocardial border of the left ventricle at the level of the papillary muscles at end-diastole
3. Measure the length of the left ventricle in the apical 4-chamber view at end-diastole from the mid mitral annulus to the cardiac apex
4. The left ventricular mass is determined by subtracting the left ventricular volume enclosed by the endocardial surface (cavitary volume) from the volume enclosed by the epicardial surface (total volume). The specific weight of the myocardium is also considered.
5. Left ventricular mass divided by body surface area will determine left ventricular mass index

Right Atrial Measurements

The primary transthoracic window for the evaluation of right atrial dimensions is the apical 4-chamber view.

Right Atrial Volume

The recommended parameter to assess right atrial size is right atrial volume calculated using the single plane Simpson's method of discs or area-length method. (normal range: men $25 \pm 7mL/m^2$; women $21 \pm 6mL/m^2$) *(ASE Recommendation)* [1]

Right Atrial Area

- Right atrial area should be obtained routinely in patients with RV and/or LV dysfunction
- Right atrial area is traced at the end of ventricular systole (largest volume) from the lateral aspect of the tricuspid annulus, following the right atrial endocardium, excluding the inferior vena cava and right atrial appendage. ($>18cm^2$ is abnormal)

Superior-inferior (Major Dimension)

The maximal superior-inferior measurement of the right atrium is from the center of the tricuspid valve annulus to the center of the superior right atrial wall parallel to the interatrial septum at the end of ventricular systole. (>5.3cm is abnormal)

Medial-lateral (Minor Dimension)

The mid-minor distance is measured at end ventricular systole from the mid-level of the right atrial free wall to the interatrial septum perpendicular to the long axis of the right atrium. (>4.4cm is abnormal)

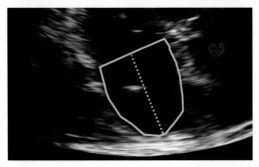

Figure 24.22: **Apical 4-chamber view of choice for evaluation of the right atrium** (ASE Recommendations) [1]

Right Atrial Pressure

Estimation of Right Atrial Pressure on the Basis of IVC diameter and Collapse

The inferior vena cava should be measured using the subcostal long axis of the inferior vena cava. The measurement should be made at end expiration and 1 to 2cm from the entrance of the inferior vena cava in to the right atrium. The change in diameter should be

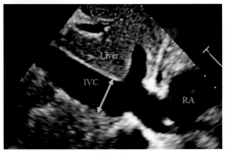

Figure 24.23: **(IVC) Inferior venacava**

evaluated during quiet respiration and with a sniff. It may be better to use the subcostal short axis of the inferior vena cava when evaluating the change in diameter during the sniff test. The left lateral position may be used to confirm a dilated inferior vena cava and improve the evaluation of the collapsibility of the inferior vena cava. The inferior vena cava may be dilated in normal young athletes. Positive pressure ventilation using the inferior vena cava dimension and collapsibility is not useful although an inferior vena cava dimension of ≤12mm in these patients suggests a right atrial pressure of <10mmHg.

Additional Indications of Increased Right Atrial Pressure

A dilated right atrium and/or interatrial septal bulge towards the left atrium throughout the cardiac cycle suggests increased right atrial pressure.

Hepatic Veins and the Estimation of Right Atrial Pressure

• With normal right atrial pressures, the hepatic vein S wave is dominant with the S wave peak velocity greater than the D wave peak velocity.

• With increased right atrial pressure, the S wave dominance is lost and the Vs/Vd is <1.0.

• With increased right atrial pressure, the hepatic vein systolic filling fraction (Vs/Vs + Vd) <55% is the most sensitive and specific sign of increased right atrial pressure.

Right Ventricle Measurements

Wall Thickness

RV free wall thickness can be measured at end-diastole with M-mode or 2D echocardiography from the subcostal window, preferably at the level of the tip of the anterior tricuspid valve leaflet or the left parasternal windows may be used. (normal: <0.5cm)

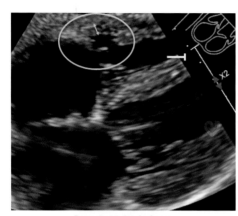

Figure 24.24: **RV thickness**
(subcostal)

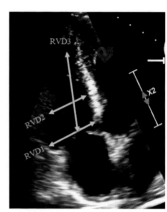

Figure 24.25: **RV dimensions**
(focused view)

Linear Dimensions

- The right ventricle can be measured from the apical 4-chamber view at end-diastole.
- Basal diameter: Maximal short axis dimension in the basal one third of the right ventricle seen in the apical 4-chamber view (RVD1) (>4.1cm abnormal)
- Mid-cavity dimension: Measured in the middle third of the right ventricle at the level of the left ventricular papillary muscles (RVD2) (>3.5cm abnormal)
- Longitudinal dimension: Measured from the mid-plane of the tricuspid annulus to the right ventricular apex (RVD3) (>8.3cm abnormal)

Right Ventricular Outflow Tract

- The right ventricular outflow tract dimension should be measured using the left parasternal or subcostal windows at end-diastole (onset of the QRS complex)
- **RVOT (proximal):** In the parasternal long axis or short axis of the aortic valve, the proximal RVOT can be measured. (>3.5cm abnormal)
- **RVOT distal:** In the parasternal short axis of the aortic valve, the distal RVOT diameter just proximal to the pulmonary valve annulus is the most reproducible and should be generally used (>2.7cm abnormal)

Right Ventricular Area and Right Ventricular Fractional Area Change

Right ventricular area may be acquired using the apical 4-chamber view by tracing from the tricuspid annulus along the free wall to the apex back to the annulus along the interventricular septum. Tracing at end-diastole and end-systole will allow calculation of the right ventricular area change (abnormal <35%).

Right Ventricular Ejection Fraction

- The method of discs has been used to determine the right ventricular "body" volume using the apical 4-chamber view. RV volumes are underestimated because of exclusion of the right ventricular outflow tract. The lower reference value of the right ventricular ejection fraction is 44%.

- Two dimensional derived estimation of right ventricular ejection fraction is not recommended because of the heterogeneity of methods and the numerous geometric assumptions. *(ASE Recommendation)* [1]

- Three dimensional right ventricular volumes and ejection fraction have been calculated. The upper reference limit for indexed right ventricular end diastolic volume is 89 mL/m^2 and for end systolic is 45 mL/m^2 (10% to 15% lower in women than men).

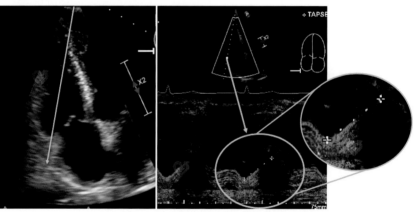

Figure 24.26: **Tricuspid annular plane systolic excursion (TAPSE) or tricuspid annular motion (TAM)**

- TAPSE or TAM is a method to measure the distance of the systolic excursion of the RV annular segment along its longitudinal plane from the standard apical 4-chamber view. It is inferred that the greater the descent of the base during systole, the better the RV global systolic function. It assumes that it is representative of the entire right ventricle and may be invalid in many disease states or in the presence of RV segmental wall motion abnormalities

- TAPSE is acquired by placing an M-mode cursor through the tricuspid annulus from the apical 4-chamber view and measuring the amount of longitudinal motion of the tricuspid annulus at peak systole.

- TAPSE should be used routinely as a simple method of estimating RV function. (≥1.7cm normal) *(ASE Recommendation)* [1]

Tissue Doppler Imaging

RV S' (systolic excursion velocity)

To obtain the RV S' velocity, an apical 4-chamber is acquired, the TDI sample volume is placed in either the tricuspid annulus or the middle of the basal segment of the RV free wall. The velocity S' is read as the highest systolic velocity without overgaining the Doppler envelope. (<9.5cm/s abnormal) *(ASE Recommendation)* [2]

RV dP/dt

The rate of pressure rise in the ventricles (dP/dt) is an index of ventricular contractility or systolic function (abnormal <400mmHg) *(ASE Recommendation)* [1]

Mitral Valve Area (MVA) by 2D Planimetry

1. Obtain a parasternal short-axis view of the mitral valve using the zoom mode. Angle the short-axis scan plane in a superior-inferior arc until the smallest anatomic valve orifice is recorded during maximal initial diastolic leaflet distention.

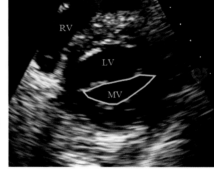

2. Planimeter (trace) where the tissue meets the blood pool during mid-diastole on a frozen image. The instrument will determine the mitral valve area. This represents the true anatomic valve

Figure 24.27: **Short axis mitral valve level**

area and will be larger than the Doppler determined valve area. Several measurements may be required in patients with atrial fibrillation.

3. Proper gain settings and care in measuring the true valve orifice is required.

4. Real time 3D and 3D guided biplane imaging may be useful in optimizing the position of the measurement plane improving reproducibility.

Aortic Valve Area (AVA) by 2D Planimetry

Aortic valve area can be determined by planimetry using either 2D, 3D or TEE 3D. Planimetry may be an acceptable alternative when Doppler estimation of the flow velocities are unreliable.

Doppler Wave Form Tracings

Mitral Valve Doppler Tracings

Normal

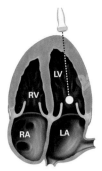
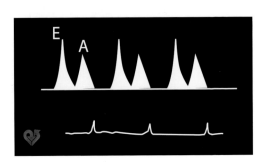

- Utilize apical window (slide transducer lateral and tilt posterior)
- Flow in diastole
- Biphasic ("M" configuration)
- Flow toward the transducer (above the baseline)
- Normal peak velocity range 0.6 to 1.3 m/s; mean 0.9 m/s
- Color flow Doppler will demonstrate red with yellow at mitral valve leaflet tips

Abnormal

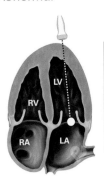

Pulsed Wave Doppler (PW)
MR (aliasing)

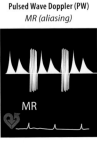

Continuous Wave Doppler (CW)
MS / MR

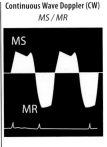

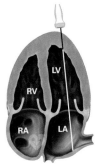

Tricuspid Valve Doppler Tracings

Normal

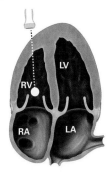

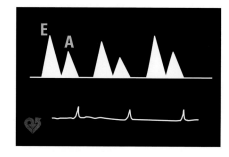

- Utilize apical window (slide transducer medially)
- Flow in diastole
- Biphasic ("M" configuration)
- Flow toward the transducer (above the baseline)
- Normal peak velocity range 0.3 to 0.7 m/s; mean 0.5 m/s
- Color flow Doppler will demonstrate red at tricuspid valve leaflet tips

Abnormal

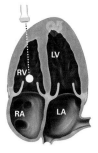

Pulsed Wave Doppler (PW)
TR (aliasing)

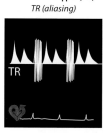

Continuous Wave Doppler (CW)
TS and TR

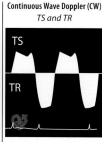

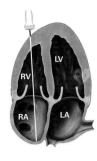

LVOT/Aortic Valve Doppler Tracings

Normal

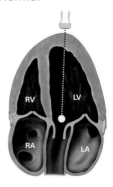

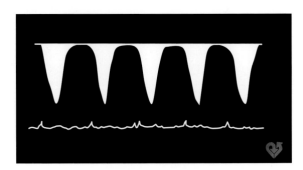

- Utilize apical window (may need to slide transducer lateral)
- Flow in systole
- Bullet shaped
- Flow away from the transducer (below the baseline)
- Normal LVOT peak velocity range 0.7 to 1.1 m/s; mean 0.9 m/s
- Normal aortic valve peak velocity range 1.0 to 1.7 m/s; mean 1.35 m/s
- Color flow Doppler will demonstrate blue with aliasing to yellow, orange and red

Abnormal

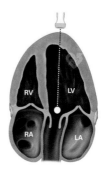

Pulsed Wave Doppler (PW)
AR (aliasing)

Continuous Wave Doppler (CW)
AR and AS

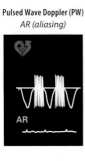

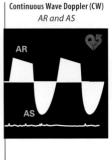

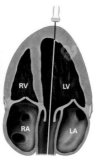

RVOT/Pulmonary Valve Doppler Tracings

Normal

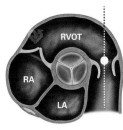

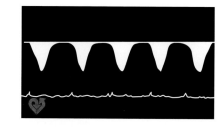

- Utilize parasternal short-axis of the base or subcostal
- Flow in systole
- Bullet shaped
- Flow away from the transducer (below the baseline)
- Normal peak velocity range 0.6 to 0.9m/s; mean 0.75m/s
- Color flow Doppler will demonstrate blue with aliasing to yellow, orange and red

Abnormal

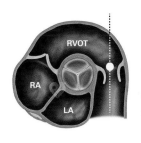

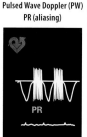

Pulsed Wave Doppler (PW)
PR (aliasing)

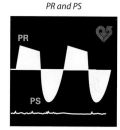

Continuous Wave Doppler (CW)
PR and PS

Doppler Measurements and Calculations

Bernoulli Equation (Simplified)

$$P_1 - P_2 = 4 \times (V^2)$$

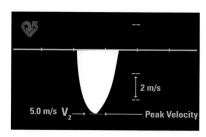

$$P1 - P2 = 4 \times (V^2)$$
$$P_1 - P_2 = 4 \times (5^2)$$
$$P_1 - P_2 = 4 \times (25)$$
$$P_1 - P_2 = 100 \text{mmHg}$$

Bernoulli Equation (Lengthened)

$$P_1 - P_2 = 4 \times (V_2^2 - V_1^2)$$

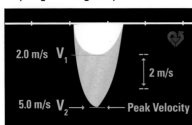

$$P_1 - P_2 = 4 \times (V_2^2 - V_1^2)$$
$$P_1 - P_2 = 4 \times (5^2 - 2^2)$$
$$P_1 - P_2 = 4 \times (25 - 4)$$
$$P_1 - P_2 = 4 \times (21)$$
$$P_1 - P_2 = 84 mmHg$$

Bernoulli Equation Mean Pressure Gradient

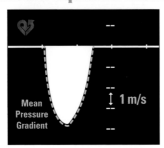

The mean pressure gradient is calculated by measuring the velocity at equally spaced points, squaring each velocity, averaging the velocity values and multiplying the average by 4.

RV Systolic Pressure (RVSP)

$$RVSPmmHg = 4 \times (TR\ peak\ velocity^2) + RAP$$

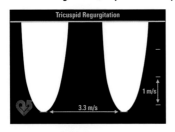

$$RVSPmmHg = 4 \times (TR\ peak\ velocity^2) + RAP$$
$$RVSPmmHg = 4 \times (3.3^2) + RAP$$
$$RVSPmmHg = 43.5 + 5mmHg$$
$$RVSPmmHg = 49mmHg$$

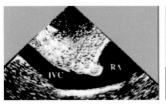
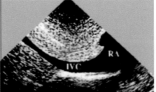

Figure 24.28:
RAPmmHg = 5mmHg
(IVC appears normal in dimension and collapses >50% with inspiration

Important to Note

- RVSP equals systolic pulmonary artery pressure (SPAP) in the absence of RVOT obstruction.
- To approximate the RAP, examine the IVC by the 2D and substitute one of the following values for the actual RAP
- Ranges are provided for low and intermediate categories, but for simplicity, midrange values of 3mmHg for normal and 8mmHg for intermediate are suggested. Intermediate (8mmHg) RA pressures may be downgraded to normal (3mmHg) if no secondary indices of elevated RA pressure are present, upgraded to high if minimal collapse with sniff (<35%) and secondary indices of elevated RA pressures are present, or left at 8mmHg if uncertain.
- A dilated IVC in a mechanically ventilated patient may not indicate an elevated RAP.
- Athletes may have dilated IVC with normal collapsibility.

24

Echo/Doppler Measurements and Calculations / Doppler Wave Form Tracings / RVSP in the Presence of a Ventricular Septal Defect

Table 24.6: Inferior Vena Cava Collapsibility Index			
Variable	**Normal** (0–5 [3]mmHg)	**Intermediate** (5–10 [8]mmHg)	**High** (15mmHg)
IVC diameter	≤2.1cm	≤2.1cm	>2.1cm
Collapse with sniff	>50%	<50%	>50%
Secondary indices of elevated RAP			• Restrictive filling • Tricuspid E/e' >6 • Diastolic flow predominance in hepatic veins (systolic filling fraction <55%)

RVSP in the Presence of a Ventricular Septal Defect

$$RVSPmmHg = SBP - 4 \times (VSD\ peak\ velocity^2)$$

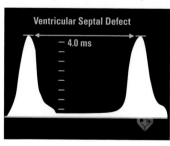

Ventricular Septal Defect

— 4.0 ms

(Assuming a SBP of 124mmHg)

$$RVSPmmHg = SBP - 4 \times (VSD\ peak\ velocity^2)$$

$$RVSPmmHg = SBP - 4 \times (4^2)$$

$$RVSPmmHg = 124mmHg - 64mmHg$$

$$RVSPmmHg = 60mmHg$$

Important to Note

RVSP equals systolic pulmonary artery pressure (SPAP) in the absence of RVOT obstruction.

Systolic Pulmonary Artery Pressure (SPAP) in the Presence of a PDA

$$\text{SPAP mmHg} = \text{SBP} - 4 \times (\text{PDA peak velocity}^2)$$

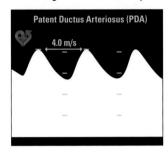

Patent Ductus Arteriosus (PDA)

4.0 m/s

(Assuming a SBP of 124mmHg)

$$\text{SPAP mmHg} = \text{SBP} - 4 \times (\text{PDA peak velocity}^2)$$
$$\text{SPAP mmHg} = \text{SBP} - 4 \times (4^2)$$
$$\text{SPAP mmHg} = 124\text{mmHg} - 64\text{mmHg}$$
$$\text{SPAP mmHg} = 60\text{mmHg}$$

Important to Note

SPAP equals right ventricular systolic pressure (RVSP) in the absence of RVOT obstruction.

MPAP Utilizing RVOT Acceleration Time

$$\text{MPAP mmHg} = 80 - 0.5 \times \text{acceleration time}$$

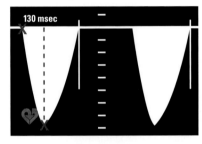

130 msec

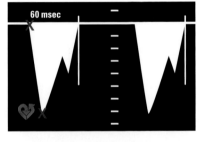

60 msec

Normal RVOT

$$\text{MPAP mmHg} = 80 - 0.5 \times \text{accel. time}$$
$$\text{MPAP mmHg} = 80 - 0.5 \times 130 \text{ msec}$$
$$\text{MPAP mmHg} = 80 - 65 \text{ msec}$$
$$\text{MPAP mmHg} = 15\text{mmHg}$$

Pulmonary Hypertension

$$\text{MPAP mmHg} = 80 - 0.5 \times \text{accel. time}$$
$$\text{MPAP mmHg} = 80 - 0.5 \times 60 \text{ msec}$$
$$\text{MPAP mmHg} = 80 - 30 \text{ msec}$$
$$\text{MPAP mmHg} = 50\text{mmHg}$$

MPAP Utilizing Pulmonary Regurgitation Jet

MPAPmmHg = 4 x (PR early-diastolic velocity^2) + RAP

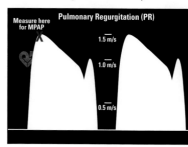

(Assuming a RAP of 3mmHg)

MPAPmmHg =

4 x (PR early-diastolic velocity^2) + RAP

MPAPmmHg = 4 x (1.5^2) + RAP

MPAPmmHg = 9 + RAP

MPAPmmHg = 9 + 3mmHg

MPAPmmHg = 12mmHg

Pulmonary Artery End-Diastolic Pressure (PAEDP)

PAEDPmmHg = 4 x (PR end-diastolic velocity^2) + RAP

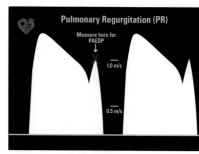

(Assuming a RAP of 3mmHg)

PAEDPmmHg =

4 x (PR end-diastolic velocity^2) + RAP

PAEDPmmHg = 4 x (1^2) + RAP

PAEDPmmHg = 4 x (1) + RAP

PAEDPmmHg = 4 + 3mmHg

PAEDPmmHg = 7mmHg

Important to Note

• The PAEDP estimates the pulmonary wedge pressure.

• The mean pulmonary pressure may be estimated by the formula:

MPAPmmHg = 4 x (PR peak velocity^2)

Pulmonary Vascular Resistance (PVR) Utilizing Tricuspid Regurgitation and RVOT VTI

$$PVR\ (WU) = \frac{Tricuspid\ regurgitation\ peak\ velocity\ (TRV)}{RVOT\ VTI\ (VTI_{RVOT})} \times 10 + 0.16$$

24

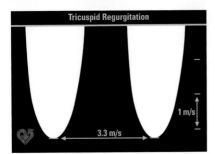

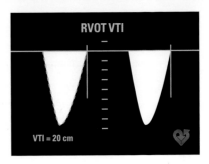

PVR ratio = 3.3 m/s / 20cm = 0.17

PVR (WU) = 0.17 x 10 + 0.16 = 1.86

Important to Note

A TRV/VTI$_{RVOT}$ ratio >0.2 may indicate a PVR >2 Wood units (WU)

LV Stroke Volume Cardiac Output Cardiac Index

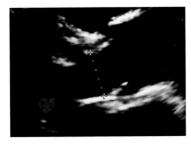

SV = CSA x VTI

SV = .785 x D^2 x VTI

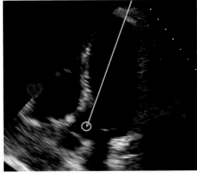

Figure 24.29: CSAcm^2 = .785 x D^2
CSAcm^2 = .785 x (2^2)
CSAcm^2 = .785 x (4)
CSAcm^2 = 3.14cm^2

5. Determine the cross sectional area of the left ventricular outflow tract (LVOT) in the parasternal long-axis by measuring the LVOT diameter during early to mid ventricular systole from inner edge to inner edge where the right aortic valve coronary cusp meets the interventricular septum to where the noncoronary aortic valve cusp meets the anterior mitral valve leaflet in a line parallel to the aortic annulus. Using the zoom feature will aid in acquiring this measurement.

6. From the apical 5-chamber view or apical long axis view, place a pulsed wave Doppler sample volume near the aortic valve annulus and determine the LVOT velocity time integral (VTI$_{LVOT}$). Increasing the sweep speed to 100mm/s may aid in acquiring this measurement. An aortic valve closing click should be obtained to ensure accuracy.

7. Multiply stroke volume times heart rate to determine cardiac output

8. Divide cardiac output by body surface area to determine cardiac index

Aortic Valve Area (AVA) by the Continuity Equation

AVA (cm^2) = CSA$_{LVOT}$ (cm^2) x VTI$_{LVOT}$ (cm) ÷ VTI$_{AoV}$ (cm)

AVA (cm^2) = .785 x LVOT Diameter^2 x VTI$_{LVOT}$ ÷ VTI$_{AoV}$

1. Determine the cross sectional area of the left ventricular outflow tract (LVOT). The left ventricular outflow tract diameter (LVOTd) is measured in a zoomed parasternal long axis view in mid-systole from the white-black interface (inner to inner) of the septal endocardium to the anterior mitral valve leaflet, parallel to the aortic valve plane. Some experts prefer to measure within 0.3 to 1.0cm of the valve orifice whereas others prefer the measurement at the annulus level. Note that in many patients, the left ventricular outflow tract is relatively rectangular within 1cm of the aortic annulus.

CSA$_{LVOT}$ (cm^2) = .785 x LVOT Diameter^2

2. The LVOT velocity is recorded with PW Doppler in either the apical 5-chamber view or apical long axis view. The PW Doppler sample volume is positioned just proximal to the aortic valve so that the location of the velocity recording matches the LVOT diameter measurement. When the sample volume is optimally positioned, the recording demonstrates a smooth velocity curve with a well defined peak, narrow band of velocities throughout systole. This may not be the case in many patients due to flow convergence resulting in spectral dispersion. In this case, the sample volume is then slowly moved towards the apex until a smooth velocity curve is obtained. The VTI is measured tracing the dense modal velocity throughout systole.

SV = .785 x D^2 x VTI$_{LVOT}$

3. Utilizing CW Doppler from multiple windows (e.g., apical, right parasternal, suprasternal, subcostal) obtain the maximal aortic velocity and measure the aortic valve velocity time integral (VTI$_{AoV}$). Increasing the sweep speed to 100mm/s may help in acquiring this measurement.

Aortic Valve Area (AVAcm^2) = .785 x LVOT Diameter^2 x VTI$_{LVOT}$ ÷ VTI$_{AoV}$

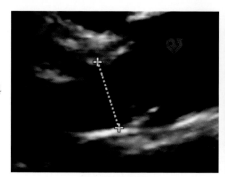

Figure 24.30: **LVOT**

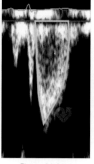

Figure 24.31:
PW Doppler LVOT

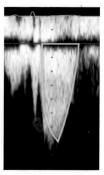

Figure 24.32:
CW Aortic Valve

Case Example

Measurements

- LVOT Diameter: 2.0cm
- VTI_{LVOT}: 15cm (V_1)
- VTI_{AoV}: 45cm (V_2)

Calculations

- Aortic Valve Area ($AVAcm^2$) = .785 x LVOT Diameter^2 x VTI_{LVOT} ÷ VTI_{AoV}
- Aortic Valve Area ($AVAcm^2$) = .785 x 2.0^2cm x 15cm ÷ 45cm
- AVA (cm^2) = $47cm^3$ ÷ 45cm
- AVA (cm^2) = $1.0cm^2$

Important to Note

- The peak velocities of the left ventricular outflow tract (V_1) and aortic valve (V_2) may be substituted for the velocity time integrals:

$$AVA \ (cm^2) = CSA_{LVOT} \ x \ LVOT \ Peak \ Velocity \div Aortic \ Valve \ Peak \ Velocity$$

- Using the peak velocities instead of the velocity time integrals does eliminate information concerning left ventricular stroke volume, cardiac output and cardiac index.

Pulmonary Valve Area (PVA)

Pulmonary valve area can be determined by the continuity equation by measuring the RVOT diameter, VTI_{RVOT} and $VTI_{pulmonary \ valve}$ in the parasternal short-axis of the aortic valve, parasternal long axis of the RVOT and/or subcostal short axis at the base

Mitral Valve Area (MVA) by the Continuity Equation

$MVA\ (cm^2) = CSA_{LVOT}\ (cm^2)\ x\ VTI_{LVOT} \div VTI_{MV}$

$MVA\ (cm^2) = .785\ x\ Left\ Ventricular\ Outflow\ Tract\ Diameter^2 \div VTI_{MV}$

1. Determine the cross sectional area of the left ventricular outflow tract (LVOT) in the parasternal long-axis by measuring the LVOT diameter during early to mid ventricular systole from inner edge to inner edge where the right aortic valve coronary cusp meets the interventricular septum to where the noncoronary aortic valve cusp meets the anterior mitral valve leaflet in a line parallel to the aortic annulus. Using the zoom feature will aid in acquiring this measurement.

$CSA_{LVOT}\ (cm^2) = .785\ x\ LVOT\ Diameter^2$

2. From the apical 5-chamber view or apical long axis view, place a pulsed wave Doppler sample volume near the aortic valve annulus and determine the LVOT velocity time integral (VTI_{LVOT}). Increasing the sweep speed to 100mm/s may aid in acquiring this measurement. An aortic valve closing click should be obtained to ensure accuracy.

$CSA_{LVOT}\ x\ VTI_{LVOT}$

3. Utilizing CW Doppler from the apical window, obtain a Doppler tracing of the mitral valve inflow and determine the mitral valve velocity time integral (VTI_{MV}). A sweep speed of 100mm/s may aid in acquiring this measurement.

4. Calculate the mitral valve area (MVA):

$MVA\ (cm^2) = CSA_{LVOT}\ x\ VTI_{LVOT} \div VTI_{MV}$

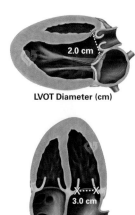

LVOT Diameter (cm)

MV Diameter

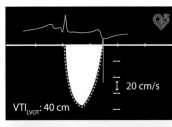

VTI_{LVOT}: 40 cm

20 cm/s

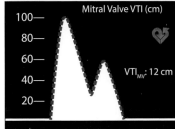

Mitral Valve VTI (cm)

VTI_{MV}: 12 cm

24

Echo/Doppler Measurements and Calculations / Doppler Wave Form Tracings / Mitral Valve Area (MVA) by the Continuity Equation

Case Example

Measurements
- LVOT diameter (cm) = 2.0cm
- VTI LVOT (cm) = 40cm
- Mitral valve annulus (cm) = 3.0cm
- VTI MV (cm) = 12cm
- VTI AR (cm) = 180cm

Calculations
- SVLVOT (cc) = .785 x 2.0^2cm x 40cm
- SVLVOT (cc) = 126 cc
- SVMV (cc) = .785 x 3.0^2cm x 12cm
- SVMV (cc) = 85 cc
- RVAR (cc) = 126 cc – 85 cc = 41 cc
- RFAR (cc) = 41 cc/126 cc = 33%
- EROAR (cm^2) = 41 cc/180cm = .23cm^2 or 23mm^2

Tricuspid Valve Area (TVA)

Tricuspid valve area can be determined by the continuity equation by measuring the RVOT diameter distal, VTI_{RVOT} and $VTI_{tricuspid\ valve}$.

Important to Note

The continuity equation is recommended when determining the effective valve orifice area in a mitral valve prosthesis.

Color Flow Analysis

Mitral Regurgitation

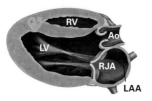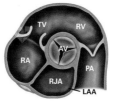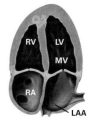

Jet Area (JA)

1. Obtain parasternal long-axis view, parasternal short-axis view of the aortic valve and apical 4-chamber view with color flow Doppler on
2. Outline the RJA and the area will be measured by computerized planimetry

Jet Area/Left Atrial Area (JA/LAA)

1. Outline the LAA and the ultrasound machine computer software will calculate the area
2. Divide the RJA by the LAA

Important to Note

- The systolic blood pressure, heart rate and duration of flow should be known.
- The color flow Doppler gain should be set appropriately (increase color gain until speckling appears then decrease color gain until color speckling disappears)
- The color flow Doppler velocity scale should be set between 50 to 70cm/s.
- Choose the largest ratio.

Tricuspid Regurgitation (JA/RAA)

The same approach may be used for tricuspid regurgitation when determining JA and JA/RAA using the parasternal long-axis of the right ventricle, parasternal short-axis of the aortic valve, apical 4-chamber and subcostal 4-chamber.

Vena Contracta

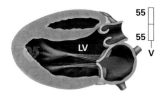

Figure 24.33: **Mitral regurgitation in the parasternal long-axis**

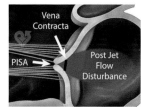

Figure 24.34: **Components of a turbulent jet**

1. Parasternal long-axis view with color flow Doppler velocity scale set at between 50 to 70cm/s
2. Zoom the mitral valve and the mitral regurgitation jet (narrowest sector width which allows visualization of the flow acceleration zone (PISA), vena contracta and a portion of the regurgitant jet should be chosen)
3. Angulate the transducer until the regurgitant flow proximal to, through and distal to the mitral valve is well visualized
4. Freeze and scroll until the largest diameter of the vena contracta is found
5. Measure the vena contracta of the regurgitant flow immediately downstream from the flow convergence zone (PISA). Three to five beats should be measured and averaged.

Important to Note

• Multiple views (e.g., apical 4-chamber view, apical long-axis view) may be required to be perpendicular to the commissural line but the vena contracta is usually best imaged in the parasternal long-axis view. The long-axis plane may be used in multiplane transesophageal echocardiography.

• The apical 2-chamber view, which is oriented parallel to the line of leaflet coaptation, generally demonstrates a wide vena contracta in mild mitral regurgitation and should not be utilized to measure the vena contracta.

Tricuspid Regurgitation

The same approach may be used for tricuspid regurgitation by using the parasternal long-axis of the right ventricle, parasternal short-axis of the aortic valve, apical 4-chamber view or subcostal 4-chamber view.

PISA (Proximal Isovelocity Surface Area) Method

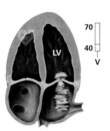 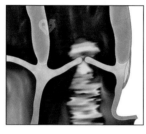 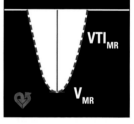

1. Optimize the color flow Doppler image of the mitral regurgitation utilizing the apical 4-chamber view

2. Zoom the regurgitant mitral valve

3. Shift the color flow Doppler zero baseline downward (upward for TEE) to an aliasing velocity of between 20 to 40cm/s

Image courtesy of Brad Roberts

4. Freeze the image and cine loop to identify the optimal hemispheric ("golf ball on a tee") which should occur in midsystole

5. Measure the radius

6. Obtain the peak velocity and velocity time integral (VTI) of the mitral regurgitation utilizing CW Doppler

7. Calculate the effective regurgitant orifice area (EROA) by the formula:

$$EROA mm^2 = \frac{6.28 \times r^2 \times \text{Aliasing Velocity (cm/s)}}{\text{Mitral Regurgitation Peak Velocity (cm/s)}}$$

8. Calculate the regurgitant volume (RV) by the formula:

RV (cc) = EROAcm² x Mitral Regurgitation Velocity Time Integral (VTI) (cm)

Case Example

Measurements
- Radius (cm): 1.0cm
- Aliasing velocity (cm/s): 40cm/s
- Mitral regurgitation peak velocity 500cm/s
- Mitral regurgitation VTI (cm): 150cm

Calculations

EROA (mm2) = 6.28 x (12cm) x 40cm/s ÷ 500cm/s

EROA (mm2) = 251cm³ ÷ 500cm/s

EROA (mm2) = .50cm² or 50mm²

RV (cc) = .50cm² x 150cm

RV (cc) = 75 cc

Table 24.7: Grade Regurgitation		
Grade	**Radius Diameter (assumes holosystolic duration)**	**ASE Recomendations**
Mild	<4mm	≤3mm
Moderate	5 to 7mm	
Moderately Severe	8 to 10mm	≥10mm
Severe	>10mm	

Simplified PISA Methods

Method 1

EROA (mm²) = r²/2

(ASE Recommendation [1] – Does not hold at extremes of blood pressures but the vast majority of patients have jets between 4 m/s to 6 m/s for which this approximation is valid.)

Method 2

PISA radius ≥1cm = EROA ≥35mm²

Method 3

RV (cc) = 2 x r² x alias velocity

Method 4

RV (cc) = 6.28 x r^2 x aliasing velocity (cm/s)/3.25

Method 5

r^2 x aliasing velocity:

> **<10cm^3/s = mild MR**
>
> **>20cm^3/s = significant MR**

Method 6

RV (cc) = 6.28 x r^2 x V x (MR_{VTI} ÷ MR_{PFV})

- **r** is the maximum aliasing radius on one beat
- **V** is the aliasing velocity
- **MR_{VTI}** is the velocity time integral of the mitral regurgitant jet from a continuous wave Doppler recording
- **MR_{PFV}** is the corresponding peak flow velocity of the MR jet

Method 7

Qualitatively evaluate the PISA with the color velocity scale set at between 50 to 70cm/s

Important to Note

- A common error in calculations is to forget to convert the peak mitral regurgitation velocity from m/s to cm/s.
- Effective regurgitant orifice area (EROA) is reported in mm^2 instead of cm^2. Multiply cm^2 times 100 to obtain mm^2.

Tricuspid Regurgitation

For tricuspid regurgitation, the velocity scale should be set at 28cm/s in order to determine the PISA radius.

Regurgitant Volume (RV)
Regurgitant Fraction (RF)
Effective Regurgitant Orifice Area (EROA)

1. Determine the cross sectional area of the mitral valve annulus from the apical 4-chamber during mid-diastole. The annulus diameter should be measured from inner edge to inner edge at the base of the mitral valve leaflets. Using the zoom feature will aid in acquiring this measurement.

CSA_{MV} (cm^2) = .785 x Mitral Valve Annulus Diameter^2

2. From the apical 4-chamber view, place a PW Doppler sample volume at the level of the mitral valve annulus and determine the velocity time integral (VTI_{MV}). Using a sweep speed of 100mm/s may aid in acquiring this measurement.

3. Calculate the mitral valve stroke volume:

SVMV (cc) = CSAMV x VTIMV

4. Determine the cross sectional area of the left ventricular outflow tract (LVOT) in the parasternal long-axis by measuring the LVOT diameter in early to mid systole. The LVOT diameter should be measured from inner edge to inner edge where the right aortic valve cusp meets the interventricular septum to where the noncoronary aortic valve cusp meets the anterior mitral valve leaflet in a line parallel to the aortic annulus. Using the zoom feature will aid in acquiring this measurement.

CSA_{LVOT} (cm^2) = .785 x LVOT Diameter^2

5. From the apical 5-chamber view or apical long axis view, place a PW Doppler sample volume at the level of the left ventricular outflow tract (LVOT) and determine LVOT velocity time integral (VTI_{LVOT}). A sweep speed of 100mm/s may aid in acquiring this measurement. A closing valve click should be included in the PW Doppler tracing.

6. Calculate the left ventricular outflow tract stroke volume:

SV_{LVOT} (cc) = CSA_{LVOT} x VTI_{LVOT}

7. Calculate regurgitant volume (RV):

RV_{MR} (cc) = SV_{MV} (cc) – SV_{LVOT} (cc)

8. Calculate regurgitant fraction (RF):

RF (%) = RV_{MR} (cc) ÷ SV_{MV} (cc)

9. From the apical window, obtain a CW Doppler tracing of the mitral regurgitation and determine a velocity time integral (VTI_{MR}) by tracing the mitral regurgitation signal. Using a sweep speed of 100mm/s may aid in acquiring this measurement.

10. Calculate effective regurgitant orifice area (EROA):

EROA (cm^2) = RV_{MR} ÷ VTI_{MR}

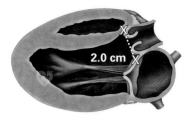

Figure 24.35: **LVOT diameter**

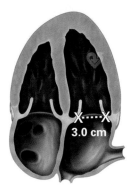

Figure 24.36: **MV diameter**

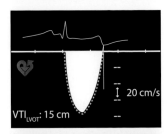

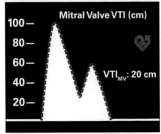

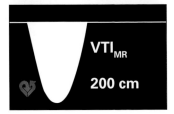

Case Example

Measurements

- Mitral valve annulus diameter = 3.0cm
- VTIMV = 20cm
- LVOT diameter = 2.0cm
- VTILVOT = 15cm
- VTIMR (cm) = 200cm

Calculations

- SVMV = (cc) .785 x 3.0^2cm x 20cm
- SVMV (cc) = 141 cc
- SVLVOT (cc) = .785 x 2.0^2cm x 15cm
- SVLVOT (cc) = 47 cc
- RVMR (cc) = 141 cc – 47 cc = 94 cc
- RFMR (cc) = 94 cc/141 cc = 67%
- EROMR (cm^2) = 94 cc/200cm = .47cm^2 or 47mm^2

Left Ventricular Systolic Performance (dP/dt)

1. Optimize mitral regurgitation jet by CW Doppler.
2. On screen or paper, draw horizontal lines at 1 m/s and 3 m/s
3. Draw a vertical line from intercept of mitral regurgitation jet at 1 m/s and 3 m/s
4. Measure time (msec)
5. dP/dt = (32mmHg x 1000) ÷ change in time in msec

dP/dt Values

- Normal   >1200mmHg/sec or <27 msec
- Borderline   1000 to 1200mmHg/sec
- Abnormal   <1000mmHg/sec or ≥32 msec

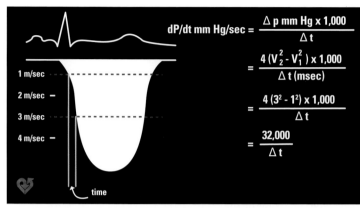

$$dP/dt \text{ mm Hg/sec} = \frac{\Delta p \text{ mm Hg} \times 1,000}{\Delta t}$$

$$= \frac{4(V_2^2 - V_1^2) \times 1,000}{\Delta t \text{ (msec)}}$$

$$= \frac{4(3^2 - 1^2) \times 1,000}{\Delta t}$$

$$= \frac{32,000}{\Delta t}$$

Right Ventricular Systolic Performance (dP/dt)

Right ventricular dP/dt is calculated similar to left ventricular dP/dt by measuring the time required for the tricuspid regurgitation jet to increase in velocity from 1 to 2 m/s. This represents a 12mmHg increase in pressure. The dP/dt is calculated as (12mmHg x 1000)/(the time in milliseconds) yielding a value in millimeters of mercury per second. An RV dP/dt of <400mmHg/sec is abnormal.

Aortic Regurgitation

Jet Width/Left Ventricular Outflow Tract Width (JW/LVOTW)

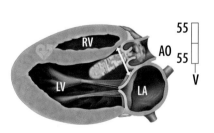
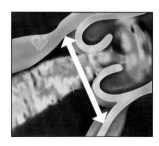

1. Measure the maximal anteroposterior diameter (width) of the regurgitant jet at the junction of the LVOT and aortic annulus within 1cm of the aortic valve using the parasternal long-axis view (JW) (zoom with color flow Doppler velocity scale set at between 50 to 70cm/s)

2. Measure the maximal width of the LVOT at the same location (LVOTW)

3. Divide the jet width (JW) by the LVOT width (LVOTW) and the resultant ratio can be expressed as a percentage

Jet Cross-Sectional Area/Left Ventricular Outflow Tract Cross-Sectional Area (Jet CSA/LVOT CSA)

1. Planimeter the regurgitant jet as visualized in the parasternal short-axis view of the aortic valve and the ultrasound machine software will calculate the jet short-axis area (Jet CSA) (zoom with color flow Doppler velocity scale set at between 50 to 70cm/s)

2. Planimeter the LVOT area in the parasternal short-axis view of the aortic valve and the ultrasound machine software will calculate the LVOT area (LVOT CSA).

3. The Jet CSA can then be divided by the LVOT CSA and the resultant ratio can be expressed as a percentage

Vena Contracta

1. Parasternal long-axis view with color flow Doppler velocity scale set at 50 to 70cm/s

2. Zoom the aortic valve and the aortic regurgitation jet (narrowest sector width which allows visualization of the flow acceleration zone (PISA), vena contracta and a portion of the regurgitant jet should be chosen)

3. Angulate the transducer until the regurgitant flow proximal to, through and distal to the aortic valve is well visualized

4. Freeze and scroll until the largest diameter of the vena contracta is well visualized

5. Measure the vena contracta of the regurgitant flow immediately downstream from the flow convergence region (PISA) (three to five beats should be measured and averaged)

6. The apical 5-chamber or apical long-axis may be substituted when the parasternal long-axis is suboptimal

Important to Note

Not valid in the presence of multiple jets

Proximal Isovelocity Surface Area (PISA)

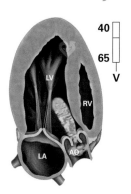
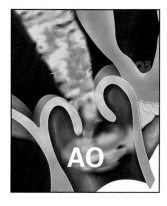

1. Optimize the color flow Doppler image of the aortic regurgitation utilizing the apical long-axis view, apical 5-chamber view or parasternal long-axis
2. Zoom the aortic valve
3. Shift the color flow Doppler baseline upward until the flow convergence region (PISA) is clearly visualized
4. Freeze the image and cine loop to identify the optimal hemisphere which should occur in early diastole
5. Measure the radius (between the first aliasing color (red-blue interface) and the regurgitant aortic orifice
6. Obtain a peak velocity and velocity time integral (VTI) of the aortic regurgitation utilizing CW Doppler
7. Calculate the effective regurgitant orifice area (EROA) by the formula:

$$\text{EROAmm}^2 = \frac{6.28 \times r^2 \times \text{Aliasing Velocity}}{\text{Aortic Regurgitation Peak Velocitycm/s}}$$

8. Calculate the regurgitant volume (RV) by the formula:

$$\text{RV (cc)} = \text{EROAcm}^2 \times \text{aortic regurgitation velocity time integral (VTI)cm}$$

Case Example

Measurements

- Radius (cm): 1.0
- Aliasing velocity (cm/s): 40cm/s
- Aortic regurgitation peak velocity (cm/s): 400cm/s
- Aortic regurgitation VTI (cm): 230cm

Calculations

- EROA (mm^2) = 6.28 x (1^{2}cm) x 40cm/s ÷ 400cm/s
- EROA (mm^2) = 251 ÷ 400cm/s
- EROA (mm^2) = .628cm^2 or 62.8mm^2
- RV (cc) = .628cm^2 x 230cm
- RV (cc) = 144 cc

Regurgitant Volume (RV)
Regurgitant Fraction (RF)
Effective Regurgitant Orifice Area (EROA)

1. Determine the cross sectional area of the mitral valve annulus from the apical 4-chamber during mid-diastole. The annulus diameter should be measured from inner edge to inner edge at the base of the mitral valve leaflets. Using the zoom feature will aid in acquiring this measurement.

$$\text{CSA}_{MV} \text{ (cm}^2\text{)} = .785 \times \text{mitral valve annulus diameter}^2$$

2. From the apical 4-chamber view, place a PW Doppler sample volume at the level of the mitral valve annulus and determine the velocity time integral (VTI$_{MV}$). Using a sweep speed of 100mm/s may aid in acquiring this measurement.

3. Calculate the mitral valve stroke volume:

$$SV_{MV} \text{ (cc)} = CSA_{MV} \times VTI_{MV}$$

4. Determine the cross sectional area of the left ventricular outflow tract (LVOT) in the parasternal long-axis by measuring the LVOT diameter in early to mid systole. The LVOT diameter should be measured from inner edge to inner edge where the right aortic valve cusp meets the interventricular septum to where the noncoronary aortic valve cusp meets the anterior mitral valve leaflet in a line parallel to the aortic annulus. Using the zoom feature will aid in acquiring this measurement.

$$CSA_{LVOT} \text{ (cm}^2) = .785 \times LVOT \text{ diameter}^2$$

5. From the apical 5-chamber view or apical long axis view, place a PW Doppler sample volume at the level of the left ventricular outflow tract (LVOT) and determine LVOT velocity time integral (VTI_{LVOT}). A sweep speed of 100mm/s may aid in acquiring this measurement. A closing valve click should be included in the PW Doppler tracing.

6. Calculate the left ventricular outflow tract stroke volume:

$$SV_{LVOT} \text{ (cc)} = CSA_{LVOT} \times VTI_{LVOT}$$

7. Calculate aortic regurgitant volume (RV):

$$RV_{AR} = SV_{LVOT} \text{ (cc)} - SV_{MV} \text{ (cc)}$$

8. Calculate aortic regurgitant fraction (RF):

$$RF\% = RV_{AR} \text{ (cc)} \div SV_{LVOT} \text{ (cc)}$$

9. From the apical window, obtain a CW Doppler tracing of the aortic regurgitation and determine a velocity time integral (VTI_{AR}) by tracing the aortic regurgitation signal. Using a sweep speed of 100mm/s may aid in acquiring this measurement.

10. Calculate effective regurgitant orifice area (EROA):

$$EROA \text{ (cm}^2) = RV_{AR} \div VTI_{AR}$$

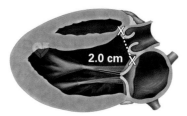

Figure 24.37: **LVOT diameter**

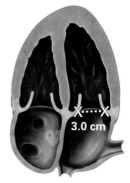

Figure 24.38: **MV diameter**

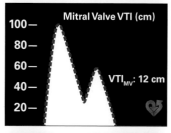

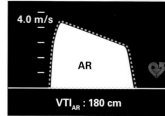

24

Echo/Doppler Measurements and Calculations / Doppler Wave Form Tracings / Qp/Qs

Case Example

Measurements

- LVOT diameter (cm) = 2.0cm
- VTI_{LVOT} (cm) = 40cm
- Mitral valve annulus (cm) = 3.0cm
- VTI_{MV} (cm) = 12cm
- VTI_{AR} (cm) = 180cm

Calculations

- SV_{LVOT} (cc) = .785 x 2.0^2cm x 40cm
- SV_{LVOT} (cc) = 126 cc
- SV_{MV} (cc) = .785 x 3.0^2cm x 12cm
- SV_{MV} (cc) = 85 cc
- RV_{AR} (cc) = 126 cc – 85 cc = 41 cc
- RF_{AR} (cc) = 41 cc/126 cc = 33%
- ERO_{AR} (cm^2) = 41 cc/180cm = .23cm^2 or 23mm^2

Qp/Qs

1. Determine the cross sectional area of the right ventricular outflow tract (RVOT) during early to mid ventricular systole. The RVOT diameter should be measured from inner edge to inner edge at the base of the pulmonary valve leaflet using the best two-dimensional picture (e.g., parasternal short-axis of the aortic valve, parasternal long-axis of the right ventricular outflow tract, subcostal short-axis of the aortic valve). Using the zoom feature will aid in acquiring this measurement.

$$CSA\ (cm^2) = .785 \times RVOT\ diameter^2$$

2. Utilizing the best two-dimensional view (e.g., parasternal short-axis of the aortic valve, parasternal long-axis of the right ventricular outflow tract, subcostal short-axis of the aortic valve), place a PW Doppler sample volume at the level of the right ventricular outflow tract and determine the velocity time integral (VTIRVOT). Increasing the sweep to 100mm/s may aid in acquiring this measurement.

3. Calculate the right ventricular stroke volume:

$$SV_{RVOT}\ (cc) = CSA_{RVOT}\ (cm^2) \times VTI_{RVOT}\ (cm)$$

4. Determine the cross sectional area of the left ventricular outflow tract (LVOT) in the parasternal long-axis by measuring the LVOT diameter during early to mid ventricular systole from inner edge to inner edge where the right aortic valve coronary cusp meets the interventricular septum to where the noncoronary aortic valve cusp meets the anterior mitral valve leaflet in a line parallel to the aortic annulus. Using the zoom feature may aid in acquiring this measurement.

$$CSA_{LVOT}\ (cm^2) = .785 \times LVOT\ diameter^2$$

5. From the apical 5-chamber view or apical long axis view, place a pulsed wave Doppler sample volume at the level of the left ventricular outflow tract (LVOT) and determine the LVOT velocity time integral (VTILVOT). A closing valve click should be included in the PW Doppler tracing. Using a sweep speed of 100mm/s may aid in acquiring this measurement.

6. Calculate the left ventricular stroke volume:

$$SV_{LVOT}\ (cc) = CSA_{LVOT}\ (cm^2) \times VTI_{LVOT}\ (cm)$$

7. Calculate Qp/Qs: (ASD, VSD)

$$SV_{RVOT}\ (cc) \div SV_{LVOT}\ (cc)$$

Important to Note

- For patent ductus arteriosus, the SV_{LVOT} represents Qp and SV_{RVOT} represents Qs. For patent ductus arteriosus:

$$Qp/Qs = SV_{LVOT} \text{ (cc)} \div SV_{RVOT} \text{ (cc)}$$

- A normal Qp/Qs is 1:1.
- A Qp/Qs of >1.5:1 is a significant shunt.

Case Example

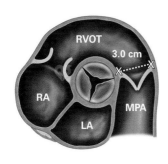

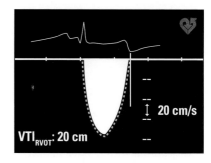

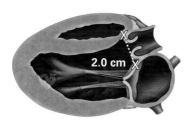

Figure 24.39: **LVOT diameter**

Measurements
- RVOT diameter (cm) = 3.0cm
- VTI_{RVOT} (cm) = 20cm
- LVOT diameter: 2.0cm
- VTI_{LVOT} (cm) = 15cm

Calculations
- SV_{RVOT} (cc) = .785 x 3.0^2cm x 20cm
- SV_{RVOT} (cc) = 141 cc
- SV_{LVOT} (cc) = .785 x 2.0^2cm x 15cm
- SV_{LVOT} (cm) = 47 cc
- Qp/Qs = 141 cc/47 cc = 3:1

Mitral Valve Area (MVA)

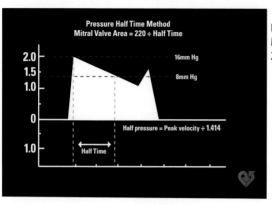

Figure 24.40:
Mitral Valve Area =
220 ÷ Pressure Half-Time

Pressure Half-time (PHT) Method

1. Optimize a CW Doppler tracing of the mitral valve inflow signal.
2. Increase sweep speed to 100mm/s
3. Measure the mitral valve E wave velocity (Vmax)
4. Divide the mitral valve E wave velocity by 1.4 to determine VPHT
5. Draw a vertical line to baseline at Vmax and VPHT
6. Measure the time interval between Vmax and VPHT
7. MVAcm^2 = 220/PHT

Important to Note

220 is an empirical derived constant and may not accurately predict mitral valve area in mitral prosthetic heart valves. The mitral valve area continuity equation may be utilized in mitral prosthetic heart valves to predict effective orifice area.

Tricuspid Stenosis

The same steps may be used to determine tricuspid valve pressure half-time and tricuspid valve area.

Deceleration Time (DT) Method

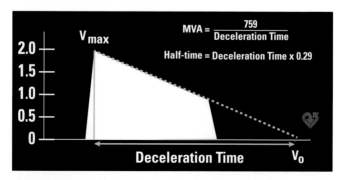

1. Optimize a CW Doppler tracing of the mitral valve inflow signal
2. Increase sweep speed to 100mm/s
3. Draw a vertical line to baseline at Vmax
4. Draw a line from VMAX following the deceleration slope to baseline (Vo)
5. Measure the time interval between Vmax and Vo. This equals the deceleration time (DT)
6. Pressure half-time (PHT) = 0.29 x DT
7. MVAcm^2 = 220/PHT = 220/0.29 x DT msec = 759/DT msec

Tricuspid Stenosis

The same steps may be used to determine tricuspid valve pressure half-time and tricuspid valve area

Case Example

Measurements

Mitral valve deceleration time (msec) = 700 msec

Calculations

Pressure half-time (msec) = 0.29 x 700 msec = 203 msec

Deceleration time (DT) method:

Mitral valve area (cm^2) = 759/700 msec = 1.08cm^2

Pressure half-time (PHT) method:

Mitral valve area (cm^2) = 220/203 msec = 1.08cm^2

PISA (Proximal Isovelocity Surface Area) Method

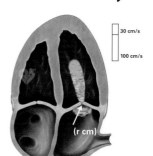 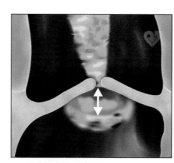

Figure 24.41: Mitral valve area (Pisa Method)

1. From the apical 4-chamber view with color flow Doppler on, zoom the area of the mitral valve
2. Shift the color flow Doppler zero baseline upward (downward for TEE) to between 30 to 45cm/s aliasing velocity
3. Freeze the image, cine loop to identify and measure the radius (rcm)

4. Utilizing CW Doppler, obtain the mitral valve inflow Doppler tracing and determine the mitral valve E wave velocity (Vmax) (not shown)

5. Determine mitral valve area (MVA) by the formula:

$$MVAcm^2 = \frac{6.28 \text{ x } r^2 \text{ x Aliasing Velocity}}{\text{Mitral Valve E Wave Velocity } (V_{max})}$$

Case Example

Measurements

- Aliasing velocity (cm/s): 30cm/s
- Radius (cm): 1.0cm
- Mitral valve E wave velocity (Vmax): 188cm/s

Calculations

- MVA (cm^2) = 6.28 x (1^2)cm x 30cm/s ÷ 188cm/s
- MVA (cm^2) = 1.0cm^2

Left Ventricular Diastolic Function

Mitral Valve Inflow

The filling of the left ventricle can be likened to filling a glass of water. The optimal way to fill a glass with water is to pour the water along the side of the glass. The optimal way to fill the left ventricle is to pour the blood along its side (lateral). That is why the anterior mitral valve leaflet is longer than the posterior leaflet. It is important to note that as the ventricle dilates, the lateral filling of the ventricle is accentuated. From the apical 4-chamber view slide the transducer lateral and tilt posterior. This will assure the ultrasound beam is parallel to the mitral valve inflow.

Utilizing a small PW Doppler sample volume size (1 to 2mm) to assure a clean Doppler spectral tracing, place the sample volume between the mitral valve leaflet tips during diastole.

Measure the following:

- Mitral valve peak E wave velocity (E)
- Mitral valve A wave velocity (A)
- Mitral valve deceleration time (Mdt)
- Mitral valve E at A velocity

To improve the measurement of the mitral valve A wave duration, move the PW Doppler sample volume slightly toward the mitral valve annulus and measure the mitral valve A wave duration.

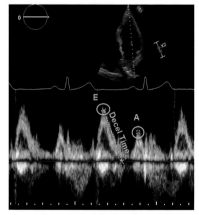

Figure 24.42: **Pulse Doppler and mitral valve inflow**

Important to Note

• Placing the sample volume too close to the mitral valve annulus or in the body of the mitral valve leaflets will result in lower mitral valve peak velocities and shorter mitral valve deceleration times (Numbers 1, 2, 3). The E wave will decrease more than the A wave as the sample volume is moved closer to the mitral valve annulus (Numbers 1, 2, 3).

• Placing the sample volume below the mitral valve leaflet tips towards the left ventricle (Numbers 5, 6) will result in lower mitral valve peak velocities and longer deceleration times and longer A wave durations. (see figures above).

• CW Doppler may be utilized to confirm the E/A ratio.

Isovolumic Relaxation Time (IVRT)

Method 1

1. Aim the CW Doppler beam between the aortic valve and the mitral valve and with fine angulation record the closing click of the aortic valve and the opening click of the mitral valve

2. Measure the time interval between these two valve clicks

Method 2

1. Place the sample volume of the PW Doppler in the LVOT, increase the sample volume size and record the closing click of the aortic valve and the opening click of the mitral valve

2. Measure the time interval between these two valve clicks

Method 3

1. Obtain a TDI of the mitral annulus

2. Measure from the end of the S' wave to the onset of the e' wave

Important to Note

• An IVRT of less than 60 suggests increased left atrial pressure.

• An IVRT greater than 100msec suggests impaired relaxation.

Isovolumic Contraction Time (IVCT)

The isovolumic contraction time (IVCT) can be measured by obtaining a TDI of the mitral annulus and measuring from the end of the mitral valve A' wave to onset of the S' wave.

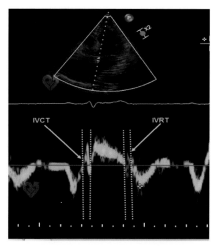

Figure 24.43: **Doppler tissue imaging**

24

Echo/Doppler Measurements and Calculations / Doppler Wave Form Tracings / Left Ventricular Diastolic Function

The following method is recommended for obtaining a high quality tissue Doppler imaging (TDI) of the mitral annulus:

1. Review the ultrasound manufacturer's tissue Doppler imaging presets

2. Acquire an apical 4-chamber and optimize the frame rate by decreasing the image depth and sector width

3. Align the tissue Doppler cursor as parallel as possible (<20°) to the mitral annulus (lateral annulus and medial (septal) annulus)

4. The sample volume should be positioned at or 1cm within the septal and lateral insertion sites of the mitral leaflets and the sample volume size should be adjusted as necessary (approximately 5mm for the lateral annulus and 3mm for the septal annulus) to cover the longitudinal excursion of the mitral annulus in both systole and diastole.

5. Decrease the tissue Doppler velocity scale to less than 25cm/s

6. Set the sweep speed to 50 to 100mm/s

7. Have patient hold their breath at end-expiration and measurements should reflect the average of ≥3 consecutive cardiac cycles

8. Measurements include the S' wave, e' wave, a' wave, e'/a' ratio, mitral PW Doppler E/e', $T_{E-e'}$(onset of QRS complex to onset of PW Doppler mitral E velocity — onset of QRS complex to the onset of TDI e' wave)

9. The average of the septal and lateral e' velocities should be used when calculating the E/e' ratio

10. The E/e' is not accurate as an index of filling pressures in normal subjects or in patients with heavy annular calcification, mitral valve disease and constrictive pericarditis.

11. The above optimization techniques can be used for the apical 2-chamber view and right ventricle

Pulmonary Vein Flow

1. Utilizing a large (2 to 3mm) PW Doppler sample volume (SV) from the apical 4-chamber view, tilt the transducer slightly anterior (almost to an apical 5-chamber view) and place the sample volume (SV) >0.5cm into the right upper pulmonary vein.

2. Measure the following:

   • PV_s1

   • PV_s2

   • PVd

   • PVa (pulmonary vein peak velocity of the atrial reversal flow)

   • PV ARdur (pulmonary vein atrial reversal duration)

Important to Note

• A diagnostic pulmonary vein tracing may be difficult to obtain on every patient. Having the patient hold their breath at end expiration, moving the transducer up the chest wall ("closer" to the pulmonary vein), changing the Doppler wall filter settings, setting the sweep speed to 50 to 100mm/s and/or increasing the PW Doppler sample volume may be useful. An average of three or more consecutive cycles should be measured.

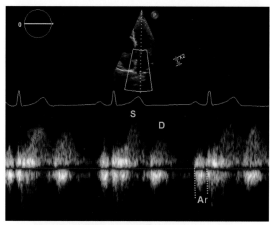

Figure 24.44: **Pulmonary vein PW Doppler wave form.**
(S) systolic wave velocity. (D) Diastolic wave velocity.
(Ar) Atrial reversal wave velocity.

• In atrial fibrillation, there is no "a" wave and the systolic wave is blunted.

• Sinus tachycardia and first-degree AV block may make the measurement of the pulmonary vein ARdur difficult.

• A pulmonary vein ARdur - mitral valve Adur of >30 msec indicates an elevated LVEDP (≥15mmHg) and remains accurate in patients with a normal ejection fraction, mitral valve disease and hypertrophic cardiomyopathy. It is age independent and may be the first or earliest indication of diastolic dysfunction.

• In patients with reduced ejection fraction, a pulmonary vein systolic filling fraction (S wave$_{VTI}$/S wave$_{VTI}$ + D wave$_{VTI}$) of <40% suggests an increased mean left atrial pressure.

Valsalva Maneuver

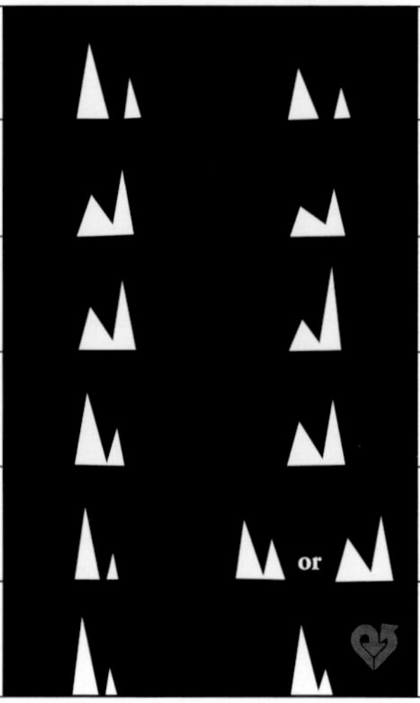

Grades	Baseline	Valsalva	Interpretation
Normal			Normal
Grade I			Normal Pressures
Grade I A			Increased Left Ventricular End-diastolic Pressure
Grade II			Pseudonormal
Grade IIIa		or	Preload Sensitive Partially Reversible
Grade IIIb			Fixed Restrictive

Figure 24.45: The PW Doppler mitral valve flow pattern in normals as well as in Grades I through III expected to be acquired during the strain phase of the Valsalva maneuver.

Important to Note

• The contraindications of the Valsalva maneuver include:
  - Unstable angina/recent myocardial infarction
  - Valvular aortic stenosis
  - Severe mitral regurgitation
  - Recent stroke
  - Recent transient ischemic attack (TIA)
• There is a decrease in venous return (decrease in preload) during the strain phase of the Valsalva maneuver and a corresponding decrease in stroke volume, cardiac output, cardiac index and filling pressures.
• The strain phase of the Valsalva maneuver is considered effective if there is at least a ≥10% decrease in the mitral valve E wave velocity and/or at least a decrease of >20cm/s in the mitral valve E wave velocity.
• Merging of the E and A wave velocities during the Valsalva maneuver may suggest normal filling pressures.
• An increase in the mitral valve A wave duration as compared to baseline during the Valsalva maneuver may indicate increased left ventricular end-diastolic pressure (LVEDP).
• When calculating the mitral valve E/A ratio with Valsalva, the absolute A velocity (peak A minus the height of the E at the onset of the A) should be used.

- In cardiac patients, a decrease of ≥50% in the E/A ratio is highly specific for increased filling pressures, but a smaller magnitude change does not always indicate normal diastolic function.

- The use of the Valsalva maneuver in the evaluation of diastolic function has decreased with the introduction of tissue Doppler of the mitral annulus.

Hepatic Vein Flow

The hepatic vein provides important diastolic information. The diagram below demonstrates the normal hepatic vein flow pattern and the hepatic vein patterns seen in restrictive cardiomyopathy, constrictive pericarditis and cardiac tamponade.

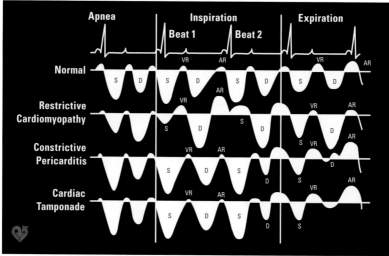

From Bansal, R. C. and Chandrasekaran, K.: "Role of echocardiography in Doppler techniques in evaluation of pericardial effusion." Echocardiography, 6:313, 1989 with permission.

Important to Note

The hepatic vein Doppler tracing is best obtained in the subcostal window utilizing PW Doppler. The sample volume is set at 1 to 3mm and placed 2 to 3cm in the vein from the inferior vena cava junction. The Doppler wall filter is best set at between 200 to 400 Hz.

Superior Vena Cava

The superior vena cava flow pattern is similar to the hepatic vein pattern. Superior vena cava flow is obtained by placing the transducer in the right supraclavicular fossa region. With PW Doppler, the sample volume is placed 5 to 8cm from the transducer with sample volume size set at 1 to 3mm and the Doppler wall filter is set between 200 to 400 Hz. Tissue Doppler Imaging (TDI)

Color M-mode (CMM)

Mitral E-wave Flow Velocity Propagation (Vp cm/s)

Table 24.8: Mitral E-wave Flow Velocity Technique	
Transducer Location	Apical 4-chamber using color flow Doppler
Modality	Color M-mode
Alignment	M-mode scan line is placed through the center of the LV inflow blood column from the mitral valve to the cardiac apex
Velocity scale	Color flow baseline is shifted to lower the Nyquist limit so that the central highest velocity jet is blue
Sweep speed	50 or 100mm/s
Flow propagation	Velocity is measured as the slope of the first aliasing velocity (approximately set at 45cm/s) from the mitral annulus in early diastole to 4cm distally into the left ventricular cavity (preferred measurement)

- In patients with a low peak E velocity (lower than aliasing velocity) measure the slope of the transition no color/to color (black/red)
- In patients with a low peak E wave velocity (<45cm/s), where no aliasing may be seen, baseline shift is adjusted to alias at approximately 75% of the peak E wave velocity
- Vp ≥50cm/s is considered normal
- A E/Vp of ≥2.5 predicts a PCWP >15mmHg
- Patients with normal volumes and EF but increased filling pressures can have misleading normal Vp

Basics of Calculating Index of Myocardial Performance

3. Optimize pulsed wave (PW) atrioventricular inflow signal. May use continuous wave (CW) atrioventricular regurgitant signal

4. Measure interval between atrioventricular valve (AV) closure and AV valve opening (AVCO)

5. Optimize pulsed wave semilunar outflow signal. May use semilunar CW signal

6. Measure the ejection time (ET)

7. Calculate the IMP:

   IMP = (AVCO - ET) ÷ ET

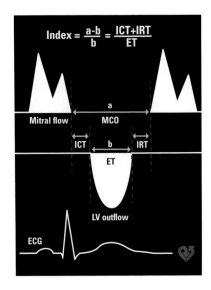

$$\text{Index} = \frac{a-b}{b} = \frac{ICT+IRT}{ET}$$

Calculation of IMP of Left Ventricle (LIMP):

1. Optimize PW mitral inflow signal. May use CW mitral regurgitant signal
2. Measure interval between mitral valve closure (MVC) and mitral valve opening (MVO)
3. Optimize pulsed wave left ventricular outflow tract (LVOT) signal
4. Measure the LVOT ejection time (ET_{LVOT})
5. Calculate the Index of Myocardial Performance (IMP_{LV})

$$IMP_{LV} = \frac{(MVC \text{ to } MVO) - ET_{LVOT}}{ET_{LVOT}}$$

Calculation of IMP of Right Ventricle (RIMP)

1. Optimize PW tricuspid inflow signal. May use CW tricuspid regurgitant signal
2. Measure interval between tricuspid valve closure (TVC) and TV opening (TVO)
3. Optimize pulsed wave right ventricular outflow tract (RVOT) signal
4. Measure the RVOT ejection time (ET)
5. Calculate the Index of Myocardial Performance (IMP_{RV})

$$IMP_{RV} = \frac{(TVC \text{ to } TVO) - ET_{RVOT}}{ET_{RVOT}}$$

Table 24.9: Index of Myocardial Performance (IMP) Values	
LIMP	**RIMP**
0.39 ± 0.05 (normal)	>0.43 adults (abnormal) (PW Doppler)
0.59 ± 0.10 (moderately abnormal)	>0.54 (abnormal) (Tissue Doppler)
1.06 ± 0.24 (severely abnormal)	0.32 ± 0.03 children (normal)

Important to Note

- Myocardial contractility and relaxation are energy dependent (related to SV, CO, EF).
- Myocardial dysfunction results in prolongation of isovolumic intervals.
- Increased IMP consistent with LV dysfunction.
  - Increase in IVCT and IVRT
  - Decrease in ejection time
- Tissue Doppler imaging may be utilized to determine IMP

References

1. Lang RM, Badano LP, Mor-Avi V, et al. Recommendations for cardiac chamber quantification by echocardiography in adults: an update from the American Society of Echocardiography and the European Association of Cardiovascular Imaging. J Am Soc Echocardiogr 2015;28:727-54.)

2. Rudski LG, Lai WW, Afilalo J, Hua L, Handschumacher, Chandrasekaran K, Solomon SD, Louie EK, Schiller NB. Guidelines for the Echocardiographic Assessment of the Right Heart in Adults. J Am Soc Echocardiogr 2010;23:685-713.)

24

Echo/Doppler Measurements and Calculations / Color M-mode (CMM) / Mitral E-wave Velocity Flow Velocity Propagation (Vp cm/s)